Editors' Commentary

EC Mulkerrin, B Carey, R Liston

As a conseq...   -increasing majority
of patients   hts the marvellous
opportunit   on of older patients
using mod   es the clinical aspect
of the prob   numerous real case
histories, w   workers in the field
of gerontol

Relevant r   an opportunity for
the knowle   chapter using data
interpretati

There are m   to the attractiveness
of the publi   ems of older people.
Many of the   on problems such as
stroke, hyp   priate management
of commor   anagement such as
oncology ar

This public: rs hoping to become
specialists i   s a useful summary
of common   ons particularly the
Membershi   Geriatric Medicine.
Finally Ger   olved in the care of
older patie

Contributors

Dr Barry Moynihan, MRCPI, Consultant Geriatrician, St George's Hospital, London

Dr Catherine O'Sullivan, MRCPI, SpR Geriatric Medicine, Cork University Hospital

Professor Tim O'Brien, PhD, FRCPI, National University of Ireland, Galway and Consultant Physician and Endocrinologist, University Hospital Galway

Dr Claire O'Brien, MRCPI, Lecturer in Medical Education, University College Cork

Dr Colm Henry, MRCPI, MRCGP, Consultant Physician and Geriatrician, Mercy University Hospital, Cork

Dr Denis O'Mahony, MD, FRCPI, Consultant Physician and Geriatrician, Cork University Hospital

Dr Hiliary Hamilton, MRCPI, Clinical Tutor in Medicine, Cork University Hospital

Dr Kieran O'Connor, BMed, MSc, MRCPI, Consultant Physician and Geriatrician, Mercy University Hospital, Cork

Professor Eamon Mulkerrin, MD, FRCP (Edin.), FRCPI, National University of Ireland, Galway and Consultant Physician and Geriatrician, University Hospital, Galway

Dr Luke O'Donnell, MD, FRCPI, Consultant Gastroenterologist, Mayo General Hospital

Dr Michael O'Connor, MRCPI, Consultant Physician and Geriatrician, Cork University Hospital

Dr Paul Gallagher, MRCPI, SpR Geriatric Medicine, Cork University Hospital

Dr Richard Liston, DGM, FRCPI, FRCP (Lond), Consultant Physician and Geriatrician, Kerry General Hospital

Dr Rosa McNamara, MRCSEd, MCEM, SpR in Emergency Medicine, Cork University Hospital

Dr Shane O'Hanlon, MRCPI, SpR in General and Geriatric Medicine, Kerry General Hospital

Dr Suzanne Timmons, MD, FRCPI, Consultant Physician and Geriatrician, Mallow General Hospital

Dr Branislav Bystricky, Consultant Medical Oncologist, Mercy University Hospital, Grenville Place, Cork

Dr Brian J Carey, MD, FRCPI Consultant Geriatrician, Department of Geriatric Medicine, Bantry General Hospital, Bantry, Co. Cork

Dr Fionnuala McSweeney, MRCPI Special Lecturer in Medicine, Mater University Hospital and University College Dublin

Dr Gerard Flaherty, BSC, MRCPI, MFTM, MM ED, SC, MSFEM, MSC, ITH, Lecturer in Medical Education and Clinical Skills, Department of Medicine, Clinical Science Institute, University Hospital, Galway

Dr John Carey, MB, FACR, CCD, Consultant Rheumatologist, Merlin Park Hospital, Galway

Dr K Afridi, MB, Research Registrar in Rheumatology, Merlin Park Hospital, Galway

Dr Marcia Bell, Consultant Endocrinologist, University Hospital Galway

Dr Mary Horgan, MD, FRCP, FRCPI, Consultant in Infectious Diseases and Senior Lecturer in Medicine, Cork University Hospital and University College Cork

Dr Michelle Murphy, MRCPI Consultant Dermatologist, South Infirmary/Victoria University Hospital, Cork

Dr Mohd Syahizul, Nuhairy Mohd Sharial, MRCPI, Registrar, Mercy University Hospital, Grenville Place, Cork

Dr Patricia Sheahan, Consultant in Palliative Medicine, Kerry General Hospital, Tralee, Co. Kerry

Dr Seamus O'Reilly, MD, PhD, Consultant Medical Oncologist, Oncology Department, Cork, Mercy & South Infirmary/Victoria University Hospitals, Cork

Dr Shane O'Hanlon, Specialist Registrar in Geriatric Medicine, Kerry General Hospital, Tralee, Co. Kerry

Dr Sinead Field, MRCPI, Specialist Registrar in Dermatology, South Infirmary/Victoria University Hospital, Cork

Professor Cillian Twomey, FRCPI, Consultant Physician and Geriatrician, Cork University Hospital

Sinead Dennehy, RGN, HDip TVN, Staff Nurse, South Infirmary/Victoria University Hospital, Cork

Dr Norman Delanty, MSc, FRCPI, Consultant Neurologist, Beaumont Hospital, Dublin

Dr John Lynch, MRCPI, Consultant Neurologist, Royal Free Hospital, London and Watford General Hospital

Professor Desmond O'Neill, MD, FRCPI, Aois agus Eolas, MANCH Hospital, Tallaght, Dublin 24

Mr Michael Corcoran, MCh, FRCSI, Consultant Urologist, University Hospital, Galway

Mr Frank Kinsella, MCh, FRCS(Opth), Consultant Ophthalmologist, University Hospital, Galway

Mr Peter K. Gormley, MCh, FRCSI, Consultant ENT Surgeon, University Hospital Galway

Dr Rosaleen Lannon, MRCPI, SpR in Geriatric Medicine, University Hospital, Galway

Dr Bláithín Ní Bhuachalla, MRCPI, SpR in Geriatric Medicine, University Hospital, Galway

Dr Shaun T. O'Keeffe, MD, FRCPI, National University of Ireland, Galway, Consultant Physician and Geriatrician, University Hospital, Galway

Contents

Assessing older patients

R Liston, S O'Hanlon

'There are no diseases of the aged, but simply diseases among the aged.' Leonard Larson, 1960

Introduction

The specialty of Geriatric Medicine traces its origins back to the 17th century when older patients were treated together with psychiatric patients in asylums. In the UK these asylums later developed into infirmaries which were run by local councils. Voluntary hospitals grew in tandem but avoided admitting older patients as they were concerned that aged patients would 'block beds' and they were considered less interesting for teaching medical students. The name 'Geriatrics' emerged after a paper by Nascher in the New York Journal of Medicine in 1909. It is derived from two Greek words, 'iatros' meaning healer and 'geros', an old man. Nascher drew comparisons with Paediatric Medicine as a specialty and suggested that Geriatrics should also be a branch of medicine in itself. He also considered the dangers of drug prescribing for older patients and in this respect, as well as in many others, he was ahead of his time. Several years later in the UK, Marjory Warren founded the first geriatric unit. She suggested in a paper in the BMJ that elderly people should be segregated and treated in separate units whilst in the hospital where they could be properly and thoroughly assessed. This approach had origins in Paris in the late 19th century where Charcot had already recognised that this approach could improve health and wellbeing. Warren is described as the 'Mother of Geriatrics' and her approach included such practical measures as improving the look of the wards with bright colours and strongly encouraging patients to get out of bed and mobilise. Warren also developed the idea of a discharge plan and shortened hospital stays. She educated medical and nursing staff to respect older patients and to be aware of their different requirements compared to younger patients. She developed and streamlined the process of rehabilitation and overall was responsible for many achievements in the relatively new specialty. In 1969 Michael Hyland became the first fully trained and substantively appointed Geriatrician in

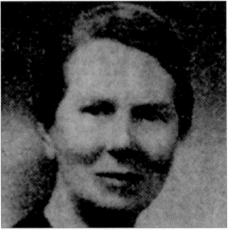

Figure 1: Marjorie Warren

Ireland and the specialty has gone from strength to strength since.

Present day Geriatric Medicine

Since Marjory Warren's time there are significant parallels but also some differences when compared to today's specialty, now sometimes called Medicine for the Elderly or Age Care Medicine. The specialty has continued to develop and grow. In many ways the climate has improved but the challenges are as great as ever. Pejorative terms such as 'bed blockers' still exist and some societies still deem older people to have a less valuable contribution to make than others. However notable strides have been made in evaluation and treatment of older patients and in most countries life expectancy has increased dramatically especially in the last hundred years. Though there are still a great many challenges, the practice of Geriatric Medicine is very rewarding. Simple assessment and treatment can transform outcomes, in some cases far more so than for their younger counterparts. For example, a simple intervention to manage urinary incontinence may completely change a person's life, reinstating their ability to leave the house and reinvigorating their social contacts. Such a problem can be a huge

TABLE I
FACTORS ACCOUNTING FOR INCREASED LONGEVITY

- Improved social conditions and housing
- Reduction in infectious diseases and epidemics
- Reduction in wars and famines
- Reduced peri-natal mortality
- Reduced lethality of degenerative diseases
- Improved medical care and therapeutics

burden on a patient and their family but is often easily alleviated with the correct management.

Demographics

Because the population of 65 years and over is increasing and is not due to peak until well into the next century, the challenge of providing care for older patients is going to increase significantly over the next number of years. The group that is increasing at the fastest rate in Western societies is the 'older old', those aged 85 years and above and this group is likely to be the greatest user of future services. As such, difficult organisational and financial decisions will need to be faced. With these increasing numbers of older people surviving into their 80s and beyond the requirements for acute hospital services will increase significantly. Strategies to keep older people living independently at home are difficult to implement without finances and political goodwill. Unfortunately these patients were in the past less likely to have their voices heard although this may now be changing. Older people are also less likely to have family members who are willing or able to care for them at home compared to previous times and in turn carers themselves are older today than they were a generation ago.

The increase in the projected number of older persons is due in no small part to the almost doubling of life expectancy that has occurred during the 20th century and longevity is probably still increasing and may even be accelerating.

The consequence of these demographic shifts, the so-called *'greying of the population'*, is that large increases in the number of older patients presenting to health services in developed countries will continue well into the future. These increases may impact in one of

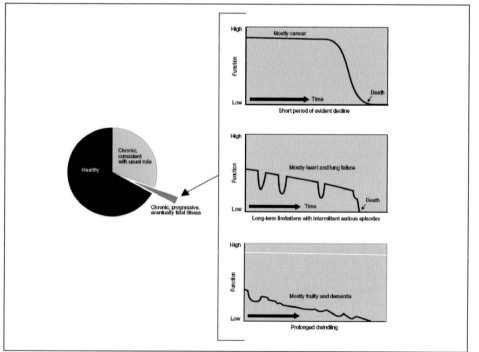

Figure 2: Chronic illness in older patients typically follows three trajectories
(Figure adapted from "Living Well at the End of Life" by Joanne Lynn and David Adamson, used with permission of the author and RAND corporation)

two ways; the first is that a cohort of older patients may present to health services with better health, with postponement of disease and disability until late in life, the so-called *'compression of morbidity'* theory. Within this theory all our illnesses would be compressed into the final few months of life with relative good health and independence up until then; a highly attractive proposition. The second is more worrying; the presentation of a higher proportion of frail older patients with worsening health, highly dependent on medical interventions and services. The hope is that the first scenario will prevail without the progression to chronic illness and disability of a large number of older patients that the second scenario would inevitably lead to. Figure 2 demonstrates the varying trajectories of the resultant chronic illness which may occur in older patients.

The challenge to health professionals and to society at large is to manage the increased population such that older individuals, who may have followed lifestyle and preventative medical advice all their lives and who may indeed have paid taxes all their lives are made actively welcome in our health care systems, when the need arises.

Comprehensive Geriatric Assessment
One of the main features that distinguishes Geriatric assessment from other medical assessments is that it is holistic – the patient is considered in his or her entirety and not simply by organ system or complaint. Geriatricians are trained to take cognisance of multiple co-morbidities and atypical presentations. They consider the patient's physical and mental state, their family and social supports. Aspects of assessment involve psychological and psychiatric considerations, functional status, environment and level of activity including exercise, transportation and social outlets. The comprehensive geriatric assessment (CGA) is defined by the British Geriatrics Society as 'a multidimensional interdisciplinary diagnostic process focused on determining a frail older person's medical, psychological and functional capability in order to develop a co-ordinated and integrated plan for treatment and long term follow up'. Frail older people are most likely to benefit from this type of assessment.

Two or more of the following are markers of frailty:
- Inability to perform one or more basic ADLs in the three days prior to admission
- A stroke in the past three months
- Depression
- Dementia
- A history of falls
- One or more unplanned admissions in the past three months
- Difficulty in walking
- Malnutrition
- Prolonged bed rest
- Incontinence

The importance of comprehensive geriatric assessment is that it may reduce short term mortality and increase functional level. This may allow a patient to live independently at home for a longer period.

Organisation of services
In general terms medical services for older patients should include the following elements:
- Acute care – ideally on a dedicated inpatient ward
- Rehabilitation – on a ward staffed by a range of skilled nurses and therapists
- Day hospital or ambulatory care unit for patient follow-up and rapid outpatient assessment
- Outpatient service for assessment of other conditions such as dementia
- Community Geriatrics service including community hospitals and continuing care
- Respite care

Some patients have complained that health services in general are too sub-specialised, and are not organised in a joined-up way. Geriatric services aim to be fully integrated so that a patient's journey from one point to another is smooth and the quality of care is impeccable throughout. Figure 3 shows how this flow should ideally occur.

Acute care
Availability of resources, however, has not always allowed the specialty to develop or function in this fully comprehensive way. As a consequence three main models of admission of older patients under the care of Geriatricians in the acute setting have evolved:
- Secondary take-over admission policy
- Age-related admission policy
- Integrated (with General Medicine) admission policy

Firstly, patients can be transferred under the care of a Geriatrician after their main presenting illness has been dealt with by another medical team; *secondary take-over of patients*. This practice is now very unusual and most departments are keen to take patients during their initial acute illnesses for reasons that will be addressed later in this chapter. The second

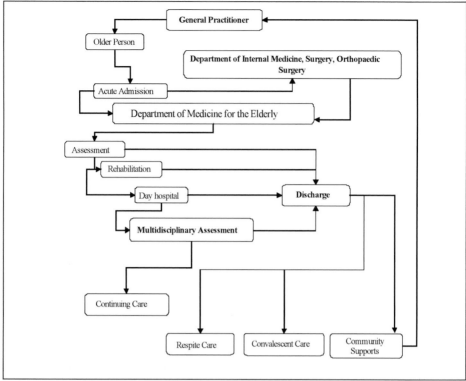

Figure 3: Organisation of Geriatric Services

method is an age-related admission policy, where all patients above a certain age are admitted under the care of a Geriatrician. This policy has the significant advantage of being clear to all with little potential for disputes between admitting teams. There is however significant potential for suitable patients to be excluded because of their age, particularly if the age of admission is set too high and also for older patients, with relatively straight forward problems to be admitted who may not require the attention of the full multi-disciplinary team. The third model is one in which Geriatric Medicine is integrated with General Medicine, with suitable admissions being directed to the Geriatric Services on a *'needs-related basis'*. This method has the advantage of allowing many patients to be assessed based on their need but has the clear disadvantage of diluting the effectiveness of a Geriatrician's time because younger general medical patients may also be admitted to what is primarily a Geriatric service.

Regardless of the type of admission policy employed the acute care of older patients, particularly those

who are frail and debilitated, has specific aims and principles, which should be the framework upon which all assessments take place. Assessment of functional status is central to the practice of Geriatric Medicine. This involves a clear understanding of the patient's pre-morbid functional abilities both in terms of mobility and in terms of the patient's activities of daily living such as dressing, washing, shopping, driving etc. It also involves obtaining a clear picture of the patient's environment and social supports. It is essential to know this information because *'goal setting'* as part of the rehabilitation process is highly dependent on good collateral information. The aim of therapy is critically dependent on the patient's pre-morbid abilities and the whole process is directed towards returning the patient to their baseline functional status.

Because of reduced physiological reserve organ failure may occur quicker than in younger patients following similar insults and the process of assessment and treatment takes longer, sometimes involving prolonged hospitalisation. It is however important to realise that these physiological changes do not occur uniformly

TABLE 2
PRINCIPLES OF ACUTE CARE

PRINCIPLE	POSSIBLE EFFECTS AND EXAMPLES
Assessment of functional status essential	Assessment of abilities in activities of daily living central to assessment of older adults – both pre-admission and pre-discharge
Chronological versus biological age	Age itself has no relevance to disease presentation or functional status
Reduced functional and physiological reserve	Organ failure occurs quicker and is slower to recover in older individuals Drug handling is altered
Multiple pathology	'Divergent' diagnostic assessment required unlike 'convergent' in younger adults
Atypical presentation of illness	No chest pain in myocardial infarction Septicaemia presents as confusion Drug toxicity presents as falls
Polypharmacy	Multiple potential drug side effects and drug interactions
'Geriatric Giants' • Incontinence • Falls • Cognitive impairment • Immobility	Multiple causes Atypical presentation means the 'giants' are no more specific than pyrexia in younger patients
Multi-disciplinary assessment	Essential for functional recovery
Rehabilitation	Essential for functional recovery
Appropriate placement	Must follow multidisciplinary review at the end rather than at the beginning of the process of assessment

across all older individuals and there is a difference between chronological and biological ageing, with some older patients functioning at a much 'younger' age than their peers and vice versa. Age, per se, should therefore never be the sole discriminator as to whether a treatment should or should not be given and each patient must be assessed individually. To do otherwise is 'ageism'. Younger patients often present with multiple symptoms but standard medical assessment will attempt to unite these symptoms into a single diagnosis; convergent assessment. The opposite is true of assessing older adults where multiple pathology is the norm and multiple symptoms and physical signs may need to be separated out as part of a more divergent assessment.

One of the most difficult aspects of assessing older individuals is that many disease processes present in an atypical fashion. Presentations with falls, acute cognitive impairment, incontinence or immobility have almost infinite differential diagnoses and will be dealt with in detail later in this book. The important point is that these 'Geriatric Giants' as described by Isaacs are not specific diagnoses in themselves

TABLE 3	
SOCIAL SUPPORTS AND LOCALLY AVAILABLE SERVICES	
1	Meals on wheels
2	Home help
3	Night sitting
4	Sheltered housing
5	Warden controlled environment
6	Day centre
7	Day hospital
8	Respite admissions
9	Public Health Nurse
10	Community physiotherapy
11	Community occupational therapy
12	Chiropody
13	Primary care team co-ordinated by the General Practitioner

TABLE 4
PRINCIPLES OF REHABILITATION
• Assessment of pre-morbid functional status
• Recognition of potential for functional recovery
• Aggressive treatment of active intercurrent illnesses and restoration of homeostasis
• Institution of preventative measures including medication and lifestyle changes
• Enhancement of mobility predominantly with physiotherapy
• Enhancement of activities of daily living with occupational therapy
• Enhancement of communication and swallowing with speech and language therapy
• Enhancement of nutritional status with nutritional advice and supplementation
• Enhancement of sensory function
• Social and psychological support
• Discharge planning

but rather an indication that further evaluation is necessary. Absent or atypical pain, for instance, is well recognised in patients with ischaemic heart disease and peptic ulcer disease and may be due to a reduction in pain sensitivity with age. Altered drug pharmacokinetics and pharmacodynamics also occur with ageing and are compounded by multiple drug prescription; polypharmacy, which will be addressed later in this book. The importance of multi-disciplinary assessment, rehabilitation and appropriate placement will be discussed later in this chapter. Some of the important principles of Geriatric Medicine are outlined in Table 2.

Rehabilitation

Rehabilitation of older adults aims to recognise potential for functional recovery, both in terms of mobility and activities of daily living and to use the expertise of doctors, nurses and the multi-disciplinary team to achieve this recovery. Prolonged hospitalisation is often required and inexperienced health professionals will often recommend continuing care too readily if the patient is perceived not to be recovering speedily enough. Accurate medical diagnosis is however a prerequisite to rehabilitation for obvious reasons – a therapist for instance must know whether it is a stroke or a peripheral neuropathy they are dealing with. Tight homeostasis is also essential as it is pointless attempting to rehabilitate patients in whom active infection, electrolyte disturbance or medication side effects have not adequately been addressed and reversed if possible. It must be recognised that due to reduced physiological reserve, time will be required for recovery to occur or at least

TABLE 5		
REHABILITATION DEFINITIONS AND EXAMPLES		
DEFINITION		**EXAMPLE**
Disease:		Stroke
Impairment:	any loss or abnormality of psychological, physiological or anatomical structure or function	Dysphasia
Disability:	any restriction or lack, due to impairment, of the ability to perform an activity in the manner or within the range considered normal for a human being	Inability to communicate
Handicap:	a disadvantage resulting from an impairment or disability, that limits or prevents the fulfillment of a role appropriate to a person's age, sex, social and cultural circumstances	Social isolation

for the patient to reach their maximum potential functional status. The co-ordinated multi-disciplinary team provides this service and usually comprises;

- Consultant and team
- Ward sister and team
- Physiotherapy
- Occupational therapy
- Speech and language therapy
- Dietician
- Social worker
- Discharge co-ordinator and/or continuing care placement officer

The rehabilitation environment should encourage independence, with personal effects, wardrobes and bedside lockers placed to encourage patients to do things for themselves and to allow the team to work harmoniously in a suitable environment. Therapists, doctors and nurses should have easy access to a gymnasium, a kitchen and bedroom for activities of daily living training and a day room for social events and group therapy. The team has been traditionally led by the Consultant Geriatrician and good communication and clear-cut shared objectives between the members of the team are essential as is mutual respect and trust in each others' judgement. Nursing care on the rehabilitation unit is critical to its overall functioning. Nurses provide round the clock care for the patients, they encourage mobilisation out of hours and at weekends and continue to assess patients' ability to swallow safely at these times. They also undertake the more traditional roles of skin and continence care and feeding as well as liaising with the medical team about intercurrent illnesses. They also usually initiate the discharge plans and liaise with community services.

When a patient is being assessed the team leader aims to achieve a consensus between the members of the team about the target level of functional ability, for instance will the stroke patient be discharged able to walk, able to use a wheelchair or is the aim to get the patients as good as is possible for admission to continuing care? Clearly the 'bar' will be set differently for each individual patient and this need to be explicitly agreed between the various members of the team. Most teams formally meet on a weekly basis and set aims for the following week. Although goal setting is essential these objectives are not written in stone and will regularly change depending on the patient's response to therapy. Other essential features are the involvement of the patient in the process,

the involvement of the relatives and accurate and early discharge planning including a mechanism for communication with the General Practitioner, public health nurse and locally available services as shown in the table 3.

Rehabilitation definitions

Table 5 shows the commonly used rehabilitation definitions. It is important to understand that there is a difference between a disease process, the impairment to anatomical or physiological systems that this causes, the consequent disruption to the activities of daily living or disability and the handicap that may arise in the patient's social and cultural environment.

The critical point to appreciate is that there is not an inevitable progression through these stages and many interventions can be applied to prevent disability or handicap. When dealing with a stroke for instance it is clear that not all dysphasia will inevitably lead to inability to communicate and not all inability to communicate will lead to social isolation. Many factors will influence whether progression will occur through these stages including factors which are intrinsic to the patient themselves and factors which are external to the patient as shown in figure 4.

Therapists

Physiotherapy

The main focus of physiotherapy is to try to improve patients' mobility through balance and gait retraining. Initially this is achieved by working on transferring from bed to chair, then to standing, through to walking and then more complex activities of daily living like climbing stairs. Because the physiotherapist is involved in the assessment of patients regarding their mobility, functional status and ability to manage in their home circumstances, it is essential that decisions regarding any changes needed are made in conjunction with other members of the multidisciplinary team. Following discharge, treatment of patients on an out-patient basis usually continues, aimed at maximising independence in mobility and functional activities, principally as a follow up to in-patient treatment on the rehabilitation ward or to those assessed in assessment units. Many of these treatments can only be performed in a dedicated and fully equipped gymnasium.

Occupational therapy

In 1989 the World Federation of Occupational

Intrinsic factors
Comorbid disease
Disease severity
Cognition
Education
Culture
Pre-morbid disability

Disease ←→ Impairment ←→ Disability ←→ Handicap

Extrinsic factors
Medical treatments
Preventative measures
Social supports
Rehabilitation
Environment
Income
Discrimination
Occupation

Figure 4: Factors determining progression to disability and handicap

Therapists defined Occupational Therapy as 'the treatment of physical and psychiatric conditions through specific activities to help people to reach their maximum level of function and independence in all aspects of life'. The purpose of Occupational Therapy is to maximise the 'fit' between what an individual wants and needs to do and his/her capability to achieve this. It aims to enable those who are temporarily or permanently disabled to be as independent as possible in the activities of their daily lives, while recovering from or adapting to disability. To keep the older person well Occupational Therapists develop approaches to treating specific disorders in the context of patients' lifestyles, physical environments and social environments. The specialty also recognises that systems need to be developed whereby medical and surgical equipment and appliances are available, based on individual assessment and need. Many of these aims can be achieved through the following:

Assessment of present functional level including
• Performance in activities of daily living (ADLs)
• Physical status
• Cognitive status
• Perceptual status
• Psychosocial status
• Home situation and supports including home visiting
• Suitability for assistive devices, wheelchairs etc.

Treatment modalities to maximise present functional status
• Perceptual retraining
• Advice on housing adaptations
• Maximising independence in activities of daily living through the use of assistive devices
• Wheelchair training
• Splinting
• Education of family and carers
• Environmental risk minimisation
• Communication between hospital and community services

Examples of group work
• Reality orientation
• Relaxation
• Reminiscence
• Social groups
• Remedial games

Speech and language therapy
The role of Speech and Language Therapy encompasses the assessment, diagnosis, management and prevention of disorders of communication. In recent years they have also become adept at assessing and treating oropharyngeal swallow disorders.

The role of the speech and language therapist in the rehabilitation of older individuals
• Assessment and diagnosis of new communication

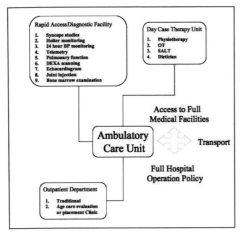

Figure 5: Elements of a day hospital

disorders
- Assessment and diagnosis of new swallowing disorders
- Ongoing monitoring of swallowing disorders and prevention of aspiration
- Treatment of communication disorders; dysarthria and dysphasia
- Treatment of swallowing disorders
- Assessment of suitability for PEG (percutaneous gastrostomy tube) insertion
- Education of family and carers
- Communication between hospital and community services

Nutrition service

Nutrition intervention in this group can be both for health promotion (including disease prevention) and therapeutic (patients with nutrition related diseases such as stroke, coronary heart disease and diabetes as well as many others). Dietetic intervention in the care of the older adult therefore encompasses screening, assessment, and formulation of protocols of treatment, monitoring, education, audit and research. Research has shown that close attention to nutritional status may help to optimise stroke patients' rehabilitation potential and use of healthcare resources. The role of the service is wide but for example, the type of treatment given to a stroke patient who is returning to the day hospital is given below. The aim of management of the post-stroke patient can be divided into 3 areas:

• Prevention of malnutrition and maintenance of nutritional status
There is a high risk of malnutrition in this group

due to dysphagia, anorexia, inability to self feed, cognitive impairment, immobility and depression. The consequences of malnutrition include delayed functional recovery, impaired immunocompetence and organ function, depression and increased morbidity and mortality. In addition malnourished patients incur large health care costs. To prevent or reverse the effect of malnutrition early dietetic intervention is essential.

• Nutritional management
Nutritional intervention will involve full assessment of nutritional status and determination of individual requirements, developing a plan of nutritional care, and prescription of appropriate diet eg. artificial nutrition support or modified textures diet. Note is also made of dentition and the use of artificial dentures as this may influence ability to masticate.

• Reassessment
Follow-up and reassessment is vital to ensure maintenance of optimal nutritional status. This includes alteration of mode of feeding according to patients' progress and monitoring transition from one type of nutrition support to another e.g. transition from PEG to modified texture diet. Expert dietary advice is an important component in preventing the reoccurrence of stroke, particularly those at high risk – diabetes, obesity, hypertension, hyperlipidaemia or renal impairment. The participation of a clinical nutritionist/dietician is therefore essential in the multidisciplinary team management of older patients recovering from complex medical problems such as stroke.

Day hospital or ambulatory care unit

The value of an Ambulatory Care Unit to the management of sick older patients has been firmly established. It is a way of providing a total package of care incorporating medical, nursing and rehabilitation (physiotherapy, occupational therapy, speech and language therapy and nutritional advice) services without an overnight stay in hospital. Rapid outpatient investigation, diagnosis, treatment and rehabilitation of older patients may forestall the need for hospital admission altogether or it may facilitate earlier discharge of hospitalised patients. The provision of services within the ambulatory care unit encompasses three main elements as shown in Figure 5.

The frequency and duration of attendance will vary reflecting each patient's individual needs. Ambulatory care units usually open five days per week with no

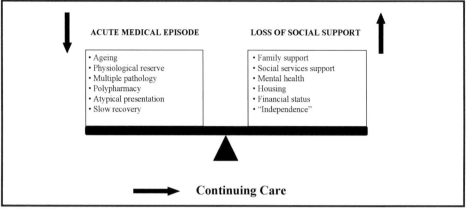

Figure 6: Factors affecting admission to continuing care

weekend activity. These units will function best if they are fully integrated with the hospital-based Department of Geriatric Medicine and are thus best developed on the acute hospital site.

The benefits of an Ambulatory Care Unit are thus obvious;
- Rapid assessment of semi-acutely ill patients with the potential to avoid hospital admission
- Follow-up of post-discharge patients with the potential to significantly reduce length of stay in hospital
- Integration with inpatient rehabilitation facilities

Transport
Because patients accessing the ambulatory care unit will be older and often frail, transport to and from the unit is critical to its successful functioning. For instance patients may not, because of health reasons or otherwise, be able to drive a car or they may simply not own a car. Public transport may not be available to them if they live in an isolated area or may not coincide with the hours of operation of the unit. Some patients will be too frail to use public transport, even if it is available. In order to provide a service to all patients, many units operate their own transport in the form of mini-buses, which are wheel chair friendly. A small proportion of patients will be severely incapacitated and will need ambulance transport.

Access to full hospital medical facilities
The ambulatory care unit needs to have easy access to full medical facilities in order to be efficient and safe. Although much of the necessary equipment

for investigation and treatment will be available in the unit, the unit will still depend on some services already provided in the hospital. For example, patients attending the ambulatory care unit will have blood testing performed as part of their investigation. Blood results should ideally be available before the patient leaves the unit at the end of the day. Some tests require multiple samples, taken over a period of several hours. Furthermore, certain bloods need to be analysed immediately, such as arterial blood gases. The laboratory therefore has to be easily accessible from the unit. Radiology facilities must also be easily accessible to the unit for similar reasons.

Continuing care
Following the inpatient and outpatient assessments and therapies described above there will be a small number of patients who will require ongoing institutional care. The likelihood of this does not just depend on the disease process but also on a large number of external factors that influence whether or not the patients will be able to return home as shown in figure 6. When admission to long-term care has been decided upon recognition that this event is traumatic to both the patient and carers must be understood. The patient should continue to have full access to medical services and the environment must be conducive to ensuring the patients' dignity, rights as a human being and privacy are maintained. In appropriate cases patient advocates need to be encouraged particularly in cases where cognitive impairment is present.

Community Geriatrics
Most geriatricians now have responsibility for some

community services including community hospitals, community day hospitals or continuing care. This is an expanding area and in the UK the advent of community geriatricians has paved the way for a more formal organisation of these services. Recent research suggests that community hospitals may be as effective for rehabilitation as acute hospitals at similar or less cost. Careful patients selection is however critical to ensure that patients who require full hospital based facilities are not prematurely discharged to these units.

Respite care

Carers often spend 7 days a week looking after their loved one and this impacts in a negative way on their physical and psychological wellbeing. The availability of respite care helps to alleviate this. A revolving programme of regular respite is beneficial for carers and also offers an opportunity for contact with medical services for the patient. Respite is intended as short term, planned stays, sometimes in community hospitals or rehabilitation units.

The future of Geriatric Medicine

Changing demographics and longer lifespans indicate clearly that in the future Geriatric services will be in more demand than ever before. Patients today rightly have higher expectations of well-being and disease-free survival. New investigations are revolutionising diagnostics and the introduction of screening programmes will increase the requirement for hospital based services. Similarly older people are benefiting from a range of new treatments and more aggressive approaches, for example in malignancy and with the advent of new surgical interventions. Further subspecialisation within Geriatric Medicine itself has also occurred in recent years with orthogeriatrics, stroke teams, TIA clinics, falls assessment units and community geriatrics being developed. Unfortunately Ireland still lags behind in terms of facilities, with a particular shortage of stroke units. Further development of services should allow geriatricians to respond to these needs but service demands may continue to grow requiring ongoing reassessment of the structure of service delivery. Development of future services will certainly be done with more input from patients and it may be possible that patients will soon be able to choose where and when they see a specialist. In this setting equity of access actively needs to be preserved and it is important to consider geographical separation when new services are developed. The main challenge will still be to deliver appropriate care in the optimum environment for patients with the aim of prolonging independent living. Whilst we cannot turn the clock back, health care professionals involved in the care of older patients should always strive to maintain or improve quality of life; an aim which is the key outcome of successful Geriatric assessment and intervention.

Suggested further reading

- Barton A, Mulley G. History of the development of geriatric medicine in the UK. Postgrad. Med. J. 2003; 79; 229-234.
- Grimley Evans J. Geriatric Medicine: a brief history. BMJ 1997; 315: 1075-1077.
- British Geriatrics Society, http://www.bgs.org.uk
- Merck Manual of Geriatrics, http://www.merck.com/ mkgr/mmg/home.jsp
- Rockwood K, Song X, MacKnight C, et al. A global clinical measure of fitness and frailty in elderly people. CMAJ 2005; 173(5): 489-95.
- Avorn J. Benefits and cost analysis in geriatric care. Turning age discrimination into health policy. N Engl J Med 1984; 310: 1294-1301.
- Coakley D. Introduction: The elements of a geriatric service. In: Coakley D ed. Establishing a Geriatric Service, London: Croom Helm ,1982, pp 9 -15.
- Clinch D, Banerjee AK, Ostick G. Absence of abdominal pain in elderly patients with peptic ulcer. Age Ageing 1984; 13: 120-123.
- Gamble E, Liston R. Conference report: Increasing longevity - medical, social and political implications. J R Col Phys Lon 1997; 31: 563-564.
- Liston R, Clinch D. Use of an age related admission policy in establishing a new department of medicine for the elderly. Ir Med J 1994; 87: 47-50.
- Pathy MS. Clinical presentation of heart disease in the elderly. Br Heart J 1967; 29: 190-197.
- Procacci P, Bozza G, Burelli G, Dellacorte M. The cutaneous pricking pain threshold in old age. Gerontologica Clinica 1970; 12: 213-218.
- Report of the working party on services for the elderly. The years ahead... A policy for the elderly. Dublin: The stationary office, Government Publications, 1988.
- Rowe JW. Health care of the elderly. N Engl J Med 1985; 312: 827-35.
- Rubenstein LZ, Josephson KR, Wieland GD, English PA, Sayre JA, Kane RL. Effectiveness of a geriatric assessment unit - A randomised controlled trial. N Engl J Med 1984; 311: 1664-70.
- Schneider EL, Brody JA. Ageing, natural death, and the compression of morbidity: another view. N Engl J Med 1983; 309: 854-55.
- Sherman ED, Robillar E. Sensitivity to pain in the aged.

Can Med Assoc J 1980; 83: 944.

- Tallis RC, Fillit HM, Broncklehurst JC (Eds) *Geriatric Medicine and Gerontology*. 5th Ed. Churchill Livingstone 1999.

Case Study 1

An 83 year old man was admitted to his local hospital following a fall. When he arrived into the busy Emergency department he was acutely confused and tachypnoeic. He was assessed by the Medical SHO as having pneumonia on a background of probable dementia with a possible recent transient ischaemic attack. Benzodiazepine sedatives were prescribed. He was admitted to the ward and was commenced on intravenous antibiotics and fluids. Two days later a Geriatric consultation was obtained, as the patient had not improved. It was noted that no collateral history had been obtained but a phone call to the next of kin revealed that the patient had been well prior to admission, was actively involved in a retirement group, walked on a daily basis and continued to drive. Examination of the patient revealed bi-basal crackles consistent with heart failure and the cardiograph showed changes consistent with an anterior myocardial infarction. The patient was transferred to the CCU and his infarct and failure were appropriately treated with aspirin, ACE inhibitors and diuretics. Benzodiazepines were weaned and after a two week period he had returned back to his baseline, his confusion resolved and there was no evidence of dementia.

This case illustrates the atypical presentation of disease in older adults and the importance of a good collateral history. Confusion in this case indicated hypoxia secondary to left ventricular failure secondary to an acute myocardial infarction. The SHO erroneously equated confusion with dementia, an error compounded by his failure to obtain a collateral history. There was no evidence of a transient ischaemic attack with no focal neurological symptoms or signs. The fall was most likely secondary to the myocardial infarction which presented silently with no pain. The patient was biologically better than his 83 years suggested as indicated by his pre-morbid lifestyle. With appropriate treatment he returned back to his normal activities following a short abstinence from driving.

Case Study 2

A 66 years old man was admitted to his local hospital having sustained a left hemiparesis. There was a background history of type 2 diabetes and hypertension. The patient lived alone and was somewhat socially isolated. He drank over 50 units of alcohol per week and was a lifelong heavy smoker. On admission there was evidence of aspiration pneumonia confirmed on chest x-ray and his glucose readings were high, varying between 11 and 15mmol/l. His CT brain scan showed evidence of a large right middle cerebral artery territory infarct. The patient was initially treated with intravenous fluids and antibiotics along with insulin to keep his sugars less than 12mmol/l. He also received aspirin, a statin and an ACE inhibitor for secondary prevention. Following stabilisation he was transferred to the Rehabilitation Unit. The occupational therapist assessed him as having no evidence of cognitive impairment and no evidence of visuospatial problems or sensory inattention often associated with left hemiparesis and thus from these points of view the prognosis was good. A left homonymous hemianopia was however present and the patient was positioned in the ward such that both his visual fields were stimulated. As expected in patients with left hemiparesis, the speech and language therapist assessed him as having no evidence of dysphasia but swallowing was impaired. Avoidance of free fluids was recommended and all other foods were thickened. A videofluroscopy was not deemed necessary. With these measures no further aspirations occurred and no artificial feeding with either nasogastric or percutaneous gastrostomy was contemplated. The nutritionist altered his diet in view of his diabetes and hypercholesterolemia. With physiotherapy he regained mobility with a Zimmer frame but required the supervision of one person at all times. His 10 week stay on the unit was complicated by crying episodes and low mood which was only partially responsive to anti-depressants and ongoing psychiatric review. Despite his young age successful discharge home was not achieved and he was discharged to continuing care but continued to be monitored on a regular basis there.

This case illustrates the importance of multi-disciplinary team work in assessing older patients. It also demonstrates the importance of discharge planning. In this case a successful discharge home was not achieved because of the patient's incomplete functional recovery which required the patient to be supervised by at least one person on a 24 hour basis. His poor social networks made it unsafe to discharge him home and he was therefore admitted to long term care.

Case Study 3

A 74 year old woman was admitted with acute cognitive impairment on a background of possible Lewy body dementia which had presented with visual hallucinations, mild cognitive impairment and parkinsonism six months previously. Medical assessment revealed profound confusion but multiple blood tests and septic screens were normal. CT brain scan showed degenerative changes only and a lumbar puncture was clear. The patients remained confused for a number of weeks and began to significantly deteriorate physically due to poor nutritional intake. A diagnosis of encephalopathy was entertained and an EEG examination was ordered which showed non-convulsive status epilepticus. The patient improved on sodium valproate but was very debilitated for a prolonged period of time. Signs of aspiration were apparent and a percutaneous gastrostomy tube was inserted and only thickened fluids and soft diet allowed orally. The decision to insert the percutaneous gastrostomy tube was taken after in-depth discussion between the speech and language therapist, the nutritionist and the other members of the rehabilitation team.

Despite the anti-convulsant, episodes of profound and fluctuating cognitive impairment continued and repeat EEG during these episodes showed evidence of degenerative brain disease only with no further seizure activity. A cholinesterase inhibitor, rivastigmine was introduced and the patient had a dramatic improvement. The percutaneous gastrostomy tube was left in situ for 12 weeks and was removed following significant weight gain. The patient was discharged home on valproate and rivastigmine.

This case demonstrates the importance of multi-disciplinary assessment particularly in the context of atypical presentation of epilepsy as in this case.

Case Study 4

A 78 year old woman was referred to the ambulatory care unit with recurrent dizzy spells, unsteadiness and one fall. The General Practitioner had initially requested admission but was assured that the patient would be rapidly assessed as an outpatient and an appointment for the following week was given. The patient had a background history of type 2 diabetes and hypertension which was proving difficult to control. The patient was on metformin, a diuretic, an ACE inhibitor and an alpha blocker. Clinical examination revealed a broad based gait and evidence of significant postural hypotension on bedside testing and tilt testing was not deemed to be necessary. A 24 hour blood pressure monitor showed reasonable readings during the day and a normal nocturnal dip indicating that it was probably safe to rationalise the patient's anti-hypertensive medication and the alpha blocker was stopped. An urgent CT brain scan showed a cerebellar infarct and the patient was commenced on a statin and aspirin for secondary prevention. A DEXA scan showed osteopaenia and calcium and vitamin D replacement was commenced. The dietician reviewed her in view of her diabetes and hypercholesterolemia. The patient continued to visit the ambulatory care unit on a twice-weekly basis for physiotherapy in view of the cerebellar infarct. Postural hypotension improved and although the patient continued to be occasionally unsteady she was deemed by the multi-disciplinary team to have reached her maximum potential and was discharged from the unit. Prior to discharge the patient was given advice regarding getting out of bed and standing up slowly. A letter was written to the General Practitioner asking that the patient be reviewed regularly and indicating that the patient would be seen again as a matter of urgency for consideration for midodrine or other measures if the postural hypotension recurred.

Data Interpretation

Question 1

A 78 year old man presents to the emergency department with confusion. His blood results are as follows:

Na^+	125mmol/l
K^+	5.2mmol/l
CRP	10mg/l
WCC	12×10^9/l
Hb	9.5g/dl
Ca^{++}	2.3mmol/l

What is the likely cause of his confusion?

a.   Hyperkalaemia
b.   Hyponatraemia
c.   Infection
d.   Hypercalcaemia
e.   Anaemia

Question 2

A 65 year old lady is admitted to hospital with transient right sided weakness. The weakness lasted for 2 hours then resolved completely. On examination the next day she has normal power but seems confused. Her answers are un-intelligible though she appears to understand instructions. What is the diagnosis?

a.   Stroke
b.   Transient ischaemic attack
c.   Seizure
d.   Transient global amnesia
e.   Acute delirium

Question 3

A 90 year old man who lives alone with a good level of function presents to the emergency department with symptoms consistent with a respiratory tract infection. After successful treatment he has difficulty mobilising after spending several days in bed and requires assistance with hygiene needs. What is the most appropriate plan of action?

a.   Discharge home
b.   Admit to nursing home
c.   Rehabilitation
d.   Respite
e.   Discharge to sheltered housing

Best of five questions

Question 1

Which of the following is not a factor accounting for increased longevity?

a.   Reduction in wars and famines
b.   Reduced peri-natal mortality
c.   Congregation of people in cities
d.   Reduced lethality of degenerative diseases
e.   Improved medical care and therapeutics

Question 2

Which of the following is not a marker of frailty?

a.   Depression
b.   A history of falls
c.   Incontinence
d.   Recent stroke
e.   Polypharmacy

Question 3

Dysphasia is an example of:

a.   Disease
b.   Impairment
c.   Disability
d.   Handicap
e.   Syndrome

Answers are on page 311

The emergency department

R McNamara, S O'Hanlon, R Liston

Introduction

Older patients make up between 15 - 18% of presentations to Accident and Emergency Departments (A&E) in the United Kingdom. They are more likely to require admission, more likely to re-attend and more likely to have serious morbidity and mortality than younger groups. In the UK 48% of older people are admitted to hospital from the A&E compared with 20% of patients overall. Older patients often present with non-specific symptoms such as confusion, falls, acute mobility impairment and dizzy spells. Any of these presentations may be the result of occult infection, myocardial ischaemia, cardiac failure, intracranial pathology or a large number of other differential diagnoses. It is not uncommon for a myocardial infarct or acute appendicitis to be painless. The reasons for this are unclear but may be related to altered physiology, altered mental and physical reserves, reduced perception of visceral pain or pre-existing pain masking new disease processes. In addition, communication difficulties caused by cognitive impairment, hearing impairment or dysphasia may make it impossible for a patient to give an account of their presenting problem. A&E is often the first contact that many older patients have with formal medical care. Although many of these patients present acutely unwell and require a high level of medical intervention it can be an opportunistic place for screening those at risk of falls, pressure sores or cognitive impairment. It also provides an opportunity to initiate contact with primary care services; GP, public health nurses, occupational therapists and social workers. It is clear therefore that older individuals presenting to A&E require special consideration and all staff involved in their assessment should be well versed with their special requirements;

- The majority of diseases increase in prevalence with increasing age so that older patients regularly have multiple co-morbid conditions
- Atypical presentations are common
- Patients may minimise their symptoms and sometimes have difficulty in communicating their problems
- Presentation with acute confusion is easily precipitated and older patients are more prone to sudden deterioration in the A&E
- Patients may be on numerous medications - polypharmacy - an important cause of morbidity and mortality in its own right and associated with an increased risk of adverse drug reactions
- Older patients should have particularly close follow-up on discharge from the A&E department as seemingly minor presentations such as fractures can lead to significant morbidity and dependence

Conditions which are common in younger patients, for example vasovagal syncope causing collapse, are uncommon in the elderly and should be diagnosed only when other possible diagnoses have been excluded. In addition a collapse, seizure or dizzy spell is rarely due to a TIA and this is a diagnostic label that should be reserved exclusively for those patients with a focal neurological presentation. In older patients who are acutely unwell, a comprehensive assessment must be undertaken with appropriate investigation until a cause is found. Easy diagnostic labels should be avoided. Some conditions which are easily missed in the A&E setting are shown in Table 1.

Physiological changes

Older patients often have a poor physiological reserve with less robust homeostatic mechanisms so that even minor injury may not be tolerated. Listed below are some of the physiological changes associated with ageing that are of relevance in the A&E Department:

- Poor tolerance of and response to fluctuations in blood volume
- Increased circulating catecholamines with blunted receptor response
- Vital Capacity, FEV_1, PaO_2 decrease with age
- Decreased mobility of joints
- Reduced renal blood flow, loss of nephrons and lower glomerular filtration rate
- Perception of thirst declines
- Plasma renin and aldosterone levels reduced
- Reduced response to vasopressin

TABLE I
CONDITIONS WHICH ARE UNDERDIAGNOSED IN OLDER PATIENTS IN A&E
Seizure
Stroke
Delirium
Polymyalgia Rheumatica
Vertebral fracture
Depression
Acute abdomen

- Reduced temperature sensation and delayed response to temperature change
- Delayed gastric emptying
- Reduced hepatic function

These physiological responses are also affected by the presence of pre-existing disease itself and often by medication used to treat disease. Thus older patients are at high risk for organ ischaemia when presenting with shock and this can mean that patients deteriorate rapidly and often unexpectedly. Pathophysiological changes which may be important include underlying coronary artery disease increasing risk of myocardial infarction, osteoporosis increasing risk of fractures and cerebral atrophy increasing the risk of intracranial bleeding in trauma.

Unique challenges

The differences in physiology, presentation and management of older patients in the A&E represent a source of ongoing difficulty for doctors. Training in Geriatric Medicine and in Emergency Medicine should take into account the diverse nature of pathology seen and the nuances of caring for these patients. The challenges in medical management of the acutely unwell older patient are many but with correct and timely intervention these patients often do very well. For example thrombolysis of an older patient with ST elevation myocardial infarction confers greater survival benefit than in younger patients.

Principles of emergency care

Emergency assessment of the older patient is broken down into different steps depending on the presentation and severity:

Triage

In the majority of Emergency departments patients are triaged by a dedicated nurse. They are triaged into 'major' and 'minor' cases and then assigned a triage category which determines the order in which patients are seen by medical staff. As explained above, older patients may lack the usual indicators of disease severity and so there is a risk that they may be triaged to a lower category. Triage category should be reviewed if the patient's condition changes. The history given by the patient may be affected by underlying cognitive impairment, and many patients do not wish to disclose the exact circumstances surrounding their presentation as they wish to avoid attention, embarrassment, hospitalisation, or referral to social services.

Primary survey

Initial assessment of any acutely unwell patient should follow a structured, logical sequence starting with a primary survey and resuscitation, then a directed history and progressing to full physical examination. This is in contrast to the traditional approach used in the clinic and on the wards of taking a complete history before progressing to a complete examination, and finally to ordering intervention.

The aim of primary survey is to detect life threatening problems and to resuscitate appropriately. The key components are:

A: Airway: Assessment should begin by ensuring patency of the airway, if necessary providing mechanical ventilation, giving high concentration of oxygen and appreciating the possibility of cervical spine injury. In the elderly patient airway management may be more challenging in the presence of poor dentition or cachexia. Intubation may be difficult because of decreased mouth opening and decreased neck mobility. Drug choices for rapid sequence intubation may be limited by pre-existing co-morbid disease. Older patients are at high risk for cervical spine injuries, particularly of the odontoid peg.

B: Breathing: To assess adequacy of breathing, signs of respiratory distress should be sought, as well as non-invasive monitoring of oxygen saturations.

C: Circulation: The aim of assessing circulation is to detect and treat shock. Blood pressure and pulse rate should be determined as well as jugular venous pressure and the character and nature of the carotid pulse. If hypotension is present fluid resuscitation should be commenced. Fluid and blood resuscitation may be complicated by pre-existing medical conditions, such as hypertension or anaemia. It may be difficult to measure response to resuscitation because of the effects of

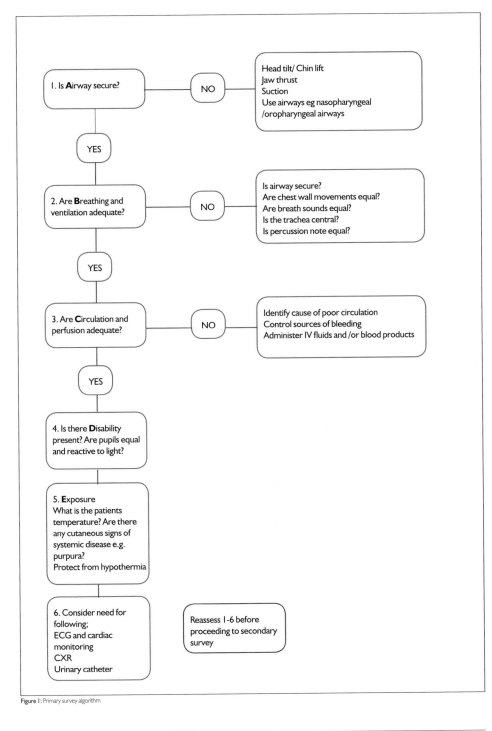

Figure 1: Primary survey algorithm

TABLE 2
PREDISPOSING FACTORS FOR TRAUMA IN OLDER PATIENTS

Hearing impairment
Reduced visual acuity
Gait disturbance
Degenerative joint disease
Reduced coordination
Muscle weakness
Impaired proprioception
Poor peripheral sensation
Muscle wasting/weakness
Cognitive impairment

medications such as beta blockers.

D: Disability (neurological evaluation): The aim is to detect any life-threatening neurological emergency. Assessment includes estimation of the Glasgow coma scale, examination of the pupillary responses and checking for signs of meningeal irritation. In the elderly pre-existing dementia may make it difficult to recognise increasing confusion associated with acute illness. Pre-existing neurological impairment may delay diagnosis of new lateralising signs. When assessing disability it is often said 'Don't forget the glucose'. Bedside blood sugar estimation is easily performed and if abnormal is easily correctable.

E: Exposure: The patient should be fully exposed so that any clues to the underlying cause of illness will be seen eg. petechial rash, jaundice or bruising. The patient's temperature should be recorded and care must be taken not to induce hypothermia while exposing the patient.

Secondary survey

The assessment continues with a full physical examination involving all organ systems in the usual manner, to ensure no abnormal findings have been missed.

Appropriate and timely disposal

After assessment and initial management, patients should be referred to the appropriate team for further care. As emergency departments develop they assume responsibility for a greater proportion of patients and admissions may decrease as a result. For example more patients with chest pain are now managed solely by emergency physicians. Discharge planning also takes place in the A&E. Some patients who are medically well but may require a temporary increase in support eg. after a wrist fracture for instance, may be appropriately discharged from the A&E after assessment and planning by the occupational therapist, social worker or discharge co-ordinator.

Shock in older patients

Shock is a physiological reaction to a variety of conditions usually characterised by hypotension and inadequate tissue perfusion. Compensatory mechanisms attempt to maintain tissue perfusion by controlling circulation, oxygen uptake and blood flow within the vital organs. However, as discussed above these mechanisms become impaired with advancing age making clinical assessment and resuscitation of the older patient more challenging. In older patients who present early with shock, invasive haemodynamic monitoring to aid volume management and adequate resuscitation to avoid hypoxia and hypoperfusion has been shown to reduce mortality without increasing length of stay or reducing quality of life or independence.

Distributive shock

Distributive shock is caused by peripheral vasodilatation of blood vessels causing a decrease in systemic vascular resistance. There are three types of distributive shock; anaphylactic, septic and neurogenic. Septic shock is sepsis associated with persistant hypotension causing tissue hypoperfusion. Anaphylactic shock occurs following degranulation of mast cells in response to an allergen, resulting in a massive release of immunological mediators which cause widespread vasodilatation, bronchspasm and oedema. Neurogenic shock results from impairment of the decending sympathetic pathways of the spinal cord, causing loss of vasomotor tone and loss of innervation to the heart; the classic picture described is hypotension without tachycardia or peripheral vasoconstriction.

In any patients with sepsis the aim is to reach the following evidence-based goals within 6 hours;
• Measure serum lactate
• Obtain blood cultures prior to early antibiotic administration
• Early and aggressive fluid resuscitation
• Vasopressor use as required

Hypovolaemic shock

Hypovolaemic shock occurs when the circulating blood volume is reduced. It is the most common cause of shock and can result from haemorrhage and dehydration.

Cardiogenic shock

Cardiogenic shock is the result of inability of the heart to pump effectively and is most commonly due to myocardial infarction. Clincally it is defined by sustained hypotension with tissue hypoperfusion despite adequate left ventricular filling pressures.

Trauma

About one third of patients over 65 attending the Emergency Department do so following trauma.

In this setting older patients are at particular risk of specific injuries including subdural haematoma, vascular injuries and all fractures including cervical spine fractures. As illustrated in case 3 significant injury may result from seemingly minor trauma. Patients aged 65 years and over, when compared to younger patients with an equal injury severity score, have been shown to have a higher admission rate, a longer length of stay in hospital and a higher mortality rate. Causes of trauma must be elicited and investigated thoroughly. Why did the patient fall? What happened before they lost control of the car? Was there a prior history of syncope, TIA or CVA, MI etc, etc? The majority of older patients who fall have an underlying medical cause and claims by the patient that they tripped or slipped must not be taken at face value; patients sometimes either do not recall the exact circumstances or play them down. Significant medical conditions can be uncovered by prudent assessment and further episodes of trauma may be avoided. These are serious events and 50% of older patients requiring hospitalisation after a fall die within one year.

General principles of trauma management

The principals of trauma management are the same in all age groups, with the same emphasis on 'ABCs' as discussed above in relation to medical emergencies. Particular points to note when treating elderly patients are;
- Be aware of hypothermia
- Remember that blood pressure and heart rate responses to hypovolaemia are affected by both physiological and iatrogenic factors
- Have a low threshold to give blood product transfusion
- Be aware of pre-existing coagulopathy and electrolyte disturbance

- Ensure glucose level is checked
- Take blood sample for medication levels where appropriate
- Record 12 lead ECG
- Maintain a low threshold for ordering further radiographic studies where there is any question of fracture, head injury or vascular injury from clinical findings. Do not rely on normal plain film studies - remember that many fractures including hip fractures can be very subtle, liaise with orthopaedic surgeons and consider MRI, CT or bone scan.

Elder abuse

It is estimated that 2-10% of older people are victims of elder abuse. The term includes psychological abuse, neglect, sexual abuse, physical abuse or financial abuse. In the A&E, history taking is important, and a high index of suspicion is required when there is evidence of neglect or the age or pattern of the injury does not fit with the history of events described. It is likely that many cases are missed and injuries such as fracture, falls and bruising should be red flags for health professionals to consider abuse. It is important to note that the abuser is often a family member or carer and may have accompanied the patient to the A&E.

Alcohol-related problems

Alcohol-related problems are an under-recognised presentation of older patients to the emergency department. Alcohol may be the direct underlying precipitant for a number of clinical scenarios including falls, syncope, various injuries and delirium or it may be associated with other primary presentations leading to erroneous and excessive investigation of elevated liver function tests, elevated MCV or hypertension. Alcohol misuse can be masked by non-specific health problems such as various GI complaints, tiredness, insomnia or can be misdiagnosed as dementia.

Studies have shown that between 5 and 12% of men older than 60 years have alcohol problems. Other studies have found that up to 17% of men over 65 years exceed 'sensible limits' of consumption. There is a lack of research regarding the proportion of older women with such problems but given that their risk factors are more common, including bereavement and depression, it is likely that the levels are as high or even higher than in older men. Older people are less tolerant of alcohol due to a number of physiologocial changes that occur with ageing including a fall in the ratio of body water to fat, decreased hepatic blood flow, reduced hepatic enzyme activity and enhanced effects of alcohol on neurones. These changes mean that alcolol has more profound effects on older individuals. Alcohol also alters the effects of other drugs including warfarin and sedatives, especially benzodiazepines.

However alcohol problems are most likely to present with injuries. Doctors need to be aware of alcohol as a major health concern for older patients and appropriate assessment and referral is essential. As a simple rule of thumb older patients will rarely volunteer their true level of consumption and the clinician may need to probe deeper, cognisant of all the above issues, in the assessment of these at-risk patients.

Recurrent falls

Falls are the commonest cause of trauma presentations in older patients and are associated with significant morbidity and loss of function. Some patients are labelled as 'recurrent falls' but caution should be exercised as this does not offer an explanation as to why the patient is falling. Thorough investigation is needed if a definite diagnosis has not been made. The A&E offers an opportunity to initiate investigation with routine blood investigations, cardiac monitoring and detailed examination including lying and standing blood pressure measurements. However where the cause of a fall is not determined referral to a falls specialist may be required.

Heat illness

Heat illness includes a spectrum of disease from prickly heat to heat stroke. Heat stroke occurs in the elderly more commonly and is seen in epidemic proportions during heat waves such as occured in France in 2004.

Heat stroke

Heat stroke is characterised by a failure of the body's thermo-regulatory system in the presence of high core body temperature. The core temperature necessary for the condition to be classified as heat stroke is rectal temperature exceeding 40.6°C. Heat stroke is divided into exertional and non-exertional (classical) heat stroke. Classical heat stroke occurs during extreme heat waves, the elderly being particularly vulnerable because of faulty homeostatic mechanisms. When therapy is delayed, the mortality rate may be as high as 80%; however, with early diagnosis and immediate

cooling, the mortality rate can be reduced to 10%. Mortality is highest among the older population, patients with pre-existing disease, those confined to bed and those who are socially isolated.

The management of heat stroke includes; cooling with the aim to reduce core body temperature to 39°C, continuous invasive temperature monitoring, IV fluids and catheterisation, cold-water immersion and transfer to ICU. There is no role for anti-pyretic drugs as the hypothalamus is not the problem. Seizures can be controlled with benzodiazepines, augmented by barbiturates. Failing this the patient should be paralysed and ventilated and continuous EEG monitoring instituted.

Hypothermia

Hypothermia is the failure of the body's thermo-regulatory system in the presence of low core body temperature. It is classified as accidental or intentional, primary or secondary and by the degree of hypothermia. Again, mortality rate increases with increasing age and older patients are more likely to present with chronic or secondary hypothermia. Over 50% of all reported mortality from accidental hypothermia has occurred in individuals aged 65 years or older.

In the absence of cardiac arrest the aim is to increase core body temperature by 0.5°C per hour.

In the presence of cardiac arrest raising the core body temperature to 32°C as rapidly as possible stabilises the myocardium to allow defibrillation. Continuous invasive temperature monitoring is required as well as passive rewarming by removing wet clothes or blankets. Active external rewarming may be necessary using warm air blankets. Active internal re-warming techniques starting with warm IV fluids is sometimes appropriate.

Suggested further reading

- *Geriatric Emergency Medicine. Meldon SR, Woolard R. McGraw-Hill Professional, 2003.*
- *Geriatric Emergency Medicine. Gideon Bosker. Mosby, 1990.*
- *Geriatric Emergency Medicine. Magauran, Kahn, Olkshaker. Saunders, 2006.*
- *Advanced Trauma Life Support Course Book. American College of Surgeons Published by American College of Surgeons, 1997.*
- *Wass A, Zoltie N. Changing patterns in accident and*

emergency attenders. *Emerg Med 1996; 13: 269–71.*

- Downing A, Wilson R. *Older people's use of Accident and Emergency services. Age Ageing 2005; 34: 24-30.*
- British Geriatrics Society, *The Older Person in the Accident & Emergency Department BGS Compendium document 3.2 (Revised March 2008 http://www.bgs.org. uk/Publications/Compendium/compend_3-2.htm)*
- Eagle J, Rideout E, Price P, McCann C, Wonacott E. *Misuse of the emergency department by the elderly population: myth or reality. J Emerg Nurs 1993; 19: 212–18.*
- Bentley J, Meyer J. *Repeat attendance by older people at accident and emergency departments. J Adv Nurs 2004; 48: 149–56.*
- Surviving Sepsis Campaign Guidelines. *http://www. survivingsepsis.org/implement/resources/guidelines.*
- Department of Health. *Transforming emergency care in England , 2004 http://www.dh.gov.uk/en/Publicationsa ndstatistics/Publications/PublicationsPolicyAndGuida nce/DH_4091775.*
- McCoy GF, et al. *Injury to the Elderly in Road Traffic Accidents. J Trauma 1989; 29: 494.*
- Evans R. *Trauma and falls. In: Sanders AB (ed). Emergency Care of the Elder Person. St. Louis: Beverly Cracom Publications, 1996.*
- Lachs, Mark S, Pillemer K. *"Elder Abuse," The Lancet, 2004, 364: 1192-1263.*
- British Geriatrics Society *Abuse of Older People Compendium document 4.10, published April 2005 http://www.bgs.org.uk/Publications/Compendium/ compend_4-10.htm*

Case Study 1

An 87 year old lady presented to the Emergency Department with a one day history of abdominal pain and anorexia. There was a past history of atrial fibrillation and angina. On examination she was tachycardic and hypotensive. She was given analgesia, commenced on intravenous fluids and referred to the surgical SHO on call, who saw her 2 hours later. By that time she had no pain and her blood pressure was normal. Her abdomen was soft and non-tender. Investigations revealed a WCC of 17 with normal Hb and U&E. Her chest x-ray showed some non-specific shadowing in the right base. The surgical team discharged her as she did not have an acute abdomen, but she did not feel well enough to go home. She now had a temperature and so was referred to the medical team on call for review. The medical SHO noted that she had nitrites on her dipstick urinalysis. On further questioning she reported longstanding urinary frequency. She was diagnosed with a UTI and treated with IV antibiotics. She also had an ABG performed due to her chest x-ray findings, and this was normal apart from a very raised lactate. 8 hours later the patient suffered a cardiac arrest. She did not survive resuscitation attempts. A post mortem revealed extensive ischaemia of the small bowel.

This case demonstrates the importance of obtaining a clear history and of being aware of atypical presentations in older patients. This patient's acute abdomen was essentially painless but the presence of atrial fibrillation and a raised lactate should have alerted the A&E team to the possibility of bowel ischaemia.

Case Study 2

An 89 year old male dairy farmer is found collapsed at home in a rural area. He is discovered by a neighbour who has not seen him for days. His past medical history is unavailable but frusemide, biosoprolol, glucophage and multivitamin tablets are found in his house. However most of the packets are full despite being dispensed three weeks previously.

On examination:

A - Airway patent

B - Breathing laboured, RR 36, O_2 Saturations 92% (on 100% O_2)

C - BP 90/70, PR 100, skin mottled and cool to touch, capillary refill 6 seconds

D - GCS 8 (E2 M4 V2), PEARL, blood glucose meter at bedside reads 'hi'

E - Patient fully undressed – noted to have significant bruising and swelling over right hip and buttock with a shortened externally rotated right lower limb. Temp 32 °C. The patient was intubated and given fluid resuscitation. IV antibiotics were promptly commenced for suspected sepsis. Re-warming was initiated using external blanket and warmed IV fluids. ABG showed acidosis and an elevated lactate. ECG was suggestive of hyperkalaemia and chest x-ray revealed a right basal pneumonia. Urinary myoglobin was elevated confirming that the patient had rhabdomyolysis. The patient was transferred to the ICU. A hip x-ray confirmed right intertrochanteric hip fracture.

The above case is not an uncommon one. Patients who are socially isolated may have delayed presentation for emergency care. In the comatose patient, past history may not be available immediately but ambulance personnel are excellent at describing the scene where the patient was found. In the above case they found the patient's medication; information that was invaluable in the patient's initial assessment; the patient is diabetic, possibly has a history of hypertension and his compliance is a serious concern given the full packets of medications found. In addition to the initial injury (a fractured hip) the patient is now in septic shock. In older patients sepsis often presents as hypothermia. This patient is also likely to be profoundly dehydrated and at high risk for rhabdomyolysis. He is also at risk for hyperosmolar non-ketotic acidosis. Management here is focused on the ABC's as discussed above, aiming to provide early goal directed therapy, which has been shown to reduce morbidity and mortality. Treatment commenced before a firm diagnosis was made and this is a critical point. Antibiotics should be given as quickly as possible and always within the first hour.

Case Study 3

A 76 year old ambulatory female arrives at the A&E, complaining of chest pain for 2 days getting progressively worse. It is 7/10 in severity, non-radiating and there are no associated symptoms. Her past medical history includes osteoporosis and hypertension. She also had a previous fractured distal radius and vertebral fracture. She was taking calcium & vitamin D supplementation and alendronate. At triage her vital signs are recorded (BP 100/70, PR 110, RR 28, afebrile) and she is transferred to the corridor of emergency department. An initial cursory exam is performed by the A&E SHO whilst the patient is fully clothed on the corridor. The patient continues to complain of chest pain. She is prescribed aspirin, clopidogrel and GTN as an acute myocardial infarction is suspected. An IV cannula is inserted and bloods are sent. She is prescribed morphine sulphate IV for the pain. An ECG shows T-wave inversion in the anterior leads and she is commenced on low molecular weight heparin. A 'routine' chest x-ray is ordered and the medical SHO on call is contacted. 30 minutes later the patient's son arrives and gives a collateral history. The patient was a belted passenger involved in a 40 kph side-on collision on the passenger side of a car 2 days previously. There was no passenger space intrusion, and no broken glass. The air bag was deployed. The patient then complains of worsening shortness of breath and chest pain and is

moved to the resuscitation area. On primary survey:

A – Patent

B – RR 36, using accessory muscles of respiration, sat 94% (28% O_2)

C – PR 130, BP 90/70, second IV cannula inserted; bolus 250 mls crystalloid given, then infusion of 150 mls/hr commenced. A type and cross match is added to blood samples.

D – GCS 15, PEARL

E – Patient is fully undressed, a large anterior chest wall bruise is noted, the sternum is tender with an obvious step deformity.

The BP is rechecked 10 minutes post fluid administration; 105/80, PR 130. CXR – AP study markedly widened mediastinum, multiple left sided rib fractures, no pneumothorax and no haemothorax. A sternal view shows a displaced sternal fracture. A CT scan is requested for further evaluation, and the working diagnosis is a suspected cardiac contusion with cardiogenic shock. Meanwhile her lab results reveal an elevated troponin T, but are otherwise normal. The patient continues to complain of chest pain, additional morphine is given and a GTN infusion is commenced. The vital signs are BP 70/50, PR 140, RR 30. A further bolus of 250mls crystalloid is given, but there is no response. The patient is transferred to CT, found to have aortic disruption on CT scan and minor cardiac contusion. She is admitted by the cardiothoracic team and transferred to theatre for surgery.

This case illustrates the importance of history taking and the value of a collateral history. In this case it completely altered the working diagnosis and initial management. It also demonstrates the need for proper and thorough examination of any patient prior to commencing a course of treatment. This patient's large bruise should have easily been seen and prompted the SHO to a directed history. This patient seemed well on arrival but deteriorated rapidly which is not uncommon in older patients. Although she was the victim of relatively minor trauma she suffered significant injury as a result of her underlying osteoporosis.

Case Study 4

A 68 year old female presents with sudden shortness of breath. It began at 8 am that morning when it woke her from sleep. She denies chest pain or cough. Her past medical history is type 2 diabetes mellitus and polymyalgia rheumatica. She is taking rosiglitazone and low dose prednisolone.

A - Patent.

B - Patient in obvious respiratory distress using accessory muscles of respiration, RR 22, Sats 88% (on 100% O₂), widespread crackles are heard throughout both lung fields on auscultation and there is an audible third heart sound.

C - BP 70/60, PR 40, vomiting

D - GCS 15, PEARL

E - Afebrile

ECG showed an inferior ST elevation myocardial infarction. IV access was obtained and she was given nitrates, aspirin, clopidogrel and frusemide. A urinary catheter was inserted. As primary PCI is unavailable she was thrombolysed with tPA. She was also commenced on continuous non-invasive positive pressure ventilation (CPAP) and commenced on inotropic support. She was transferred to the CCU for further management.

Silent myocardial infarction is not uncommon in older patients, particularly older women. This woman's course was further complicated as she developed pulmonary oedema as a result of acute heart failure. Indeed were it not for this she may not have had any symptoms at all. The sudden onset of dyspnoea in the absence of chest pain can be considered a 'chest-pain equivalent' in terms of reperfusion therapy. Acute pulmonary oedema was managed with nitrates, diuretics and CPAP augmented by inotrope therapy. In the absence of hypotension, morphine sulphate also has a beneficial effect in acute pulmonary oedema, even in the absence of pain.

Data Interpretation

Question 1

Mr S, an 87 year old retired plumber, presents to the emergency department complaining of right sided abdominal pain and confusion over the last 24 hours. He has no significant medical history and is not on any medication. Examination reveals some mild tenderness in the right iliac fossa. He also has sinus tachycardia (100 bpm) and clinically he is dehydrated. Bedside urinalysis is positive for blood. CXR is performed and shows pneumoperitoneum.

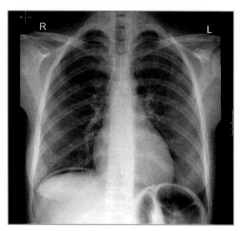

What is the diagnosis?

Question 2

Mr Murphy is a frail elderly gentleman who presents to the emergency department following a head injury. He is confused. He is accompanied by his son who reports that the confusion started after the head injury. He tells you that his father has had several falls over the last 12 months and is very accident prone. Today's presentation was the result of a fall downstairs. On examination Mr Murphy is frail, cachetic and unkempt; he has a large laceration on his forehead above his left eye which requires suturing. Further examination reveals several clinically fractured ribs but no overlying bruising and a large abdominal bruise which appears to be healing. You also note that he is missing front teeth and is not wearing dentures. During the examination Mr Murphy becomes very agitated and starts to demand that he be discharged, he is upset at the thought of being admitted and shouts that he '... will not be put in a home'. His son, who has remained with you throughout the examination, tells you that his father is often like this.

What features in the examination would alert you to the possibility of elder abuse?

Best of five questions

Question 1
In the management of sepsis which one of the following is true;

a.   Inotrope administration should be delayed until ICU admission is arranged
b.   Antibiotic therapy should be delayed until the source of infection is determined
c.   Antibiotics administration should be delayed until blood cultures are taken
d.   Serum lactate is predictive of mortality
e.   Platelets should only be given when there is risk of bleeding

Question 2
Which one of the following physiological changes are not associated with ageing?

a.   Decreased circulating catecholamines
b.   Decreased lung compliance
c.   Reduced GFR
d.   Cerebral atrophy
e.   Osteoporosis increases risk of fractures

Question 3
Which one of the following statements is false?

a.   Up to 10% of elderly patients are victims of elder abuse
b.   Fever in the elderly is defined as an oral or tympanic temperature above 37.6 °C or a rectal temperature above 37.2 °C
c.   The mortality rate of elderly A&E patients with fever is up to 10% at one month
d.   Up to 30% of elderly patients are affected by falls each year
e.   50% of elderly patients who require hospitalisation following a fall die within 12 months

Answers on page 311

Memory problems

Shaun T O'Keeffe

Introduction

In this chapter, 'cognitive impairment' will be used rather the phrase 'confusion' beloved of lay people, nurses and surgeons. 'Confusion' is not a diagnosis, obscures more than it illuminates and often implies chronicity and hopelessness.

There are a number of important questions to be considered when an older person is described as 'confused':
• Is cognitive impairment present?
• Is it causing any functional problems?
• Is impairment acute, chronic or acute on chronic?
• What is the cause?
• What can be done?

The patient presenting with memory problems

There are a number of questions to be considered when a patient is referred with memory problems. The first is whether there is indeed a memory problem. The usual concern of the patient, family and family doctor is whether the patient might have early Alzheimer's disease (AD) or another dementia. The differential diagnosis in this setting includes anxiety (often the 'worried well'), depression and isolated memory impairment. In general, those who refer themselves are less likely to have serious problems than those who are brought reluctantly by concerned family members.

Cognitive testing

Although formal cognitive testing will be required in all these patients, much information can be gleaned by listening carefully to how well the patient tells their story and their use of language. A lack of detail and frequent head-turning to consult with a relative are often ominous features.

The 30-item Folstein Mini-Mental State Examination (MMSE) has become the standard brief test of cognitive function, although some prefer the 10-item Abbreviated Mental Test (AMT). There are a number of good reasons

for the popularity of the MMSE. (1) It can be completed in 3 - 4 minutes; (2) It covers the cognitive aspects frequently affected by dementia; (3) It is widely used and understood so facilitates communication; and (4) Normative data are available to indicate appropriate cut-off points for detecting the presence and severity of dementia. The availability of a validated version for an Irish population is also very useful.

The very popularity and ubiquity of the MMSE does, however, create some problems. The MMSE was developed as a screening test and not a diagnostic test. The use of a cut-off of <24 for detecting dementia works very well in epidemiological studies, but education and previous intellectual capacity and visual and hearing deficits may all influence individual scores.

Other simple tests that may be useful in the clinic include the clock drawing test and asking the patient to generate word lists. The former tests visuospatial function in addition to planning. My practice is to draw a circle, ask the patient to fill in the clock numbers and then place the hands of the clock at a specified time, such as 10 minutes after 11. A number of formal scoring systems are available, but abnormalities are usually obvious and can be followed with serial testing. The most common word list test is to ask the patient to generate the names of as many animals as possible in a minute. Most normal people can generate 15 names or more, although allowance must again be made for prior education and linguistic skills. More detailed neuropsychological testing is useful for research purposes and is clinically valuable in people with unusual patterns of cognitive decline who may have an uncommon form of dementia.

Does the patient with memory impairment have dementia?

Memory impairment is a cardinal feature of dementia, but a diagnosis of dementia also requires another deficit of higher cortical function, such as language, apraxia (inability to carry out previously learned

TABLE I
FEATURES THAT SUGGEST NON-ALZHEIMER DEMENTIA

FEATURE	CONDITION	
• Age of onset < 60 years	FTD	
• Rapid progression	CJD, strokes	FTD – frontotemporal dementia
• Early gait disorder	NPH, VD, MSA	CJD – Creutzfeldt Jacob disease
• Early urinary incontinence	NPH	NPH – normal pressure hydrocephalus
• Early parkinsonism	LBD, MSA, PSP	VD – vascular dementia
• Pyramidal signs	VD, brain tumour	MSA – multiple system atrophy
• Early hallucinations	LBD, VD	PSP – progressive supranuclear palsy
• Disinhibition	FTD	LBD – Lewy body disease
• Myoclonus	CJD	
• Loss of vertical eye movements	PSP	

motor tasks despite intact motor function and comprehension), agnosia (failure to identify objects despite intact sensory function), visuospatial function, judgment and abstract thinking. Also, the deficits must be of sufficient severity to interfere with social or occupational functioning.

Ageing itself can be associated with mild slowing of cognitive function and of retrieval of information, but a change in cognition with functional consequences should not be attributed to 'old age'. It is not uncommon to encounter patients with isolated memory problems but without other deficits. By definition, such patients do not have dementia. A number of terms are used to describe such patients, including mild cognitive impairment, age-associated memory impairment and age-related cognitive decline. It is clear that a proportion of such patients will progress to clear-cut dementia. Time is the best test, and follow-up is essential.

What type of dementia does the patient have?

The evaluation of the demented patient should follow the standard course of history, physical examination and laboratory and other tests. For older patients with dementia, the main issue is whether or not they have Alzheimer's disease (AD), vascular dementia or an atypical or other dementia. Knowledge of the features of AD is particularly important because it is the most common cause of dementia.

The history must include a detailed history of the onset and progression of the disease, of the impact on basic and advanced activities of daily living and on associated behavioural and sleep problems.

Medication history is also important. The impact on the carers should also be evaluated. A number of features suggest a dementia other than typical AD (table 1).

Physical examination in dementia is focussed on detection of vascular risk factors, focal neurological signs and parkinsonism. General alertness will give a good indication as to the likelihood of delirium. Heart rate, blood pressure (lying and standing) and cardiac status should be assessed. The neurological examination should include careful assessment of gait and tone. Early parkinsonism in a demented patient raises the possibility of Lewy body disease or of a parkinson-plus syndrome. The latter may be associated with postural hypotension, ataxia and pyramidal signs (multiple system atrophy) or with loss of downward gaze (progressive supranuclear palsy). Focal neurological signs point to cerebrovascular disease or to other intracranial disease.

Laboratory investigations and X-rays are directed at looking for potentially reversible causes of dementia. As shall be seen, this search is usually fruitless. Nevertheless, full blood count, ESR, urea and electrolytes, glucose, calcium, liver function tests, thyroid stimulating hormone and vitamin B_{12}, serum or red blood cell folate and, at least in those perceived to be at high risk, syphilis screening should be checked in all demented patients. Patients with typical features of AD do not require a CT brain scan. A scan is mandatory if there are unusual features such as early onset of disease, rapid progression, unexplained neurological symptoms or signs, a history of falls or head injury, treatment with anticoagulants, early gait disturbance or incontinence or focal neurological signs.

Important dementias

Alzheimer's disease

AD may develop at any age. However, onset is most common after 65 years, and there is an exponential rise in incidence up to at least 90 years. Early (before 60 years) onset AD accounts for about 5% of AD cases, and, within this group, about 10% show an autosomal dominant pattern of inheritance due to one of three known causative gene mutations. Compared with the common β3 allele of the apolipoprotein E (ApoE) gene on chromosome 19, the β4 allele increases the risk for AD (15 fold for someone with a double dose) and the β2 allele is protective. High premorbid intelligence and education seem to be protective against or at least delay the onset of AD.

The onset of AD is usually gradual, and carers often find it hard to identify precisely when they became aware there might be a problem. Sometimes, onset may seem to be sudden, as when the patient moves to a new and strange environment or when a relative visits after an absence and recognises a significant decline in cognition. An acute episode such as an episode of delirium or a stroke may also provoke clinically obvious dementia.

Progression of AD is generally gradual but there are often periods of relative stability. A good collateral history is essential as people with dementia will often minimise their problems. Initial functional impairment affects complex activities such as dealing with finances. With progression, activities of daily living such as dressing and maintaining personal hygiene become more impaired and urinary and, less commonly, faecal incontinence may develop. In severe AD, speech becomes more incoherent and may be lost, while motor function is also progressively impaired. Behavioural or psychiatric problems commonly occur in AD. Depression occurs in about 25% at some stage. Delusions, often persecutory, occur in up to 75% of patients and hallucinations, usually visual, in up to 50%. Agitation, wandering and sleep disturbance also occur and may precipitate nursing home admission. Physical examination is normal in AD, although coexisting diseases are common in older sufferers. Weight loss is common, and the causes are multifactorial.

Neuropathological diagnosis of AD is based on the

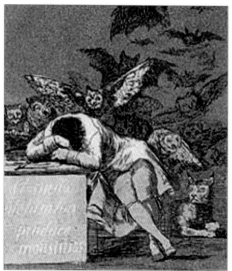

Figure 1: Goya's 'The Sleep of Reason Produces Monsters'

presence of two characteristic lesions: neurofibrillary tangles (NFT) and neuritic plaques. Both occur to a lesser degree in 'normal' ageing and NFT occur in other neurological conditions and also in non-AD dementias. NFT are intracellular and composed of abnormal cytoskeletal proteins, with a major component being the microtubule-associated protein tau. Neuritic plaques are extracellular and contain an amyloid core composed of a protein called A4/β-amyloid derived from a precursor amyloid precursor protein (APP). One major hypothesis is that AD results from an excessive generation of A4/β-amyloid which is toxic to neurons and also causes abnormalities of tau and hence formation of NFT. The almost invariable development of AD in Down's syndrome patients over 40 years supports this hypothesis since diffuse A4/β-amyloid deposits precede development of NFT and of neuritic plaques in these patients. However, other reports suggest a stronger relationship between NFT and AD and hence a primary role for early changes in neuronal cytoskeleton.

Although several neurotransmitter pathways are affected in AD, impairment of acetylcholine neurotransmission is particularly prominent, occurs early in the disease process and is relevant to characteristic neuropsychological impairments of AD, including short-term memory loss. The role of inflammatory mechanisms in the pathogenesis of AD has also attracted much attention. However, although epidemiological studies have suggested a possible protective role for non-steroidal anti-inflammatory drugs, this approach has not proven effective in clinical trials to date.

Vascular dementia (VD)

Strokes are most likely to cause or exacerbate dementia if they reach a critical threshold in size and if they are bilateral and affect critical cortical or subcortical sites. In contrast to pure AD, neurological signs and gait disturbance are early features. Most patients will have stroke risk factors. Brain imaging will usually confirm the clinical diagnosis of strokes. However, the clinical significance of the common white matter changes (leukoariosis) seen in brain scans of older people remains uncertain.

Until recently, an attempt was often made to make a clear distinction between VD and AD. This distinction is now seen as less clear-cut. Epidemiological studies have shown that traditional vascular risk factors, such as atrial fibrillation and hypertension, are also risk factors for the clinical diagnosis of AD. Isolated vascular dementia is actually uncommon at post-mortem, and many patients diagnosed with vascular dementia using standard criteria have coexisting AD. In a study of nuns who had cognitive testing before death and brain examination after death, it was found that the presence of brain infarcts was a major factor in determining whether AD pathology led to clinically apparent dementia. Finally, cholinesterase inhibitors are also useful in what would traditionally be defined as vascular dementia. On the other hand, treating typical AD patients with low-dose aspirin has no worthwhile benefit and increases the risk of serious bleeds.

It is now common to think of dementia with or without vascular risk factors. This acknowledges that modification of vascular risk factors may help prevent development and progression of all dementias, including AD.

Lewy body disease (LBD)

LBD is relatively common and has a clinical presentation different to AD and other common dementias. The psychotic symptoms of LBD are difficult to control because neuroleptic medications are dangerous. Finally, cholinesterase inhibitors seem especially useful in these patients. LBD is the most common of the disorders presenting with both cognitive impairment and extrapyramidal features. The differential diagnoses in such patients include progressive supranuclear palsy, corticobasal degeneration, striatonigral degeneration, Huntington's disease, and Wilson's disease. However, isolated extrapyramidal signs and Parkinson's disease itself are also common in older people, and dementia develops in up to a third of patients with Parkinson's disease. In autopsy series, 15% to 25% of older demented patients contain cortical and subcortical Lewy bodies with or without concomitant AD pathology.

A diagnosis of probable LBD requires two of: (1) fluctuating cognition with pronounced variations in attention and alertness; (2) recurrent visual hallucinations, often dramatic and elaborate; and (3) spontaneous motor features of parkinsonism. Supporting features include repeated falls or syncope, sensitivity to neuroleptics and troublesome delusions. Several studies have found high specificity but poor sensitivity for these diagnostic criteria.

Lewy bodies are eosinophilic intracellular structures found mainly in neurones. In LBD, by definition, there are both cortical and subcortical Lewy bodies. Generally, there are also varying degrees of AD-type changes in these patients.

Frontotemporal dementia (FTD)

FTD accounts for up to a quarter of patients with dementia presenting before 65 years and results from a non-Alzheimer degeneration of the frontal and temporal lobes. FTD includes what used be called Pick's disease. It is strongly familial and is often linked to mutations on the region of chromosome 17 that codes for the micro-tubule-associated protein tau (hence the designation of the disease as a 'familial tauopathy'). There is also an association with motor neurone disease.

Presentation with mood disturbance is common, but the characteristic feature of the disease is the development of personality change with a breakdown in social skills. Three broad patterns are apparent: disinhibition with inappropriate jocularity; apathetic, pseudo-depressive behaviour with loss of initiative; and repetitive and ritualistic behaviours similar to obsessive-compulsive disease. Lack of interest in personal hygiene and incontinence are common problems. Hyperorality with mouthing of inedible objects is characteristic, as is overeating, especially of sweet foods. Speech output is characteristically reduced. In the later stages, mutism often develops. Frontal executive functions are also very impaired. Conversely, memory may be relatively unaffected in the early stages.

Potentially reversible dementias
It is rare to find a true 'reversible dementia'. Although up to 15% of dementia patients have a potentially reversible disease, many of these are coexisting rather than causative and less than a third actually improve with a tiny proportion actually 'cured'. The most common potentially reversible conditions are drug-induced cognitive impairment, depression, vitamin B_{12} deficiency, hypothyroidism and normal pressure hydrocephalus. True depressive 'pseudodementia' or 'myxoedema madness' is very uncommon. Similarly, treatment of vitamin B_{12} deficiency rarely leads to significant changes in cognitive performance. Dramatic responses can occur with cessation of treatment with long-acting benzodiazepines.

Cognitive impairment with normal pressure hydrocephalus (NPH) sometimes reverses with neurosurgical shunt insertion. The classical triad of NPH is cognitive impairment with early gait disturbance and urinary incontinence. (A similar presentation can occur in vascular dementia and FTD). On CT scan, the ventricles are dilated out of proportion to cerebral atrophy. Because of the high frequency of shunt complications, it is important to try and identify those patients most likely to improve with shunting. A relatively short duration and mild severity of cognitive impairment predicts a better response, as does improvement in timed walk and balance tests or in cognitive performance after removing about 30ml CSF at lumbar puncture. Reversible dementia due to brain tumours is extremely rare.

Management of the patient with dementia
Co-morbid medical and psychiatric conditions, particularly depression, should be identified and treated. Polypharmacy should be minimised and anticholinergic and sedative drugs avoided if at all possible. Alcohol use should be minimised. Optimising vision, hearing, and nutrition help to promote general health. Behaviour modification, scheduled toileting, and prompted voiding can reduce urinary incontinence. Skills practice and positive reinforcement can increase functional independence in persons with dementia.

Caring for the carer
The carer role is often physically, emotionally and financially draining, and stress and depression are common problems among carers. Abuse of the patient can also occur if adequate support is not provided. Physicians should ask carers about depression and stress. Periodic respite admissions are often helpful. Caregivers need to be provided with education, encouragement, and practical advice. This includes instructing in the fundamentals of behaviour management techniques. Carers should be encouraged to contact their local Alzheimer's society.

Ethical issues
Ethical issues that occur during the care of people with dementia include:
- Telling the patient the diagnosis
- Appropriateness of tube feeding in severe dementia
- Determination of competence, for example in financial matters
- Balancing patient safety with preservation of patient autonomy
- Dealing with the demented driver

The presence, by definition, of significant cognitive impairment makes disclosure of the diagnosis difficult in many demented patients. Nevertheless, since people with mild dementia often have sufficient competence to make decisions about their own care and finances, it is important that disclosure, tailored to the capacity and needs of the individual patient, is strongly considered.

Questions about competence (capacity) are encountered when considering whether an older person with dementia should return to their own home, whether they can provide valid informed consent for surgical interventions or whether they are capable of making a will or enduring power of attorney. Competence can be defined as a state in which a patient's decision-making capacity is sufficiently intact for their decisions to be respected. There are a number of generally accepted principles:
- The presence of dementia should not create an automatic presumption of incompetence
- Cognitive deficits are only important if they interfere with decision-making
- Incompetence is situation-dependent: it depends on the degree of match between the patients' abilities and the decision making demands of the particular situation
- A person's level of competence can change even over a short period of time, for example in those with delirium

Cognitive abilities important to competence include the ability to express a choice and the ability to understand and to reason with relevant information in order to weigh up different treatment options.

The principles of respect for autonomy (what are the wishes of the patient?) and beneficence (what is in best interests of the patient?) are fundamental to medical ethics. Autonomy is a good in itself, whether or not it advances welfare. In considering what is in a patient's best interest, it must be remembered that safety is not synonymous with welfare and that quality of life is as important to many people as duration of life. Hence, for example, unless incompetence is clear-cut, patients who wish to go home must go home, regardless of whether or not healthcare professionals view this as the best or safest choice.

While very few patients with dementia of even moderate severity are safe to drive, patients with mild dementia often retain motor skills and often have well-ingrained safe driving habits. Questioning the patient and carers about driving accidents and habits and examination of vision, attention and visuospatial skills may be helpful, but ultimately a road test by an experienced driving instructor is most useful.

Patients with early dementia often have sufficient competence to make a valid Enduring Power of Attorney (EPA). This allows patients to determine who they would prefer to administer their affairs when they become incapable themselves. If there is no EPA and an incompetent patient has significant assets, it may be necessary to make the patient a Ward of Court.

End-of-life issues become important in patients with advanced dementia. Poor oral intake, perhaps related to swallowing problems and aspiration, and weight loss become increasingly common. This may lead to consideration of tube feeding. The absence of evidence that tube feeding prolongs life or improves quality of life makes the decision to withhold such interventions a medical rather than an ethical one.

Specific pharmacotherapy
Cholinesterase inhibitors, drugs that inhibit acetylcholinesterase - the enzyme responsible for the hydrolysis of acetylcholine, (donepezil, galantamine and rivastigmine) and memantine (an NMDA receptor antagonist) are currently approved for the treatment of AD. However, their effectiveness in achieving clinically relevant improvements, primarily in cognition, global function, behaviour, and quality of life, is disputed. Independent reviews have concluded that, while cholinesterase inhibitors and memantine consistently result in statistically significant improvements in cognition and in global assessment, these effects seem of marginal clinical significance. Comparisons of different cholinesterase inhibitors show no differences. The effects on behaviour and on quality of life are less consistent and are also of doubtful clinical significance, except, perhaps, in a minority of sufferers. Most studies to date have been of short duration and evidence for the rationale of combining cholinesterase inhibitors and memantine is, as yet, sparse and unconvincing.

Recently, the (uncertain) evidence of benefit from cholinesterase inhibitors has been extended to patients with vascular or mixed dementia and, somewhat more convincingly, to patients with LBD. The benefits that have been reported with cholinesterase inhibitors are dose-related as are the side effects. The latter are predominantly cholinergic in nature including nausea, vomiting, diarrhoea, abdominal pain and weight loss. Dose titration will minimise side effects. Caution is advised with patients who have severe liver disease, pre-existing bradycardia, peptic ulcer disease, asthma, chronic obstructive pulmonary disease or glaucoma.

As noted earlier, control of vascular risk factors may benefit many patients with dementia and not just those thought to have VD. This has received some support from the finding of the Syst Eur study that control of systolic hypertension reduced the number of patient developing dementia during follow up.

Treatment of behavioural disturbances
Nonpharmacological strategies to modify identifiable causes (such as pain) or environmental triggers that can be avoided should be the first approach to managing behavioural problems. Delirium should also be considered if behavioural problems develop quite suddenly. The possibility of depression should always be considered. Sensory stimulation of various types (auditory, visual, tactile) and a variety of special environments have been evaluated, usually in nursing home patients, with conflicting results.

There is now convincing evidence that both conventional and newer atypical antipsychotic (neuroleptic) medications increase mortality in older people with dementia and increased rates of stroke and myocardial infarction have been identified in some studies. Accelerated decline in cognitive function has also been reported. In view of these findings, use of these drugs should be restricted to those with the most troublesome symptoms of psychosis or aggression. The lowest effective dose should be used and the need for ongoing treatment re-examined periodically. Trazodone, which has useful sedating and anti-depressant effects, is widely used by geriatricians. Anticonvulsants are sometimes helpful in troublesome agitation.

Patients with LBD are very sensitive to neuroleptics, and death can result within weeks of starting such agents in these patients. Apart from clozapine, which can cause blood dyscrasias, quetiapine seems the least likely of the atypical neuroleptics to cause parkinsonism in these patients. However, trazodone and cholinesterase inhibitors are probably a better first choice in this condition.

Delirium (acute confusional state)

Delirium (acute confusional state) is an important condition of older people because it is common, highly unpleasant and has serious short and long-term consequences. Delirium is often unrecognised or misdiagnosed by doctors and nurses and management is frequently poor.

At the time of admission to hospital, between 10 and 22% of older medical patients are delirious. An additional 10 - 30% develop delirium after admission. Delirium develops in 5 - 10% of patients following general surgery, 33 to 50% of patients following hip fracture repair and in 20 - 40% of patients after elective joint replacement surgery. High rates of postoperative delirium have also been noted after major cardiac or vascular surgery and in patients admitted to intensive care units.

Clinical features

A diagnosis of delirium should be considered when one hears a patient described as 'confused', 'vague', 'a poor historian', 'poorly motivated' or 'uncooperative'. Delirium is characterised by a change of cognition that develops over a period of hours or days. Symptoms tend to fluctuate over the course of a day and are worst at night. Disturbed consciousness and impaired ability to attend to the environment are cardinal features. Patients are highly distractible and find it difficult to focus or sustain concentration during conversation. They are often disoriented with

TABLE 2 DISTINGUISHING DELIRIUM AND DEMENTIA		
	Delirium	**Dementia**
Onset	Acute	Gradual
Attentiveness	Impaired	Normal
Consciousness	Reduced	Normal
Perceptual disturbance	Common	Late
Fluctuations	Yes	No
Outcome	Recovery/ death	Chronic/ progressive

rambling, incoherent speech. Persecutory delusions and visual hallucinations are common. Patients may be tearful or anxious.

Two distinct clinical subtypes of delirium are recognised: agitated delirium with psychomotor overactivity; and quiet delirium in which patients appear apathetic and withdrawn. Quiet delirium is easily missed or misdiagnosed as depression.

A history from a carer of the onset and course of the cognitive disturbance is invaluable in distinguishing between dementia and delirium (Table 2). Even when such a history is unavailable, delirious patients can often be easily recognised from the bedside by their characteristic distractibility. Generalised slowing of the electroencephalographic (EEG) trace occurs in most patients with delirium but is a non-specific finding in older people.

Outcome of delirium

Although delirium is traditionally regarded as a transient disorder, 30 to 60% of delirious patients still have significant new cognitive impairment at discharge, and an increased risk of developing dementia in the years following an episode of delirium has also been noted. Delirium has consistently been associated with prolonged hospital stay, functional decline during hospitalisation and increased risk of admission to extended nursing care, even after adjusting for potential confounding factors. Hospital-acquired complications such as pressure sores, falls, infections and urinary incontinence are more common in delirious patients and may prolong the delirium.

Aetiology

Delirium is almost invariably multifactorial in older

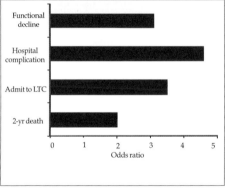

Figure 2: Outcomes of delirium, adjusted for prior dementia, functional level, severity of acute illness, comorbid burden. (Adapted from O'Keeffe and Lavan, JAGS 1997)

people, and it is important to distinguish between predisposing factors that increase the vulnerability of the patient to delirium and factors that precipitate delirium. In patients who are very vulnerable, the precipitating insult may be very mild, such as a simple urinary tract infection.

Prior cognitive impairment, older age, severity of illness and psychoactive drug use have consistently emerged as the most important risk factors for delirium. Laboratory indices of dehydration or metabolic disturbance, alcohol abuse and visual impairment have also emerged as important risk factors in some studies.

In older patients, delirium may be the presenting feature of an otherwise clinically silent myocardial infarct or pneumonia. Common causes of delirium in hospital patients include chest or urinary infections, hypoxia due to cardio-respiratory disease, medication toxicity, dehydration and electrolyte disturbance and stroke (especially involving the right hemisphere). Alcohol withdrawal should always be considered, even in the absence of a history of alcohol abuse. Thiamine deficiency, non-convulsive seizures, intracranial infections and subdural haematoma should be considered in difficult cases. Anticholinergic drugs are an important cause of delirium. The total burden of anticholinergic drugs may matter more than any single agent, and this burden may be contributed to by metabolites of drugs not usually thought of as having major anticholinergic effects such as digoxin, warfarin, nifedipine and prednisolone. Iatrogenic factors, such as use of restraints, malnutrition, polypharmacy and

bladder catheterisation, are especially important in patients who develop delirium after admission to hospital.

Pathophysiology

It appears that delirium represents the clinical manifestation of diffuse, reversible impairment of cerebral oxidative metabolism and neurotransmission. The dominant theory at present is that a state of relative cholinergic deficiency and dopaminergic excess is the final common neural pathway for delirium, although disturbances in other neurotransmitter systems have also been reported.

Treatment of delirium

The general principles of treating delirium are: make the diagnosis early; treat any precipitating factors; prevent physical and emotional harm by providing a supportive environment; maintain nutrition and hydration; and last, but not least, use pharmacological therapy judiciously.

Supportive measures

It is important to maintain the intake of fluid and nutrition. Subcutaneous fluids are a useful option in agitated patients. Multivitamin supplements, especially thiamine, are essential in obviously malnourished or alcoholic patients. Physical restraints, including cotsides, are inhumane and potentially dangerous in people who are often already distressed and paranoid. Spectacles and hearing aids should be provided to minimise sensory deprivation. Self-care and mobility should be promoted. Interventions such as bladder catheters and venous cannulation should only be used when essential. A calm and friendly approach by staff with frequent reassurance and re-orientation is necessary, especially when painful or unpleasant procedures are undertaken. It is particularly helpful if family members can sit with the patient.

Pharmacological management

Pharmacological measures are not needed in all patients. Nevertheless, while the need for medication is obvious in the agitated, hallucinating patient, even quietly delirious patients can experience considerable distress. It is kinder and less dangerous to commence regular low dose therapy early on rather than waiting for agitation or distress to increase and then resorting to a 'chemical cosh'.

Randomised trials, albeit in younger patients, have confirmed that neuroleptic agents are superior

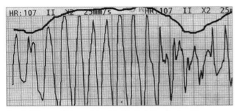

Figure 3: ECG trace with characteristic twisting (blue line) of torsades de pointes

to benzodiazepines in the treatment of delirium. Neuroleptics do not impair respiratory function and are less likely to aggravate cognitive impairment. Haloperidol is probably the best choice, although few direct comparisons with other agents have been reported. Oral haloperidol in an initial dose of 0.5 - 2.0 mg, three or four times daily, is usually adequate for older patients (Table 3). Parenteral treatment is sometimes needed in very agitated patients or in the intensive care unit.

The concerns regarding adverse effects of antipsychotic agents in dementia are also relevant to delirium, since increased mortality has been reported even within a few weeks of starting these medications. Although there is little good evidence at present, it is recommended that electrolyte abnormalities should be corrected and an ECG examined for prolongation of the (rate-corrected) QT interval before starting treatment, especially with higher or parenteral doses. A prolonged QT interval has been linked with the development of torsades de pointes ventricular arrhythmia. Avoidance, discontinuation or a reduction in neuroleptic dose should be considered if the corrected QT interval is greater than 450 msec or if there is a greater than 25 percent increase above baseline on follow-up.

Benzodiazepines are the treatment of choice for withdrawal states and for patients with extrapyramidal disease. They may also be used as an adjunct to parenteral haloperidol to reduce the frequency of extrapyramidal side effects. Lorazepam, which has a relatively short half-life and is available for parenteral use, is commonly used.

Prevention of delirium

It has proved difficult to prove that the supportive measures mentioned above are helpful in the treatment of delirium. However, there is now good evidence that a strategy comprising repeated reassurance and orientation of the patient, non-pharmacological sleep

TABLE 3
PHARMACOLOGICAL MANAGEMENT OF DELIRIUM

General principles
- Tailor doses according to age, body size, sex and degree of agitation
- Titrate doses to effect
- Increase scheduled dose if regular 'as-needed' doses required
- Maintain effective dose for a few days, then taper and stop

Neuroleptic medications
- Avoid in withdrawal states, anticholinergic toxicity and hepatic failure
- Haloperidol is usually first choice
- Oral therapy
  - Bioavailability 66%; time to peak effect 4 - 6 hours
  - Usually 0.5 - 1.0 mg b.d. with additional doses 'as-needed' 4 hourly
- Intramuscular therapy
  - Bioavailability 100%; time to peak effect 20 - 40 minutes
  - Severe agitation, give 0.5 - 1.0mg, observe for 30 - 60 minutes and repeat if needed
- Extrapyramidal side effects, especially if dose > 3mg daily or prolonged
- QTc prolongation, especially with higher or parenteral doses. Check electrolytes and baseline and follow-up ECG, and consider discontinuation or a reduction in dose if QTc greater than 450 msec or more than 25 percent increase above baseline

Atypical neuroleptics
- Less drug interactions and less extrapyramidal effects than haloperidol
- ? Similar effects on QTc
- Antipsychotic potency: Risperidone > Olanzapine > Quetiapine
- Sedation: Olanzapine > Quetiapine > Risperidone
- Extrapyramidal safety: Quetiapine > Olanazapine > Risperidone
- Usual starting doses: Risperidone 0.5mg b.d.; Olanzapine 2.5 - 5.0mg daily; Quetiapine 25 - 50 mg daily

Benzodiazepines
- Use in sedative and alcohol withdrawal, parkinsonism
- Sometimes used as adjunct to haloperidol to reduce risk of extrapyramidal side effects
- More likely than neuroleptics to cause respiratory depression and paradoxical excitement
- Lorazepam: Usual starting dose: 0.5 – 1.0 mg orally (or i.v. in emergency) with additional doses 4 hourly 'as needed'

promotion, early mobilisation, provision of visual and hearing aids and avoidance of dehydration can prevent delirium in high-risk patients.

Suggested further reading

- Gill et al. *Antipsychotic drug use and mortality in older adults with dementia. Ann Intern Med. 2007 http://www.annals.org/cgi/reprint/146/11/775.pdf.*
- Patterson et al. *Diagnosis and treatment of dementia: 1. Risk assessment and primary prevention of Alzheimer disease. CMAJ. 2008. http://www.cmaj.ca/cgi/content/full/178/5/548.*
- Feldman et al. *Diagnosis and treatment of dementia: 2. Diagnosis. CMAJ 2008. http://www.cmaj.ca/cgi/content/full/178/7/825.*
- Hoffer et al. *Tube feeding in advanced dementia: the metabolic perspective. BMJ. 2006 http://www.bmj.com/cgi/content/full/333/7580/1214.*
- Kaduszkiewicz et al. *Cholinesterase inhibitors for patients with Alzheimer's disease: systematic review of randomised clinical trials BMJ 2006. http://www.bmj.com/cgi/content/full/331/7512/321.*
- Burns A, Gallagley A, Byrne J. *Delirium. J Neurol Neurosurg Psychiatry. 2004 http://jnnp.bmj.com/cgi/content/full/75/3/362*

🗀 Case Study 1

Mrs S, a 73 year old retired teacher, is referred for assessment of possible memory decline. She feels her memory has become worse over the last year or two. Mrs S has trouble remembering names and makes lists of important tasks. She otherwise manages well, has no difficulty looking after her finances and still drives into town regularly. She has been sleeping poorly recently and says she feels a bit down at times. Her general health is excellent, and her only medication is bendrofluazide for hypertension and temazepam for insomnia. Physical examination is normal. Mrs S scores 28/30 on the MMSE examination, losing 2 points on testing short term memory. She is able to name 18 animals in 1 minute. Clock drawing is normal.

It is clear that Mrs S has memory problems, but this is not causing any major functional problem and there is no evidence of impairment in any other cognitive domain. The MMSE score is in the 'normal' range, but given her high educational status, this does not exclude significant cognitive impairment. She has a risk factor for vascular disease (hypertension), has some features of depression and is taking benzodiazepines which can contribute to cognitive problems. The working diagnosis is mild cognitive impairment, but one would wish to explore further whether she might have depression and to wean her off the benzodiazepine. It would also be important to ensure than blood pressure control was adequate and to screen for a lipid disorder. Screening blood tests should be performed. The need for CT brain scan is debatable. Mrs S should be followed up with further cognitive testing.

🗀 Case Study 2

Mr. T, an 82 year old retired farmer, is referred because of dementia with troublesome behaviour. He had progressive cognitive decline for at least 4 years, and, after a CT brain scan showed several small infarcts, the G.P. diagnosed vascular dementia and started treatment with aspirin and anti-hypertensives. At the time of presentation Mr T would forget the names of his family, was prone to wandering and had had several falls after getting up at night. He was always asking to 'go home'. In recent months, he would talk to and shout at imaginary figures in his room. Treatment with risperidone 0.5mg b.d. and temazepam 10mg nocte led to drowsiness, reduced mobility and more falls. On examination, he was parkinsonian with marked postural instability. Eye movements were normal, and one plantar was upgoing. There was no orthostatic blood pressure drop. His mood appeared low, and his MMSE score was 13. His daughter was at the end of her tether and wished, reluctantly, to admit him to extended nursing care.

The combination of dementia, visual hallucinations, recurrent falls and parkinsonism (following low dose treatment with an atypical neuroleptic) raises the possibility of Lewy body dementia. There is likely to be a vascular contribution to the dementia, and depression may also be a factor in the behavioural problems. Urgent intervention is required, not least because of the strain on the carer. The risperidone should be stopped and the benzodiazepine reduced gradually. A cholinesterase inhibitor should be commenced. Since this may not act immediately, low-dose trazodone might also be started for a more immediate effect and as a treatment for depression. Improvement in the parkinsonism may allow Mr T to walk more safely and the additional exercise might improve sleep and lessen agitation. Vascular risk factors should also be reassessed with a view to perhaps starting a statin or improving blood pressure control. The carer should be offered a brief respite or assessment admission and advised that discussion of long-term care should be delayed to see if these interventions help.

is available, one may have to request a nurse to 'special' him over the next day or two. In practice, one may find it easier to 'rescue' such a patient from the surgical ward and take him to a specialist geriatric unit.

🗁 Case Study 3

You are asked by the surgeons to see Mr B, an 80 year old man who underwent an emergency appendicectomy 5 days earlier. He has been very agitated for the last two nights. A chest X-ray showed a right basal pneumonia and he is receiving intravenous antibiotics. However, he has removed the intravenous cannula and oxygen mask on several occasions and his hands have now been tied to his chair to prevent this. He is receiving 'as required' diazepam 5 - 10mg orally and haloperidol 5 - 10mg intramuscularly each night. When you see the patient, he is drowsy yet aggressive and is pulling at his hand restraints. Formal cognitive testing is impossible. Mr B appears well nourished. Vital signs are normal, and he has basal chest crackles. There are no focal neurological signs. The abdominal wound is healing well and there is no urinary retention or evidence of a deep venous thrombosis. You contact his worried family and learn that there was no prior cognitive impairment, alcohol abuse or major medical illness.

Mr B has an agitated postoperative delirium without preceding dementia. While pneumonia and hypoxia are possible precipitants, it is important to check an ECG to rule out a myocardial infarction and to repeat basic blood tests to ensure that hydration is adequate. The immediate challenge is to provide more humane care and better pharmacological therapy. Mr B and his family should be reassured that his confusion will almost certainly improve although patience will be required. Mr B needs to wake up from his chemical cosh the night before. A regular treatment regimen should be written up, for example with 1mg of haloperidol orally at 4 and at 10 pm and additional rescue doses of 1 - 2mg IM if required. The benzodiazepine may be leading to some disinhibition and should be stopped. Since Mr B doesn't appear terribly ill from his pneumonia and can now swallow, oral antibiotics may suffice. The restraints are adding to distress and agitation and should be stopped. Instead, Mr B should be mobilised and encouraged to dress and wash himself. Family members should be encouraged to stay with him and to coax him to eat and drink. If none

Data Interpretation

Question 1

An 80 year old woman with a history of ischaemic heart disease and hypertension developed delirium 3 days ago. She had previously been physically and cognitively well. Medications on admission to hospital were aspirin 75mg daily, frusemide 40mg bd, pravastatin 40mg daily and lisinopril 5mg daily. Physical examination and chest x-ray show extensive right basal consolidation. No other abnormality was found on examination or investigation. Her delirium is now causing her distress and creating management problems on the ward. Current blood tests show the following:

FBC – normal
Na^+ – 138 mmol/l
K^+ – 2.9 mmol/l
Urea -7 mmol/l
Creatinine – 78 μmol/l

a. What investigation is needed before pharmacological treatment of delirium?
b. What interventions should be started immediately?

Best of five questions

Question 1

The surgeons ask your advice over the phone about an 80 year old woman who has become confused 3 days after elective hip replacement. Which of the following statements would be correct?

a. Postoperative confusion is rare with current surgical and anaesthetic techniques
b. It would be reasonable to presume that the anaesthetic is probably the main culprit in this case
c. The surgical team should be discouraged from arranging an immediate CT brain scan
d. Haloperidol would be the treatment of choice for this patient
e. Denial by the patient of chest pain or dyspnoea effectively rules out myocardial infarction as the cause of delirium

Question 2

The nurses ask you to see a 60kg, 85 year old man admitted with pneumonia and dehydration, who has become very agitated and who climbed over bedrails the previous night.

You diagnose delirium. Assessment reveals no obvious precipitant other than the pneumonia. The patient has some paranoid delusions that staff are trying to harm him. The family are very concerned. Which of the following would be most appropriate management option in these circumstances?

a. Continue use of bedrails
b. Catheterise the bladder to monitor fluid balance
c. Start haloperidol 1mg twice a day
d. Start a small dose of benzodiazepine at night to encourage sleep and facilitate management
e. Reassure the family that all symptoms will resolve within a few days

Question 3

An 80 year old man attends the clinic with a 1 year history of cognitive decline. MMSE is 24. He has prominent and vivid visual hallucinations of wild animals. Low dose quetiapine has not proved helpful. He has fallen several times in the last few months, and you notice that he has rigidity and poverty of movements and his walk is slowed with reduced arm swing. What is the most likely diagnosis?

a. Alzheimer's disease
b. Vascular dementia
c. Subdural haematoma
d. Lewy body disease
e. Schizophrenia

Answers are on page 311

Stroke and hypertension

S Timmons, R Liston

The WHO definition of stroke is a neurological deficit of sudden onset with focal dysfunction of a non-traumatic vascular origin, lasting for longer than 24 hours. Stroke is the third leading cause of death in the world. The incidence of stroke approximately doubles each decade after the age of 45, with a 2% annual risk over 80 years of age and a 3 - 7% annual risk over 95 years of age. This chapter aims to look at the continuum of stroke care from primary prevention and management of transient ischaemic attacks through to acute stroke, including its presentation and classification, the prediction of prognosis, the monitoring of physiological parameters, thrombolysis, neuroprotection and common complications. Stroke rehabilitation and secondary prevention will also be discussed. Finally, hypertension in older people is discussed.

Primary prevention

In people aged 65 years and older the risk factors for stroke are well recognised and include hypertension, atrial fibrillation, diabetes mellitus, left ventricular failure and carotid stenosis. Smoking, lack of physical exercise and obesity may also be important. However, current evidence suggests that treatment of atrial fibrillation and control of hypertension are probably the two most important stroke preventative strategies for older people. These two risk factors are readily identifiable and modifiable, but are not always optimally treated. Atrial fibrillation occurs in 7 - 14% of older people, and approximately 5% per year of these will develop stroke. This rate is reduced to about 1.5% with warfarin therapy so all older patients in atrial fibrillation should be considered for anti-coagulation.

Patients with asymptomatic carotid stenosis have twice the stroke risk of the general population but a stroke often occurs in a different vascular territory than the stenosed vessel. Clearly the same disease process also affects other vessels. Carotid endarterectomy may be of benefit in selected patients if the stenosis is greater than 60% on angiography (CASANOVA study) but at best, approximately 80 patients need to have surgery to prevent one stroke. Of note, perioperative mortality and morbidity is not significantly higher in asymptomatic octogenarians than younger patients, and older people should be considered for surgery. Although diabetes is a risk factor for stroke, there is no proof that normalisation of blood sugars reduces the risk of stroke although it would appear intuitive that it should do so especially if lifelong glycaemic control has been good. There is little doubt that diabetic patients with co-existing hypertension or hypercholesterolaemia should receive appropriate therapy, with ACE inhibitors or angiotensin receptor blockers and statins, as these risk factors increase their overall risk of vascular disease.

Except in carotid stenosis or atrial fibrillation, aspirin seems to be ineffective in primary stroke prevention and may increase the risk of cerebral haemorrhage (Physicians Health Study). Similarly, there is no rationale for using warfarin in patients in sinus rhythm, unless they have a specific indication such as valvular heart disease or a left ventricular thrombus. There is also no proven association between high cholesterol and ischaemic stroke risk in elderly people. However, statins may stabilise atherosclerotic plaques, increase nitric oxide bioavailability leading to vasodilatation, reduce platelet adherence to endothelium and have anti-inflammatory effects. Thus, they may help

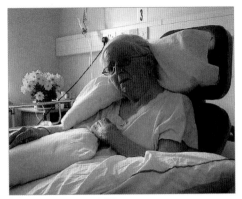

Figure 1: Patient with right hemiparesis of 5 days

TABLE I

FACTORS INDICATING HIGH RISK OF CVA WITH ATRIAL FIBRILLATION

Factors	SPAF-3 trial	Atrial fibrillation investigators	CHADS -2 index	Framingham study
Increasing age	Female > 75	Yes	>75	Yes
LVF	Clinical or EF < 25%	ECHO confirmed	Yes	Not included
Hypertension	Yes	Yes	Yes	Yes
Previous TIA / CVA	Yes	Yes	Yes	Yes
Diabetes	Not included	Yes	Yes	Yes
ECHO findings	Not included	Only LVF	Not included	Not included

prevent stroke. Statin therapy in patients with known ischaemic heart disease undoubtedly reduces stroke occurrence (4S study, CARE, LIPID, HPS, MIRACL). However, the PROSPER study specifically looked at 6000 people aged 70 - 82 with known cardiovascular disease or significant risk factors such as diabetes, smoking or hypertension and found no reduction in stroke incidence with pravastatin treatment. Vascular mortality and myocardial infarction were however reduced. The ALLHAT and WOSCOPS trials did not show a significant reduction in stroke incidence in patients without established IHD, but the CARDS study in diabetic patients, and the ASCOT study in patients with hypertension and multiple cardiovascular risk factors found convincing reductions in stroke incidence. Thus, based on current evidence, older people with diabetes and hypercholesterolaemia, with IHD, or with multiple vascular risk factors should receive statin therapy.

Barriers to stroke prevention in older people

The treatment of patients with atrial fibrillation with warfarin and control of hypertension are probably the two most important stroke preventative strategies for older people. Many studies have shown that warfarin is hugely under-prescribed because of unfounded fears of bleeding complications and over-concern about the risk of falls in older people. Hospital-based warfarin clinics are also not always suited to older people who may have inadequate transport means. Similarly, many older people are not being treated to target blood pressure, particularly systolic pressure. Three-quarters of GPs would not initiate antihypertensive therapy in older people with systolic pressures of 140 - 159mmHg, and most would not escalate treatment to achieve a goal of 140mmHg. Most doctors believed the diastolic pressure was more

important than systolic, where the opposite is the case. Another problem with treatment is that an older person may not tolerate antihypertensives at high doses or multiple medication regimes. Lowering the blood pressure excessively may precipitate postural hypotension. This may be lessened by aiming for gradual blood pressure reduction, with diastolic pressure maintained above 65mmHg. Cigarette cessation is worthwhile at any age, and reduces cardiovascular events, but again may not be pursued aggressively in older people. Finally, the evidence for benefits in carotid surgery for octogenarians is as robust as for younger patients, and age alone should not be a barrier to surgery.

The National Audit of Stroke Care, commissioned by the Irish Heart Foundation, has found that there is little organised primary prevention for stroke in Ireland and only 16% of Irish hospitals have TIA services. Stroke prevention is hindered by a lack of designated funding, leading to inadequate staff and time to dedicate to stroke prevention. Stroke prevention also requires specific protocols for the screening and management of stroke risk factors. A National Stroke Strategy is currently being drafted by the Cardiovascular Review Group, which will include stroke prevention.

Transient ischaemic attack (TIA)

A TIA is defined as a neurological deficit lasting less than 24 hours that is attributed to focal cerebral or retinal ischaemia; most however last less than ten minutes. The annual stroke risk following a TIA is usually quoted to be about 5% per year. However, this generally excludes early stroke risk, which may be as high as 10% within 3 months, with half of these occurring in the first two days. Older patients and

TABLE 2
CLINICAL EVALUATION AND INVESTIGATION OF TIA

Examination
- Blood pressure
- Pulse rate and rhythm
- Heart sounds and murmurs
- Carotid or other bruits
- Fundoscopy: hypertensive changes or visible emboli
- Detailed neurological examination, guided by symptoms

Investigations
- FBC: anaemia, polycythaemia or leukaemia
- Clotting screen
- Glucose: hypoglycaemia or hyperglycaemia
- ESR: temporal arteritis, vasculitis or endocarditis
- Biochemical profile: hyponatraemia, hypernatraemia or hypocalcaemia
- Cholesterol profile and triglyceride level
- ECG: atrial fibrillation, LVH or ischaemia
- Carotid Doppler ultrasound unless another cause of TIA is likely or patient is clearly unfit for surgery
- CT brain to exclude tumour or haemorrhage
- Echocardiogram if abnormal cardiac examination
- Holter monitor if palpitations or abnormal ECG

TABLE 3
MANAGEMENT OF TIA

- Start aspirin immediately
- Treat hypertension
- Start statin therapy if hypercholesterolaemia, diabetes or IHD
- If already on aspirin, continue it and add dipyridamole or change to or add clopidogrel
- If atrial fibrillation, start warfarin unless contra-indication, in which case give aspirin 300mg/day
- If carotid stenosis > 70%, refer for carotid endartectomy If 50-70%, discuss with vascular surgeon and explain risk / benefit to patient. If <50%, surgery is not advisable
- Address life style issues, obesity, alcohol and smoking if necessary

those with more prolonged symptoms, diabetes and dysphasia are at higher risk of stroke while retinal artery TIA or amaurosis fugax - transient monocular visual loss - carries a smaller stroke risk. Patients require prompt investigation and TIA should be viewed as an acute medical emergency. While awaiting investigations patients should receive aspirin 150-300 mg/day unless there is a contra-indication such as allergy or previous gastrointestinal bleed, in which case clopidogrel can be used. Other treatments are discussed under secondary prevention.

Aetiology of stroke
Carotid, basilar and vertebral arteries or their branches are susceptible to atheromatous plaques associated with the risk factors already described. Large vessel infarcts occur when a plaque ruptures exposing subendothelial structures, which in turn activates platelets. A clot develops and further narrows the vessel, causing ischaemia and potentially infarction of the area of the brain supplied by that vessel, unless sufficient collateral blood supply is available. Small vessel ischaemia involving penetrating cerebral arteries causes lacunar infarction - these are most common in

hypertensive and diabetic patients - and the mechanism of their production may be quite different from that involved with the large vessels and may primarily involve hypertensive arteriosclerotic changes. With respect to emboli, loosely formed clots may move distally, causing partial or total occlusion of a smaller, distal vessel. Thus an internal carotid plaque causing minor carotid stenosis may cause ischaemia in a retinal or middle cerebral artery. Emboli may also originate in the left atrium in atrial fibrillation, in a left ventricular aneurysm post myocardial infarction or in the larger thoracic arteries. Conditions causing hyperviscosity predispose to stroke by promoting thrombosis. In older people, polycythaemia, leukaemia, other malignancies and dehydration are the more common causes. Prolonged hypotension due to arrhythmia, sepsis or cardiac compromise may cause cerebral ischaemia at 'watershed' areas of the brain between two major arterial territories.

Cerebral imaging in acute stroke

CT brain
CT brain is currently the gold standard for imaging in acute stroke and should be performed within 24 hours of stroke onset. It is not reliable in suspected posterior circulation infarct, where bony artefacts can obscure infarcts in the brainstem and cerebellum. It is debatable whether CT brain is better than MRI for detecting cerebral haemorrhage, but this has not been definitively proven. CT brain may be normal in one-quarter of patients in the first three hours after an ischaemic stroke. Early changes of cerebral infarction in the middle cerebral artery territory include loss of

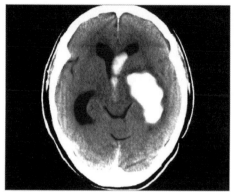

Figure 2: CT brain showing left basal ganglia haemorrhage with intraventricular blood and some midline shift

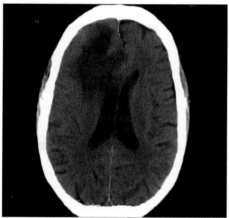

Figure 3: CT brain showing right frontal infarct

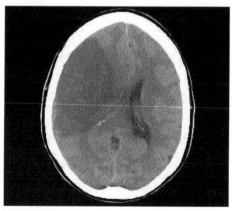

Figure 4: CT brain showing massive right middle cerebral artery infarct with cerebral oedema and midline shift

the white-grey matter distinction, loss of definition of the basal ganglia or cortical sulci (due to swelling) or focal hypodensity. These changes can be quantified using the ASPECTS score. A thrombus in the MCA may be visible as increased density within the artery, or in the more distal branches in the sylvian fissure as the dot sign.

MRI

MRI diffusion weighted imaging (DWI) is more sensitive than CT for very early infarct identification. Cerebral ischaemia causes shrinkage of the extracellular compartment, with increased DWI signal within hours. MRI with contrast administration can also give information about the perfusion of the brain (perfusion weighted image, PWI). Areas that have not yet developed ischaemia-related water changes but have reduced perfusion (DWI-PWI mismatch) have the potential to survive if circulation is restored spontaneously or through thrombolysis. This information may aid the decision making process regarding whether to administer thrombolysis to an individual. CT perfusion studies, using intravenous contrast, give similar information on blood flow to PWI and are more readily accessible than MRI based imaging in most hospitals.

Strokes are usually classified using the Bamford nomenclature from the Oxfordshire Community Stroke Project. An infarct involving an entire cerebral cortex is a Total Anterior Circulation Infarct (TACI), while one involving only some of it is a Partial Anterior Circulation Infarct (PACI). Vertebrobasilar circulation infarcts are called Posterior Circulation Infarcts (POCI) and lacunar infarcts are LACI. This classification is useful as it summarises the neurological deficit and helps predict prognosis.

Predicting outcome in acute stroke

Some indication of prognosis for individual patients can be made based on initial clinical examination and CT findings. Almost 50% of patients with primary intracerebral haemorrhage or SAH and 40% of those with TACI die in the first month. By contrast, less than 5% of patients with PACI and 2% of those with lacunar infarcts die in the first month. Brainstem dysfunction indicates a poor prognosis and worrying signs include Cheyne-Stokes respiration, dysphagia, reduced consciousness or bilateral up-going plantar responses. However, as will be discussed later, infection, metabolic disturbance, seizure or hypoxia may worsen neurological status and lead to erroneous

TABLE 4
INDICATIONS FOR URGENT CT BRAIN

Possible candidate for thrombolysis

Suspicion of subarachnoid haemorrhage (SAH)

Possible cerebellar haematoma

Head injury with suspected subarachnoid haemorrhage or

subdural haematoma

Patient on anticoagulation

Lumbar puncture required; possible meningitis or

encephalitis

Rapid worsening or fluctuation of neurological status

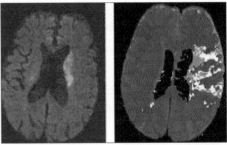

Figure 5: MRI images of a left MCA territory infarct. The ischaemic area as visualised by DWI (left image) is much less extensive than the under-perfused area on the PWI

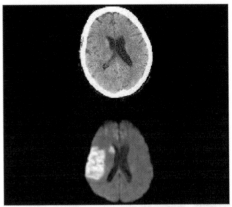

Figure 6: CT brain and MRI images of a right middle cerebral artery territory infarct. The infarct is subtle on the CT brain (top image), but readily visible on the MRI

predictions of prognosis. Most deaths within a few hours of symptom onset involve haemorrhage. Deaths in the first few days may be due to brainstem infarction or secondary compression by cerebral oedema, haemorrhagic transformation of an initial infarct, stroke progression or recurrence. Deaths after the first week are usually caused by complications: pneumonia, pulmonary embolism or pressure sores. The severity of stroke may be quantified using specific neurological scales such as the widely accepted National Institute of Health Stroke Scale or the Scandinavian Stroke Scale, which document consciousness, speech abilities, power, etc.

Thrombolysis in acute stroke

Thrombolysis aims to restore blood flow rapidly to the area of cerebral ischaemia and thereby reduce the ultimate infarct size and hence reduce functional disability. Tissue plasminogen activator (tPA) has definite benefits for functional outcome if given at a dose of 0.9mg/kg within 3 hours of symptom onset (NINDS trial) and is safe if protocols are strictly adhered to (STARS study, SITS-MOST registry). The rate of symptomatic intracerebral haemorrhage post thrombolysis is 4 - 7%. If suspected, usually due to worsened neurological status, thrombolysis is discontinued and urgent CT brain performed and fresh frozen plasma administered if needed. Thrombolysis may be beneficial if given within 3 - 6 hours of symptom onset using MRI DWI-PWI guidance to determine the risk/benefit ratio. A recently published study showed benefit from thrombolysis up to 4.5 hours after onset of symptoms in patients with acute stroke. It is important to remember however that current ACCP guidelines are based solely on the time since symptom onset and CT findings, although this may change with further studies in this area. The

National Audit of Stroke Care shows that only 5% of Irish stroke patients are admitted within 2 hours of stroke onset (compared to 40% in the UK) and less than 1% receives thrombolysis. The challenge for healthcare providers is to facilitate patients in presenting promptly to A&E departments by heightening awareness of stroke symptoms in the general public and improving pre-hospital triage by GPs and paramedics (using mnemonics such as FAST – face, arm, speech test). There also is a need for streamlining of the in-hospital process of clinical evaluation and cerebral imaging and reporting to allow a rapid decision about the indication for thrombolysis. This will require agreed thrombolysis protocols, dedicated stroke on-call teams and coordination between acute hospitals in a region. Smaller, remote hospitals may use telemedicine to avail of 24/7 expertise to facilitate decision-making and safely administer thrombolysis.

Clinical trials are evaluating other thrombolytic agents, such as desmoteplase, which may have a

TABLE 5
CLASSIFICATION OF STROKE BY VESSEL INVOLVED

Anterior Cerebral Artery (ACA): **(Frontal cortex)**	Contralateral hemiparesis, sensory loss, gait apraxia, incontinence, personality change
Middle Cerebral Artery (MCA): **(Frontal, parietal, temporal and** **part of occipital cortex)**	Contralateral hemiparesis, sensory loss, dysphasia, dyspraxia, inattention or neglect, poor concentration, memory impairment
Deep branches (lacunar): **(Internal capsule)**	Isolated hemiparesis or hemisensory loss
Posterior Cerebral Artery (PCA): **(Occipital cortex)**	Contralateral homonymous hemianopia, memory impairment
Vertebro-basilar Arteries: **(Brainstem, cerebellum)**	Contralateral hemiparesis, sensory loss, ipsilateral cerebellar signs, ipsilateral facial paresis, sensory loss, bilateral cortical blindness*, amnesia, locked in state

*Bilateral cortical blindness is sometimes called Anton's syndrome; these patients are blind but have intact pupil responses and blink to confrontation as these reflexes do not involve the occipital cortex. Patients often are unaware that they are blind.

longer therapeutic window. Glycoprotein IIb/IIIa antagonists are also under trial. Intra-arterial thrombolysis gives a lower dose of prourokinase or tPA directly into the thrombus and so has less risk of systemic haemorrhage, and a longer therapeutic window, but is mainly experimental at this time. Combined intravenous and intra-arterial thrombolysis and mechanical thrombus removal are also under investigation.

Neuroprotection

In stroke, acute cerebral ischaemia causes free radical accumulation, acidosis and accumulation of intracellular calcium, all leading to neuronal death. In the area of brain that is under-perfused, some neurones will be irreversibly damaged, while some are just 'stunned' and capable of recovery with time, the so-called ischaemic penumbra. Many neuroprotective therapies have been developed to try to protect these potentially salvageable neurones. Many glutamate, NMDA and calcium antagonists have been extensively investigated without success. Recently, NXY-059, a nitrone radical trapping agent had initial promising results, not replicated in a follow-up study (SAINT studies). Ongoing trials are investigating the effect of uric acid, an antioxidant, and magnesium, which reduces glutamate release (IMAGES trial negative, FAST-MAG trial ongoing).

Anti-inflammatory agents such as arundic acid, IL-1alpha antibodies, and erythropoietin are also in the early trial stage.

In some European countries, infusions of albumin, dextran or other starches are combined with venesection to dilute the blood. The aim of this is to improve perfusion of ischaemic brain by optimising the haematocrit. A Cochrane review found no evidence that this improves prognosis however. Controlled hypothermia reduces cerebral metabolism and so may reduce the neurological deficit in acute stroke. However, it causes many complications itself and there may be a rebound worsening of status after rewarming and so is not a standard treatment. Pyrexia should however be treated in acute stroke, with paracetamol and external cooling.

Measures to reduce cerebral oedema

Cerebral oedema post stroke occurs due to the breakdown of neuronal cell membranes, cytotoxic oedema and by disruption of the blood-brain barrier, vasogenic oedema. Cerebral oedema may in turn cause temporal lobe herniation, brainstem compression, hydrocephalus and reduced cerebral blood flow. Haemorrhages and larger infarcts are more likely to be accompanied by oedema. Glycerol and mannitol may reduce cerebral oedema by osmosis but a Cochrane review found no evidence of benefit in stroke. Steroids reduce peri-tumour oedema and have also been tried in stroke, but again with no definite benefit. Hemi-craniotomy is performed in some large centres in the US to relieve intracranial pressure in large hemispheric strokes. Two open, non-randomised studies showed a benefit but patients who responded were younger and fitter than the conservatively managed patients.

Stroke units

The Stroke Unit Trialists' Collaboration has demonstrated that patients managed in a stroke unit setting have immediate and sustained benefits in survival rates, physical independence and rate of return home. The greatest benefit in mortality is seen between one and four weeks, indicating that stroke units primarily prevent complications. Earlier mobilisation in stroke units than general wards has been shown to be an independent factor associated with discharge of patients home rather than to institutional care. The National Audit of Stroke Care, published in 2008, found that only 3% of Irish acute hospitals had a stroke unit, with only 16% of hospitals having organised stroke care. In contrast, 91% of UK hospitals have stroke units (Sentinel Audit 2006). The forthcoming National Stroke Strategy may help to secure funding for the organisation of acute stroke services in Ireland, including the designation of geographically defined and adequately staffed stroke units in each acute hospital. These units will have regular multidisciplinary team meetings. Teams should include stroke nurse specialists, stroke-specific therapists and targeted screening for the complications of stroke should be part of their core work. There should be seamless integration of acute stroke care, from thrombolysis or other hyperacute treatment to secondary prevention measures and rehabilitation.

Common early post stroke complications

Worsening neurological status

Early recurrent ischaemia occurs in approximately 4% of strokes. Some degree of haemorrhagic transformation occurs in most strokes but is not detected because it is clinically silent and CT is rarely routinely repeated. However, clinically significant secondary haemorrhage occurs in only a few percent, more commonly in larger infarcts. Other causes of worsening neurological status include cerebral

TABLE 6
INDICATIONS FOR THROMBOLYSIS

- Adult aged 18 years and over
- Neurological signs should not be clearing spontaneously or be post-ictal or be minor and isolated
- Onset of symptoms less than 3 hours before beginning treatment
- CT does not show an established infarct (hypodensity > 1/3 cerebral hemisphere) or intracranial bleed
- No history of previous intracranial bleed and no head trauma or prior stroke in previous 3 mths
- No myocardial infarction in the previous 3 mths
- No GI or urinary haemorrhage in previous 21 days and no active bleeding or acute trauma (fracture)
- No major surgery in the previous 14 days
- No arterial puncture at a noncompressible site in the previous 7 days
- Blood pressure controlled (systolic < 185mmHg and diastolic < 110mmHg)
- INR < 1.7, APTT in normal range, platelet count > 100,000mm^3
- Blood glucose > 2.7mmol/l
- Informed consent

oedema, hydrocephalus (especially with posterior fossa infarcts), extension of intracerebral haemorrhage into the cerebral ventricles, seizure, infection, metabolic disturbance, hypoxia, hypercapnea and sedating medications.

Deep vein thrombosis

A swollen hemiparetic leg in a bed-fast patient is usually due to DVT and may not always be painful. Approximately 5% of early deaths following stroke are attributed to pulmonary embolism. Low molecular weight heparin reduces the incidence of DVT but may increase the risk of cerebral haemorrhage and is not routinely used in most units. Patients with haemorrhagic stroke should not receive LMWH. All hemiparetic stroke patients should be mobilised as soon as possible and wear thromboembolism prevention stockings (TEDS) unless there is a contra-indication. If a patient with an ischaemic infarct develops a DVT, they can be treated with LMWH. In patients with intracranial haemorrhage, insertion of a Greenfield vena cava filter is an option.

Aspiration

Acute stroke care should include dysphagia screening

by trained staff. Dysphagia occurs in almost 50% of stroke patients initially and approximately one-third aspirate to a clinically significant extent, especially in the first week. Patients at risk include those with altered consciousness or confusion, poor cough, dysphasia and facial weakness. Bedside assessment utilises knowledge of the physiology of a normal swallow. Normal swallowing involves transit of a food bolus from the mouth through the pharynx to the oesophagus. The larynx elevates during the swallow to prevent food entering the larynx. Thus, the patient is observed taking a sip of water, and laryngeal elevation is directly inspected and palpated at the anterior aspect of the neck. The patient is asked to speak after the swallow, and if the water has penetrated to the level of the vocal cords, the voice is 'moist'. Throat clearing, or frank coughing, also indicates laryngeal penetration. If necessary, videofluorographic swallowing studies can verify and assess the degree of aspiration and can detect 'silent' aspiration, where there is laryngeal penetration but no coughing.

The treatment of dysphagia is multifactorial, involving the speech and language therapist (SALT), physician, nursing staff, dietician and physiotherapist. The SALT can determine at what consistency of liquids and solids patients aspirate and so guide dietary recommendations. For example, a patient may safely swallow solids, but require intravenous or subcutaneous fluid administration. Correct positioning of the patient, including using a 'chin tuck' position to direct food into the pharynx and adaptive feeding equipment can also improve swallow function. Patients at risk of aspiration at any consistency may require enteral feeding to improve nutrition and reduce the risk of aspiration, and hence improve survival and quality of life. However, there is very little robust research in this field to prove that enteral feeding actually achieves these goals. Enteral feeding is via a nasogastric tube in the short term, or via a percutaneous gastrostomy (PEG) or jejunostomy in those with persisting dysphagia.

There are two important points to remember with enteral feeding. Firstly, there are ethical issues around artificial feeding, particularly in the setting of a severe stroke. Secondly, the patient will require appropriate long-term follow-up as most dysphagia improves with time, and nutritional requirements will vary with time. Many patients will return to full or partial oral diet, and this has to be supervised and coordinated in a multidisciplinary fashion, often in the community setting, involving family and carers, nursing home staff, community dietician and SALT. There have been studies of surgical diversion procedures that bypass the pharynx (mouth directly to oesopaghus via jejunal flap), which may be developed further in the future. Similarly, lingual exercise and electrical stimulation therapy are under trial for dysphagia management.

Constipation and faecal incontinence
Constipation is common after stroke due to immobility, poor fluid or food intake and analgesic medication but is often overlooked. It causes distress, increased tone, urinary retention and eventually faecal incontinence due to overflow. Faecal incontinence is a significant barrier to a patient being cared for at home.

Urinary incontinence
Almost half of all stroke patients are incontinent in the first 48 hours, most commonly due to reduced consciousness or detrusor instability. Incontinence beyond the first few days in an alert patient should lead to the exclusion of urinary infection or constipation causing retention. Stroke patients are predisposed to urinary tract infection and unnecessary catheterisation should be avoided. Adequate fluid intake, discontinuation of unnecessary diuretics and regular toileting should be encouraged.

Dehydration
Patients at risk include those with immobility, hemianopia or visual neglect where they may not be able to reach or be aware of fluids placed near them. Communication difficulties also cause problems as patients may not be capable of asking for a drink. Reduced consciousness with associated reduction in thirst and excessive fluid losses due to tachypnoea, sepsis or hyperglycaemia with polyuria may also be important factors.

Secondary prevention post TIA or stroke
Investigations into the aetiology of stroke are similar to those for TIA. Patients should be advised to stop smoking and reduce alcohol intake if relevant. Diabetes and hypercholesterolaemia must be actively excluded. Hypertension that persists beyond the first two weeks should be treated. In patients who have had an anterior circulation stroke or TIA, (excluding those with massive stroke in whom there is little to gain) and have at least a 70% angiographic stenosis

but not total occlusion, carotid endarterectomy has a definite benefit in patients fit for surgery (NASCET, ECST studies). For patients with a 50-70% stenosis, there is a benefit only in centres with low complication rates, while stenosis less than 50% is best treated with aspirin. Carotid angioplasty and stenting have not yet been shown to be safer or more beneficial than surgery.

Patients in sinus rhythm should receive aspirin 75mg/day. Higher doses do not improve risk reduction but cause more gastrointestinal side-effects. The Antiplatelet Trialists Collaboration Group's meta-analysis of antiplatelet therapy demonstrated a 23% reduction in the risk of non-fatal stroke in patients with a previous stroke or TIA. Clopidogrel may reduce the risk of recurrent stroke slightly more than aspirin (CAPRIE trial), but is much more expensive. It is useful in patients intolerant of aspirin and as a first line agent in those with peripheral vascular disease. Aspirin combined with dipyridamole also has been found to be more effective than aspirin alone (ESPS-2) in preventing recurrent stroke with one stroke prevented per eighteen patients treated for 2 years but importantly aspirin had more favourable effects on mortality. Moreover, a recent comparison of aspirin/dipyridamole SR with clopidogrel failed to confirm any superiority of the combination in preventing events. There is no evidence that warfarin is superior to aspirin in patients in sinus rhythm. There are no evidence-based guidelines for patients who suffer a stroke while already taking aspirin but options include adding dipyridamole or changing to clopidogrel. The decision should involve assessment of the patient's bleeding risk and other concurrent vascular disease. Patients in atrial fibrillation after a TIA or stroke have a 12% annual risk of stroke. The EAFT trial showed that anticoagulation of 100 patients, with target INRs

between 2.5 and 4, prevented nine strokes while aspirin 300mg/day prevented four. Warfarin should not be commenced for at least 2 weeks post-stroke because of the risk of secondary haemorrhage. Although there is little direct trial evidence in elderly patients post TIA or stroke, it is reasonable to start statin therapy in patients with hypercholesterolaemia and diabetes or IHD. The SPARCL study showed a reduction in the rate of recurrent stroke with atorvastatin, but a small increase in haemorrhagic stroke, an effect which has been noted in other studies. The PROGRESS trial of 6000 patients with a previous TIA or stroke of whom 25% were aged 70 years or older found that patients receiving combination perindopril and indapamide therapy had a reduced rate of recurrent stroke. Fourteen people needed to be treated for 5 years to prevent one stroke. Importantly, the patients did not have to be hypertensive to benefit from the treatment.

Rehabilitation

Associated with recovery post stroke, muscle function usually improves from the centre to the periphery such that patients regain head control first, then sitting trunk control, then standing balance and finally walking. Lower limb recovery is earlier and more complete than upper limb recovery. Motor recovery plateaus 3-6 months post-stroke, but functional recovery may continue for several years. As a rule of thumb, 10% of patients achieve complete recovery within 3 months, while 10% have no recovery. Approximately 50% of stroke survivors will have some level of functional disability at six months, but less than 5% of patients with TACI will be independent at 6 months. Speech and language function may continue to slowly recover over several years. Global dysphasia has a poor prognosis, while isolated fluent dysphasia often recovers fully. When planning rehabilitation goals, co-morbid diseases and the patient's previous mobility and function need to be taken into account. For example, a patient with pre-existing severe dyspnoea may never be able to walk more than a few steps with a hemiplegic gait and equally may not be able to self-propel in a standard wheelchair so the most appropriate rehabilitation goal might be aiming for independence in an electric wheelchair. Functional scales can track improvement that occurs during the rehabilitative process; the Barthel Index is a commonly used one which looks at activities of daily living such as washing, dressing, toileting and mobility. The Rankin Score is a cruder index, which measures independence on scale from

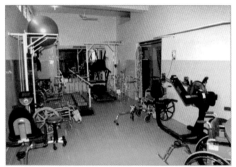

Figure 7: Stroke rehabilitation gymnasium

TABLE 7 CHARACTERISTIC FEATURES OF RIGHT HEMIPARESIS	TABLE 8 CHARACTERISTIC FEATURES OF LEFT HEMIPARESIS

• Visuomotor perception and memory intact
• Behaviours to be learned should be demonstrated step-by-step, encouraging imitation
• Dysphasia may be present with vocabulary and auditory span reduced
• Caregivers may assume that the patient comprehends much more than he does – patients may limit or eliminate words. Patients may be able to pick up ideas of conversation through body language, tone of voice and facial expression
• Patients are generally able to learn from their mistakes
• Patients are able to synthesise parts of a task
• Patients will learn from observing others
• Patients will appear cautious and unorganised when approaching an unfamiliar situation and will therefore need a lot of feedback
	• Visuomotor perceptual impairment is prominent with loss of visual memory and associated left sided neglect
	• Patients may appear impulsive or unorganised in their activities of daily living
	   • Lack insight and judgement
	   • Poor safety awareness with secondary falls
	   • Inability to follow through on instructions
	• Neglect is more common than in right hemiparesis and may involve several modalities
	   • Vision
	   • Touch
	   • Proprioception
	   • Hearing
	• Learning is impaired and performance may not improve
	• Patients may not learn from their mistakes
	• Patients and carers may not recognise the extent of subtle sensory deficits and may battle with staff for premature discharge

1 to 5, with 5 representing bed bound and totally dependent and 1 representing full independence. The Stroke Impact Scale is a stroke-specific outcome scale that incorporates cognitive, functional and social assessments.

Stroke rehabilitation includes one or more of the following methods: (1) compensatory strategies; (2) strengthening exercises; (3) facilitation and neurophysiologic techniques (Bobath); and (4) task-oriented approaches. Compensatory strategies encourage the use of the unaffected side to allow early return to self-care, but may theoretically hinder the recovery of the affected side. Conversely, facilitation focuses on improving the function of the affected side. Task-specific training may incorporate constraint of the unaffected side (CIMT), which has clinical evidence support. Treadmill retraining also promotes recovery of walking by encouraging neuroplasticity. Cochrane review shows it to improve walking speed in those with good recovery, but to have less benefit in dependent patients. From a rehabilitation point of view there are significant differences in the approach to patients with right sided and left sided hemiparesis as described in Tables 7 and 8.

Common late post stroke complications

Spasticity
Although the hemiplegic limbs are often flaccid

immediately following a stroke, over weeks or months they may become spastic. Lower limb spasticity may sometimes aid weight bearing but upper limb spasticity is usually problematic. This is most prominent in the flexor muscles and so the typical posture involves an adducted and flexed shoulder, flexed elbow and wrist and fisted hand, severely disrupting activities of daily living, such as dressing. Because fingernails become inaccessible, they can protrude into the skin of the palm, which may become macerated and prone to fungal infection. Muscles eventually become shortened as contractures develop. The key to treating spasticity involves its early avoidance or limitation. This includes avoidance of posture and activities that increase tone, passive stretching of the affected muscles and specific physiotherapy to influence local reflexes acting on the affected limb. Medications such as dantrolene and baclofen can also be considered early but cause drowsiness, which often limits their use. Botulinum toxin has the advantage of being injected into the affected muscle, thereby weakening that muscle without affecting other muscles or causing drowsiness, and should be used early in problematic spasticity. Spasticity can also be increased by pain, oedema of the affected limb and discomfort, for example due to constipation. These easily treatable causes should be actively excluded.

Depression

25 - 50% of stroke survivors suffer depression at some stage. Stroke guidelines recommend that depression is actively screened for, but this often does not happen. As well as general depression scales (e.g. the Geriatric Depression Scale, General Health Survey SF 36 or Beck's Depression Index), there are stroke-specific depression scales – the Stroke Specific Quality of Life Scale, and the Aphasic Depression Scale. Strokes that affect the right hemisphere increase the risk of depression. Frontal lobe involvement may cause personality change, including withdrawal or emotional lability. However depression can occur after any type or location of stroke, and also relates to the degree of functional impairment, social handicap and family support available to the patient. Depression interferes with rehabilitation and patients with post-stroke depression have poorer functional outcome, worse cognition and three times the mortality rate at 10 years post stroke than non-depressed stoke patients. There is a significantly increased risk of suicide in patients with stroke, especially in women and those under age 60. Treatment is with serotonin reuptake inhibitors or tricyclic antidepressants, which have been shown in the short-term to improve mood, functional outcome and cognitive status. More research into pharmacological and non-pharmacological treatment of depression particularly in the longer term is required.

Pain

Shoulder pain occurs in up to 75% of hemiparetic strokes. It is most often caused by inferior subluxation due to muscle hypotonia. Differential diagnoses include capsulitis or tendonitis, rotator cuff tears and humeral fracture or dislocation. To reduce the incidence of shoulder subluxation and also to prevent oedema, the hemiparetic upper limb should be supported while the patient is seated. A rare cause of upper limb pain is reflex sympathetic dystrophy or 'shoulder hand syndrome' which presents as upper limb swelling, dysaesthesia, heat and erythema and is due to autonomic-induced vasodilation. Another is post-stroke central pain syndrome or Dejerine-Roussy syndrome which occurs weeks or months after a stroke that involves the thalamus. Sensory fibres from the body relay to the sensory cortex through the thalamus. Patients may have unpleasant dysaesthesia on the affected side and even a gentle touch feels unpleasant or painful. For most types of pain occurring after a stroke treatment involves simple analgesia, opioids, antidepressants or anticonvulsants such as carbamazepine, gabapentin or pregabalin. Transcutaneous electrical nerve stimulation (TENS) may also be helpful.

Social consequences of stroke

Stroke survivors report high levels of psychological morbidity, disability across a range of domains and poor quality of life. The presence of handicap can affect interpersonal relationships, mobility and leisure, with social isolation as a consequence. Stroke also affects the relatives and carers of the stroke patient. One third of care-givers report carer strain, and up to one half are depressed, particularly if the stroke victims have residual cognitive impairment, dysphasia, functional deficits or abnormal behaviour. Patients in turn have worse outcomes when their caregivers are depressed. Lack of appropriate discharge planning and early discharge of stroke survivors can place increased and unrealistic demands on carers. They may find it hard to cope with the behavioural problems of stroke sufferers. Care-givers experience a profound sense of loss and have to adjust to a new relationship with their relative, taking on new responsibilities, feeling the demands of care-giving, and having to depend on the support of others. The Irish Heart Foundation provides a patient information booklet entitled 'A Guide for those affected by Stroke and their Carers', which is available on the IHF website. There may also be a financial aspect to the strain of the stroke. The stroke victim may have been employed prior to the stroke, and so suffers immediate financial loss. One third of caregivers have to reduce their work hours, resign, or retire from their jobs. Of note, caregivers employed full-time are at highest risk for depressive symptoms. Finally, many stroke patients may wish to resume driving, and should have clinical assessment of vision, attention, hearing, visuospatial skills, and motor function. This can be followed by a 'behind-the-wheel' assessment. Patients should be advised to notify the Vehicle Licensing Authority and their insurance company of their stroke. The Irish Wheelchair Association website lists the available driving assessment sites in Ireland.

Other cerebrovascular events

Primary intracerebral haemorrhage (PICH)

This accounts for approximately 10% of patients presenting with suspected stroke. PICH should be suspected when a patient is receiving anticoagulation or has reduced consciousness, drowsiness, headache, neck stiffness, vomiting or seizures. A cerebellar haematoma may be amenable to neurosurgical drainage, but other haemorrhages are usually treated conservatively. Unlike ischaemic strokes, consideration should be given to reducing hypertension acutely in PICH. Poor prognosis is indicated by a large bleed, large midline shift, intraventricular blood, deep coma and loss of brainstem reflexes. There is currently no trial evidence to support osmotic agents, steroids or nimodipine in PICH. If the patient had been receiving warfarin, this should be reversed with vitamin K and fresh frozen plasma.

Subarachnoid haemorrhage (SAH)
Primary SAH is a rare cause of stroke in older patients but traumatic SAH following a fall with head injury may occur. Patients may present with the classical sudden, severe headache with or without reduced consciousness, focal neurological abnormalities or seizures. In 90% of patients, CT is diagnostic within the first 24 hours. If CT is negative, cerebrospinal fluid should be obtained. Cochrane review recommends oral nimodipine, a calcium antagonist, 60mg every four hours orally for primary SAH to reduce associated vasospasm and potentially improve survival and neurological status.

Subdural haematoma
These are more common with increasing age because cerebral atrophy causes the brain to shrink away from the dura, stretching the dural veins and predisposing them to rupture. Patients may or may not have a history of fall with head injury. Presentation includes headache, confusion, seizures, focal neurological findings and fluctuating consciousness. CT brain is diagnostic and symptomatic haematomas are amenable to neurosurgical drainage. However an older person may be confused or drowsy after a fall due to an underlying metabolic abnormality or sepsis that may also have precipitated the fall. The decision to proceed to CT brain should be influenced by whether symptoms are significant enough to warrant drainage, whether there is focal neurology or worsening neurological status or whether there is another equally likely cause for symptoms such as significant hyponatraemia or severe infection.

Differential diagnosis of cerebrovascular event
• Hypoglycaemia: This can mimic stroke and cause irreversible neuronal damage. All patients with suspected stroke must have an immediate capillary blood glucose measured

• Migraine: This can occur de novo in an older person but is rare and is a diagnosis of exclusion
• Tumour: Usually subacute symptoms. Acute presentation suggests haemorrhage into a previously asymptomatic tumour. CT brain may show marked peri-tumour oedema, with enhancement on administration of intravenous contrast
• Intra-cerebral abscess: Rare unless there has been obvious preceding infection or immunosuppression. Sub-acute presentation is usual with seizures, fever, confusion or altered consciousness. Consider if CXR shows a cavitating lesion. Contrast CT brain shows ring-enhancement
• Encephalitis or meningitis: Rare in later life, consider if there is sub-acute onset or specific predisposition such as immunosuppression, skull fracture or current infection. HZ encephalitis is rare but may complicate acute HZ infection
• Seizure: A partial seizure may cause ipsilateral weakness post-ictally, so called Todd's paresis. Likewise, a prolonged generalised seizure or benzodiazepine administration to arrest a seizure may cause reduced consciousness, usually improving over a few hours. However patients with acute stroke may have seizures within the first 24 hours. It is important to determine whether the weakness or drowsiness preceded or followed the seizure. It is very difficult however to accurately assess neurological status immediately after a seizure and seemingly catastrophic strokes can often be followed by miraculous recoveries!

Miscellaneous causes of stroke:
• Saggital sinus thrombosis: Rare, consider if hyperviscosity, malignancy or severe dehydration. CT brain may demonstrate diffuse small superficial cortical haemorrhages. MRI, particularly MR venography is diagnostic. Treatment is with anticoagulation
• Arterial dissection: Very rare over the age of 70. May occur in carotid or vertebrobasilar arteries. Consider if minor neck trauma, excessive neck movement or neck pain preceded symptoms. MR angiography or contrast angiography are diagnostic
• Vasculitis: Rare, consider if known vasculitis, very raised ESR, or evidence of renal or lung vasculitis such as blood or casts in the urine or patchy abnormalities on CXR

Hypertension
The WHO states that hypertension is a major factor responsible for most deaths worldwide, nearly 50%

more than cigarette smoking. The lifetime risk of developing hypertension is 90% in people surviving to 80 - 85 years of age. It has been estimated that a 5mmHg reduction of systolic blood pressure in the population as a whole would result in a 14% overall reduction in mortality due to stroke, a 9% reduction in mortality due to CHD and a 7% decrease in all-cause mortality. Functional changes, including increased arterial wall tension, increased peripheral resistance, and increased arterial stiffness are associated with systolic hypertension in older people. The Framingham study showed that systolic blood pressure increases linearly with age, while diastolic pressure rises and then drops again, increasing the pulse pressure. By the age of seventy, 95% of people have isolated systolic hypertension, defined as systolic pressure > 140mmHg and diastolic pressure < 90mmHg. With advancing age, the systolic blood pressure more closely predicts cardiovascular risk than diastolic pressure. Indeed, older people with isolated systolic hypertension and diastolic hypotension and hence a large pulse pressure may have the highest rate of cardiovascular morbidity and mortality. Cardiovascular risk increases above blood pressures of just 115/75mmHg. 'Prehypertension' is a term introduced for those with pressure ranging from 120-139mmHg systolic and/or 80 - 89mmHg diastolic blood pressure. Other factors associated with a higher cardiovascular risk at any level of hypertension include increasing age, loss of the normal night-time blood pressure dip (usually about 10%) and evidence of end organ damage such as left ventricular hypertrophy, retinopathy or microalbuminuria.

Is lowering blood pressure beneficial in older people?

It has been proven beyond doubt that treating hypertension in older people reduces mortality and cardiovascular morbidity. Lowering blood pressure will reduce the risk of cerebrovascular disease, coronary artery disease, heart failure, renal failure and possibly dementia. The Framingham study indicated that control of hypertension is as beneficial in reducing stroke risk in persons over the age of 70 years as it is in younger people. Gueyffier et al performed a sub-group meta-analysis of patients aged 80 years and older in clinical hypertension trials, demonstrating that treating hypertension reduces the risk of stroke requiring 100 patients to be treated to prevent one stroke per year. The HYVET study lends further support to the importance of treating

hypertension in appropriate very elderly patients. SHEP and Syst-Eur looked specifically at isolated systolic hypertension in people over 60 years of age. Treatment prevented 3 strokes and 5 cardiovascular events per 100 patients treated for 5 years, with similar benefits among the older patients in these studies. The SCOPE trial found that candesartan reduced the risk of stroke in people aged 70 - 90 years. Thus there is very strong evidence to support treating hypertension in older people, at least up to the age of ninety. For any age person, target BP should be 140/90 mmHg, or 130/80 mmHg in diabetic patients. Lifestyle changes should also be considered in older people, such as dietary manipulation, low salt and high potassium intake, weight reduction and exercise. The Trial of Non-pharmacologic Interventions in the Elderly (TONE) study showed that weight loss and sodium restriction were very beneficial in older people.

Which agents should be used?

It is probably more important to achieve target systolic blood pressure control than be overly concerned about which agent is used to achieve it. Most patients will have co-morbidities that indicate a particular agent should be used as first line. Also, most patients will need more than one agent to achieve target and there may be less side-effects from low doses of two agents than high doses of one. The MRC trial found that diuretics but not beta-blockers reduced stroke and cardiovascular risks in hypertensive patients aged 65-74 years. ALLHAT compared doxazosin and ACE inhibitors and calcium antagonists to chlorthalidone, a thiazide diuretic, in 25,000 patients with hypertension and one other risk factor for IHD. Chlorthalidone prevented more strokes than the other agents. The STOP hypertension-2 study found no difference between diuretics, beta blockers, calcium antagonists and ACE inhibitors in patients aged 70 - 84 years of age. The LIFE study found that losartan, an angiotensin-2 receptor blocker (ARB) was superior to atenolol in patients aged 55-80 years old. An open label study of ACE inhibitors versus diuretics in General Practice found a modest reduction in cardiovascular events with ACE inhibitors rather than diuretics and an increase in fatal strokes. The INSIGHT study found calcium antagonists equivalent to diuretics, while Val-Syst found valsartan better tolerated than calcium antagonists in isolated systolic hypertension.

Thus at present diuretics remain the first line agents in older people with hypertension, although not all older people will tolerate them. Angiotensin receptor blocker/calcium channel inhibitor combinations are also well tolerated. Beta-blockers are most useful in patients with ischaemic heart disease, in particular post myocardial infarction. Alpha receptor antagonists are rarely used as first line agents but are useful in patients with side effects from other agents and in men with prostatomegaly. ACE inhibitors or angiotensin receptor blockers should be first line therapy in hypertensive diabetic patients (ABCD, HOPE trials). ACE inhibitors are indicated post myocardial infarction, and in conjunction with diuretics in both cardiac failure and post stroke. Finally, the first oral renin inhibitor, aliskerin, has recently been licensed for the treatment of hypertension. It has a long duration of action and good tolerability, and lowers blood pressure comparably to other agents. Studies of its benefits in reducing cardiovascular morbidity are underway, and will determine its place in the treatment of hypertension in older people.

Suggested further reading

- Alber G, Amarence P, Easton J, Sacco R, Teal P. Antithrombotic and thrombolytic therapy for ischemic stroke: the Seventh ACCP Conference on Antithrombotic and Thrombolytic Therapy. Chest 2004; 126(3 Suppl): 483S-512S.
- Bamford J, Sandercock P, Dennis M, et al. Classification and natural history of clinically identifiable subtypes of cerebral infarction. Lancet 1991; 337: 1521-6.
- Cornett O. Antithrombotic and Thrombolytic Therapy for Ischaemic Stroke. Cardiol Clin 2008; 26(2): 251-265.
- Dafer R, Rao M, Shareef A, Sharma A. Poststroke depression. Top Stroke Rehabil 2008; 15(1): 13-21.
- Duprez D. Systolic Hypertension in the Elderly: Addressing an Unmet Need. Am J Med 2008; 121: 179-184.
- Finley-Caulfield A. Critical care of acute ischemic stroke. Crit Care Clin 2006; 22(4): 581-606.
- Garcia D, Hylek E. Reducing the Risk for Stroke in Patients Who Have Atrial Fibrillation. Cardiol Clin 26 (2008); 267–275.
- Hofmeijer J, Van Der Worp H, Kappelle L. Treatment of space-occupying cerebral infarction. Crit Care Med 2003; 31: 617-25.
- Irish National Audit of Stroke Care, Irish Heart Foundation, Dublin, 2008.
- http://www.irishheart.ie/iopen24/pub/strokereports/stroke_report.pdf
- Kaplan R, Tirschwell D, Longstreth W, Manolio T, Heckbert S, Lefkowitz D, et al. Vascular events, mortality, and preventive therapy following ischemic stroke in the elderly. Neurology 2005; 65: 835-42.
- Muir KW. Imaging of acute stroke. Lancet Neurol 2006; 5(9): 755-68.
- National Clinical Guidelines for Stroke, 2nd edition, Royal College of Physicians, London, 2004.
- http://www.rcplondon.ac.uk/pubs/contents/70527aa8-651c-43e4-8f3e-a714872a1573.pdf
- National Institute of Neurological Disorders and Stroke (NINDS) rt-PA Stroke Study Group. Tissue plasminogen activator for acute ischaemic stroke. NEJM 1995; 333: 1581-7.
- Neutel JM, Gilderman L. Hypertension control in the elderly. J Clin Hypertens. 2008; 10 (1 Suppl 1):33-9.
- Seventh report of the Joint National Committee on Prevention, Detection, Evaluation, and Treatment of High Blood Pressure. Hypertension 2003; 42(6): 1206-52.
- Shah M, Rehabilitation of the Older Adult with Stroke. Clin Geriatr Med 2006; 22: 469– 489.
- Stroke Unit Trialists' Collaboration. Organised inpatient (stroke unit) care for stroke. Cochrane Database Syst Rev 2002; (1): CD000197.
- Zorowitz R. Rehabilitation of the stroke survivor. In ed Rakel, Conn's Current Therapy, 52nd edition, WB Saunders Co., 2000.

Case Study 1

A 72 year old man is admitted with rapid atrial fibrillation and shortness of breath. He has a background history of hypertension but his wife informed his General Practitioner recently that he has been poorly compliant with his medication. Electrocardiograph shows rapid ventricular response. Chest x-ray shows cardiomegaly and pulmonary oedema. He settles with oxygen, intravenous diuretics and digoxin. When better, his heart failure and blood pressure are further treated with an ACE inhibitor.

This patient has atrial fibrillation and evidence of left ventricular failure. He is at high risk for a stroke and therefore should commence warfarin, goal INR 2 - 3, unless he has a definite contra-indication in which case aspirin 300mg/day could be given instead. Patients under 65 years old with isolated atrial fibrillation do not need anticoagulation (annual stroke risk about 1%, similar to the population at large) but many physicians would give aspirin. Above the age of 65 years, patients with atrial fibrillation and no other risk factors (table 1) should receive aspirin 150 - 300mg/ day. Risk factors for an increased rate of stroke include age over 75 years, hypertension, left ventricular failure, enlarged left atrium on echocardiography, previous TIA or stroke and diabetes. The presence of one or more of these confers an annual stroke risk of 6 - 12% (SPAF–III trial) and all guidelines agree that these patients should receive warfarin therapy unless contraindicated. Other factors involved in the decision for warfarinisation include the patient's general fitness, co-morbidities and cognitive status, the potential for drug interactions eg. COPD patient requiring frequent antibiotic courses, the patient's ability to safely comply with a changing warfarin schedule and attend regularly for INR checks. The extent of input from relatives and carers may also be important. If this man had a clear history of palpitations of less than 48 hours duration, he could be safely cardioverted. Beyond this time limit, patients require 3 weeks of warfarin before cardioversion to reduce the risk of embolisation after restoration of sinus rhythm and 6 weeks of warfarin thereafter. Recent evidence suggests rate control and warfarin is superior to attempted cardioversion in this scenario.

Case Study 2

A 68 year old right-handed man has a six-hour history of 'being muddled'. You introduce yourself and ask him to lie on his bed but he does not cooperate. When you point to the bed and prompt him to lie on it, using your hands, he does this. He cannot answer any questions appropriately but seems happy to talk to you, although his speech is not making much sense.

This man has fluent or receptive dysphasia – he can speak well but it does not make sense and he can't answer questions appropriately. He cannot follow commands unless accompanied by a visual prompt. This indicates a lesion in Wernicke's area in the left temporal lobe, interfering with his understanding of language. The optic radiation passes through the parietal and temporal lobes en route to the occipital cortex and fibres from the superior visual field pass inferiorly through the temporal lobe so this patient may have a right superior field defect. Any lesion behind the optic chiasm causes a contralateral field defect.

Case Study 3

A 78 year old woman was admitted 6 days previously with a right hemiparesis and reduced consciousness. You approach her from the right side of the bed and introduce yourself. She looks at the nurse to your left and opens her mouth to speak. After a few seconds, she manages 'he-he-lo'. You ultimately ask yes / no type questions and she answers these appropriately. She seems very tearful at times but quickly cheers up again. She falls asleep at one point during the examination. She follows commands normally with her left limbs but has severe weakness of the right limbs, although she tries hard to move them. She nods her head to acknowledge touch on her left hand but seems unaware of touch on her right hand.

This lady has expressive or motor dysphasia – she understands well and follows commands and answers yes / no questions appropriately. She has however limited, slow, hesitant speech. She has evidence of involvement of the left frontal and parietal lobes. Frontal: emotional lability, right motor weakness, expressive dysphasia indicating damage to Broca's area. Parietal: right sided sensory loss. This indicates a TACI, with involvement of the ACA and MCA territories. She is drowsy, in keeping with this. This type of stroke has a poor prognosis.

🗁 Case Study 4

Mrs Smith is 78 years old and in the Accident and Emergency Department of her local District General Hospital. She has left hemiparesis, sensory loss and reduced consciousness. Her CT brain is normal. BP is 210/100 mmHg, respiratory rate is 28, pulse is 100 and temperature is 38°C. Her capillary blood glucose is 22mmol/l but she has not previously been diagnosed as diabetic according to her daughter. The patient cannot cooperate well with respiratory examination but you can hear widespread noisy breathing, worse on the right.

The patient has reduced consciousness and possible aspiration (fever, tachypnoea, tachycardia and noisy breathing) and will require intravenous fluids. Normal saline is the fluid of choice as dextrose may increase cerebral oedema and worsen hyperglycaemia. Normal saline at a rate of 1 litre, 10 - 12 hourly would be appropriate. The hyperglycaemia may be transient due to a stress response or infection but hyperglycaemia itself predicts a worse outcome. Animal studies have shown that insulin therapy improves brain ischaemia but this has not been proven in humans (GIST–UK trial). Over-treatment brings the risk of hypoglycaemia with potential neuroglycopaenia and worsening of neurological status. If the hyperglycaemia persists, some physicians would give an insulin infusion but she would require at least 2-hourly capillary glucose measurement, with a target glucose of about less than 11mmol/l. There is no role for oral agents in non-diabetic patients. 75% of patients with acute stroke are initially hypertensive. Aggressive lowering of blood pressure (BP) may reduce blood flow to the ischaemic area due to loss of cerebral autoregulation and should be avoided in the first two weeks post stroke. The American Heart Association recommends that BP should only be treated if persistently > 230/120mm Hg or if there is another indication to treat such as aortic dissection, hypertensive encephalopathy, intracerebral haemorrhage or myocardial infarction. Patients with known hypertension may be able to continue their medications with close BP monitoring. Hypotension worsens cerebral ischaemia and if it occurs, should be treated with intravenous fluids, inotropes or vasopressors. All stroke patients should be regularly monitored with pulse oximetry, particularly if they have reduced consciousness or are at risk for aspiration and should be given oxygen as required. One semi-randomised study found a worse prognosis in non-hypoxic stroke patients given routine oxygen, possibly due to increased free radical formation.

In the above case history there are clues to suggest aspiration but the fever may also be secondary to the stroke itself. Blood, urine and sputum cultures should be obtained if possible and parenteral antibiotics commenced. Regular rectal or nasogastric (NG) paracetamol should also be given as fever increases the metabolic rate and may worsen stroke prognosis. This patient should receive aspirin 150 or 300mg, either rectally or via an NG tube. The IST and CAST trials showed a small but definite benefit in giving aspirin within 48 hours of stroke with 1 better outcome per 100 patients treated. There are no studies looking at other anti-platelet agents in acute stroke. Several studies have found no benefit in using heparin, low molecular weight heparin or heparinoids in acute stroke. If this patient was within 3 hours of symptom onset and had no other contra-indications, she would be a candidate for thrombolysis if her systolic blood pressure settled to less than 185mmHg.

Data Interpretation

Urea   7.3mmol/l
Creatinine   78μmol/l
T4   36pmol/l
TSH   0.02mU/l

Question 1

An 80 year old woman with a history of diabetes is brought to the A&E department having being found collapsed on the floor at home. She has left hemiparesis, is confused and has been incontinent of urine. Routine blood tests show the following:

FBC - normal
Na$^+$ - 156mmol/l
K$^+$ - 5.3mmol/l
Urea – 10.2mmol/l
Creatinine - 78μmol/l
Capillary blood glucose - 1.6mmol/l

a.   Describe the abnormalities
b.   How do these relate to her clinical presentation?
c.   What would your immediate treatment be?

Question 2

A 70 year old man with a long history of hypertension is taking ramipril, bendrofluazide, aspirin, a statin and lercanidipine. He has peripheral vascular disease and a previous minor stroke. His blood pressure is 168/98mmHg and he is in sinus rhythm. Routine bloods reveal the following:

FBC   normal
Na$^+$ 132mmol/l
K$^+$ 3.2mmol/l
Urea   8.6mmol/l
Creatinine   124μmol/l
Glucose   5.4mmol/l
Full lipid profile   normal
TFTs   normal

a.   Describe the abnormalities
b.   What medications are indicated to reduce his risk of further stroke?

Question 3

An 82 year old woman had transient upper limb weakness and dysphasia during the previous week. Her ECG shows atrial fibrillation with a ventricular rate of 110 beats per minute at rest and CXR shows cardiomegaly. Medications include aspirin 75mg daily, perindopril and frusemide. Routine bloods include the following:

FBC   normal
Na$^+$ 137mmol/l
K$^+$ 3.2mmol/l

a.   What anti-thrombotic medication is indicated for this woman?
b.   How should her atrial fibrillation be rate controlled?
c.   What other non-cardiac therapy would help her rate control?

Best of five questions

Question 1

A 76 year old man presents with dysphasia, right upper limb weakness and right hemianopia. He is likely to have suffered a:

a.   left lacunar infarct
b.   left posterior cerebral artery infarct
c.   left middle cerebral artery infarct
d.   left total anterior circulation infarct
e.   left vertebral artery infarct

Question 2

A 69 year old woman with hypertension presents with a two week history of anterior neck pain and recurrent transient left upper limb weakness. She has a constricted right pupil. Her most likely diagnosis is:

a.   cervical myelopathy
b.   uncontrolled diabetes
c.   carotid artery dissection
d.   cardioembolic cerebral infarct
e.   malignant hypertension

Question 3

Which of the following has been shown to improve prognosis after a stroke:

a.   Routine oxygen therapy to keep oxygen saturation >98%
b.   Pneumatic lower limb compression
c.   Aggressive blood pressure control
d.   Early mobilisation in stroke units
e.   Achievement of normoglycaemia

Question 4

Dysphagia is diagnosed in the acute stroke setting:

a.   Only if a patient shows evidence of coughing after eating

b.   If the patient can not tolerate any consistency of fluids

c.   Only by a qualified speech and language therapist

d.   If a patient desaturates at night

e.   In about 50% of patients

Answers on page 311

Bone and joint disorders

J Carey, K Afridi, B Carey, EC Mulkerrin

Introduction

Musculoskeletal disorders and rheumatic diseases are important illnesses for physicians who care for the elderly to be aware of for several reasons:

1. They are very common in this population
2. The diagnosis can be difficult as patients may be poor historians and physical findings can be subtle or transient
3. Other diseases which can masquerade as arthritis and related conditions such as malignancy and endocarditis are more prevalent in this population
4. While treatments may help alleviate suffering, the elderly may be more prone to side effects and toxicities and may also be taking several other medications which increases the risk of potentially serious drug interactions

Rheumatology is unique in that diagnosis often relies solely on the patient's history and physical examination. Pitfalls occur at every stage of the diagnostic process especially with diagnostic tests where positive and negative predictive values can be surprisingly poor. However for the astute clinician, the diagnosis and management of these disorders can be extremely satisfying, greatly enhancing patient outcomes and their quality of life.

The aim of this chapter is to familiarise physicians and other health professionals with some of the more common disorders present in older persons, and discuss some basic strategies for systematically evaluating these entities and their differential diagnoses. Diagnostic reasoning and medical decision making for complex and rare diseases requires experience and a breadth of knowledge not easily accomplished from reading general textbooks. In-depth discussion of some of the rarer disorders is outside the scope of this chapter and the reader is referred to formal rheumatology textbooks for further details.

Symptoms

Joint pain or arthralgia is the commonest presenting complaint in elderly patients. It is imperative to ascertain the site, onset, duration and distribution of pain, provoking factors and response to interventions and treatment. Articular and periarticular pain can radiate widely, and patients' description of pain may vary including 'aching', 'throbbing' and 'stiffness' so the use of closed questions during history taking can be misleading. The location of the site of origin of the pain is crucial to the process of differential reasoning and diagnostic certainty.

Although individuals' perceptions of the nature and severity of their discomfort will vary, several features of pain may help in pointing toward certain conditions:

- Sharp, severe pain suggests fractures and gout
- Pain with use of an affected area or weight-bearing, and improvement with rest suggests mechanical problems such as fracture, degenerative arthritis or avascular necrosis
- Pain occurring with initiation of activity which gradually dissipates over several hours and recurs with periods of rest (gelling) suggests inflammatory arthritis
- Dull constant aching suggests metabolic, medication-related or neoplastic disorders

Other symptoms to elicit in history taking should include the presence of:

- Constitutional symptoms: fever, night sweats, weight loss, fatigue
- The presence of skin changes or rashes
- The presence of joint swelling, though this can be very subjective
- Whether the problems are persistent, migratory, palindromic or progressive
- Thorough systems review including medication history

Physical examination

General physical examination should be undertaken in all persons. However some specific issues should be kept in mind. The location and presence of musculoskeletal tenderness (pain with enough pressure to blanch the examiner's finger nails), deformities (kyphosis, scoliosis), gait abnormalities

TABLE I
DIFFERENTIAL DIAGNOSIS OF JOINT PAIN IN OLDER PERSONS

Diffuse	Localised to or around joints
Fibromyalgia syndrome	Arthritis (eg. osteoarthritis, rheumatoid arthritis)
Myositis (idiopathic, infectious, drug-induced)	Tendonitis (supraspinatus tendonitis)
Medications (cholesterol-lowering drugs, minocyclines, chemotherapy)	Bursitis
	Capsulitis
Infections (influenza, subacute bacterial endocarditis)	Tumors
	Injuries: fractures, cartilage or ligament tears
Malignancy (myeloma, metastatic disease)	
Metabolic disorders (eg. hypothyroidism, hypercalcemia)	

(antalgia, shuffling) and loss of function (weakness, painful limitation of movement) should be noted.

- Erythematous skin changes around nail beds, rashes, sclerodactaly and tenderness in affected joints provide clues to underlying diagnosis
- The presence of adenopathy or organomegaly while a feature of adult onset Still's disease and systemic lupus erythematosus should raise concern for malignancy
- Specific manoeuvres to elicit signs of disorders such as impingement for supraspinatus tendonitis, tendon friction rubs for scleroderma and nailfold capillaroscopy for patients with Raynaud's phenomenon
- Finally a good overall assessment of the musculoskeletal system can be gleaned from inspection of the patient:
  - Sitting in a chair
  - Rising from the chair
  - Inspection of the patient standing
  - Examination of the patient lying on the couch
  - Walking, turning, and walking on toes and heels where possible

Functional impairment

Assessment of functional impairment should be undertaken in all patients with musculoskeletal disorders. This will alert physicians to perhaps unforeseen difficulties, and whether patients can take care of their activities of daily living (eg. dressing, going to toilet unaided, and cooking), and if any handicap of personalised needs should be addressed. The importance of these assessments including patient questionnaires such as the 'health assessment questionnaire' and assessments by trained professionals such as physiotherapists and occupational therapists are essential. Such evaluations can give important insights into patients' disabilities and needs for supportive services, in addition to being useful in monitoring response to therapy and disease progression over time.

Management of musculoskeletal diseases in elderly persons can be complicated due to several factors including poor cognition, poor illness insight, non-compliance and lack of appropriate resources such as a falls prevention programme. Medications prescribed for these maladies can interact with other medications they are taking, are often more likely to cause side effects than in younger patients and can have confusing dosing instructions for elderly patients, who may also have difficulty reading them. The importance of the support of family members and allied health professionals cannot be over-emphasised in order to maximise disease management and optimise patient outcomes.

Osteoarthritis

Osteoarthritis (OA) is the commonest form of arthritis, and one of the leading causes of disability. Epidemiological studies suggest 25% of persons aged 55 years and older have some radiographic evidence of knee osteoarthritis, almost half of whom will be symptomatic, while the prevalence of radiographic hip osteoarthritis is approximately 5% in those 65 years and older. The prevalence increases with age, such that almost half the members of some Caucasian populations over 60 years of age have radiographic evidence of hand osteoarthritis, most of whom are asymptomatic. The skeletal sites for predilection of this disease may vary by race or country of residence. Risk factors for osteoarthritis include: female gender, obesity, family history, prior trauma to, or inflammatory arthritis within the joint.

There are several forms of osteoarthritis which can be simply divided into either primary or secondary. Primary osteoarthritis is seen predominantly in postmenopausal women, being 3 times more common than men. It primarily involves the distal interphalangeal joints, though other sites may also be affected including the proximal interphalangeal joints, the first carpometacarpal joints, the shoulders, neck, back, hip and knees. Secondary arthritis as its name implies is usually secondary to an inciting factor which primarily damages the joint or one of its structures and includes diseases like rheumatoid arthritis, a meniscal tear or removal or osseous fracture. Joint inflammation, defective repair mechanisms, and the complex interplay of multiple structural and biochemical factors leads to loss of joint integrity, symptoms and eventual joint failure. Although often considered one of two forms: 1) 'primary', 'nodal' or 'idiopathic' and 2) 'secondary' newer evidence from imaging and genetic studies would suggest such a classification may be out-dated.

Initially following inflammation or damage to a joint there is cartilage loss and early bone changes including eburnation and fissuring. Later, as its name implies, there is significant joint destruction and bony swelling of the joints. Although many persons remain asymptomatic, others will have pain, stiffness, sometimes swelling, and loss of function which can result in significant disability. Examination reveals crepitus, bony swelling, sometimes effusion and/or joint tenderness. Care should be taken to look for other causes of joint pain such as tissue injuries, tendonitis, bursitis or evidence of referred pain. Radiographs can be normal earlier in the disease process, later showing loss of joint space, periarticular erosion and osteosclerosis, and later joint destruction and 'gull-wing deformities'. Synovial fluid analysis when effusions are present typically reveals clear viscous yellow fluid with leukocyte counts of <1,000 and negative cultures. Laboratory tests in the absence of other disorders are usually normal and rarely helpful except perhaps to 'rule-out' other mimics. Referral to a specialist is often not necessary at this time as such practice results in increased cost, while not affecting progress.

Guidelines for the management of osteoarthritis have been published by both the American College of Rheumatology and the European League Against Rheumatism. The focus of these protocols is patient education, stepped approaches to maintaining function with analgesia, exercise programmes, education, devices, and weight loss where appropriate. Unfortunately no treatment programme to date has been shown to halt the inexorable progression of this, the most common form of arthritis. The first step in pharmaceutical treatment after the above measures is simple analgesia such as intermittent or regular paracetamol. Although justifiably touted as a potentially safer therapy for many years, newer trials would suggest that glucosamine and chondroitin sulphate have limited efficacy in this disorder. While more potent medications such as non-steroidal anti-inflammatory medications (tablets or capsules and gels) and centrally and peripherally acting analgesics have been recommended, the effectiveness of such therapies is greatly hindered by their propensity to cause unwanted side-effects in this population including peptic ulcer disease, renal failure, cardiovascular disease or dizziness and falls. Arthroscopic surgery has been used traditionally in the hope of providing relief and perhaps postponing the inevitable, but two recent studies have suggested that this is no more beneficial that usual medical care or sham surgery. Intra-articular corticosteroids may help individuals with significant acute pain or effusions but have no long-term benefit. Although approved by many government agencies for use in this disorder, the best available evidence suggests intra-articular hyaluroinc acid preparations offer no real benefit. Individuals with significant pain and functional impairment coupled with advanced radiographic evidence of joint failure who are deemed otherwise healthy should be considered for total joint replacement. Advances in total knee and hip replacements in the past 20 to 30 years have made such procedures very successful and the treatment of choice in symptomatic individuals with advanced disease.

Polymyalgia rheumatica: 'special arthritis of old age'

Perhaps nothing better encapsulates the unique aspects of inflammatory arthritis in elderly patients than polymyalgia rheumatica. Originally described as 'Senile Rheumatic Gout' in 1888 by William Bruce, more than fifty years later the term 'special arthritis of old age' was used, which finally became known as Polymyalgia Rheumatica (PMR) in 1957. Extensive reviews on this topic are available in the literature and most textbooks of rheumatology and general medicine.

Despite being described 120 years ago, diagnosis remains problematic today. The differential diagnosis includes many other diseases which are more

Therapy	Evidence of efficacy	Risks
Paracetamol	Fair – Good	Hepatotoxicity, GI distress
NSAIDs	Good	Peptic ulcer, gastritis, colitis, renal failure, rashes, cardiovascular disease
Glucosamine and Chondroitin Sulphate	Fair	Nausea, diarrhoea, constipation
Tramadol	Good	Dizziness, nausea, vomiting, delirium
Corticosteroid injections	Good	Infection, osteonecrosis, lipodystrophy
Tricyclic anti-depressants	Fair-good	Dizziness, falls, urinary retention, drowsiness
Mild narcotics	Fair	Addiction, GI distress, dizziness
Moderate narcotics	Fair	Addiction, GI distress, dizziness, drowsiness, falls, delirium
Intra-articular hyaluronic acid derivatives	None	Local injection site reactions, cost

Note: 'NSAIDs' = non-steroidal anti-inflammatory drugs

common in older persons including other forms of inflammatory arthritis, fibromyalgia syndrome, myositis, myopathies, metabolic abnormalities, drug toxicities and paraneoplastic syndromes. A careful history and physical examination is the key to making the diagnosis while excluding other causes of the patients symptoms, by screening for hypercalcaemia, myositis, thyroid disease and other metabolic disorders. Patients with PMR usually present with an insidious onset of aching or stiffness in the joints, which primarily affects the large joints and axial skeleton. There is marked morning stiffness, but synovitis of the peripheral joints is absent, though pitting oedema of the upper limbs at presentation has been described. Although elevation of acute phase reactants such as the erythrocyte sedimentation rate and c-reactive protein are commonly seen, approximately 20% of persons have normal levels of these biomarkers of inflammation. A low grade anaemia can be seen but dramatic lowering of haemoglobin should prompt consideration of other causes of the symptoms.

Treatment with corticosteroid therapy is very effective and responses to treatment are instant and often dramatic, even at low doses such as 10-20 milligrams per day of prednisolone. Unfortunately therapy is limited by the propensity of corticosteroids to cause side-effects such as myopathy, osteoporosis, cataracts and diabetes mellitus. However it is recommended that treatment is tapered over 1 - 2 years. Although earlier studies have suggested such a regimen is effective at curing many patients of their disease, newer evidence suggests many patients cannot wean off their glucocorticoids or may flare several weeks, months or years after doing so. The evidence for other therapies is anecdotal, though recent evidence has suggested that perhaps methotrexate has some benefits. To compound matters, approximately 50% of elderly patients with incident rheumatoid arthritis have been noted to have a 'PMR'-like presentation.

Giant cell arteritis (GCA) is an auto-inflammatory disorder of unknown aetiology which affects primarily the larger arteries including the aorta and its primary branches, and also has a predilection for the cranial arteries. It is the commonest form of vasculitis, whose incidence increases with advancing age. Women appear to be affected almost twice as often as men.

While occasionally a difficult diagnosis to make, classic presentations in the presence of positive histological findings of a temporal artery biopsy are common. Symptoms are outlined in table 3. It is worth noting that somewhere in the region of 50% of persons will have a history of polymyalgia rheumatica, 80% will have an elevated acute phase response and 80 - 90% have histological evidence of giant cell arteritis on biopsy of their cranial arteries. In addition, involvement of the temporal arteries by other forms of vasculitis is well described, some of which may require quite different therapy.

Therapy is aimed at relieving the potentially devastating consequences of large vessel vasculitis including visual loss, limb ischaemia, dissection and rupture of the aorta. Glucocorticoids remain the treatment of choice usually started at doses in the order of 0.5 - 1 milligrams per kilogram of body weight per day. Such therapy likely decreases the risk of visual loss, though it does not eliminate it. Recent evidence suggests the final common pathway for visual loss is in-situ thrombosis of a diseased ophthalmic artery and studies show anti-platelet therapy appears effective at decreasing this risk. Unfortunately, similar to PMR, tapering of glucocorticoid therapy in these patients is often difficult and studies evaluating the effectiveness of other therapies for this disorder have been disappointing. Although controversial, a recent meta-analysis demonstrated that methotrexate may be effective. Long-term complications of this disease are not uncommon and include therapy-related side effects which have a high morbidity and mortality.

Rheumatoid arthritis

Rheumatoid arthritis is the commonest form of inflammatory arthritis. Although prevalence rates vary, studies show it affects between 1 and 3 % of the population. Women are affected more commonly than men with peak incidence in middle-aged women. Although therapeutic advances have been made, morbidity and mortality remain high; the 5 year survival for patients with newly diagnosed rheumatoid arthritis is similar to persons with a new diagnosis of triple vessel heart disease.

Patients can present in a number of fashions, either with an acute arthritis, which can affect a single or multiple joints, fever of unknown origin, or a slower, more insidious onset. In fact up to 50% of persons will have a 'PMR-like' presentation making definite diagnosis difficult at times. The classic clinical picture is one of a symmetric polyarthritis affecting the hands and feet (proximal interphalangeal joints, metacarpal joints or metatarsal joints respectively), wrists, elbows, shoulders, hips, knees, tibio-talar and calcaneo-talar joints, although other joint involvement has been well described. Patients tend to have several hours of morning stiffness, gelling, painful restriction of activities, fatigue and malaise. Joint swelling and tenderness are usually obvious, though can be subtle at presentation. Untreated, the inflammation and tumour like pannus lead to progressive cartilage loss, bone erosion, tendon rupture and permanent deformity. Extra-articular features include uveitis, scleritis, serositis, interstitial lung disease, secondary sicca complex (xerophthalmia and xerostomia), skin nodules and less commonly vasculitis and pachymeningitis.

Investigations should be undertaken in persons with rheumatoid arthritis as these may aid diagnosis and give useful prognostic information and help decide whether therapy is working or needs to be more aggressive. A mild anaemia is common. Approximately 80% of persons have an elevated ESR and CRP. A positive rheumatoid factor is only seen in approximately 80% of cases, similar to the percentage for cyclic citrullinated peptide (CCP antibody). The presence of both increases specificity for rheumatoid arthritis, but neither is specific for this disease. Up to 10% of healthy women will have a positive rheumatoid factor, and more than 90% of Sjogren's syndrome patients have an elevated rheumatoid factor. Both tests are commonly positive in several other diseases including hepatitis C infection, endocarditis, systemic lupus erythematosus, giant cell arteritis, Wegener's granulomatosis and relapsing polychondritis. Initial radiographic findings show periarticular osteopaenia and later juxta-articular erosions followed by secondary osteoarthritis and significant bone loss. Imaging studies such as ultrasound and magnetic reasonance imaging are more sensitive for erosion and may show classical pannus, but their use is reserved for individuals where there is uncertainty about the diagnosis.

There have been two distinct advances in the management of this disease in the past decade or so

TABLE 3
FEATURES SUGGESTIVE OF TEMPORAL ARTERITIS
Headache (especially temporal)
Presence of Polymyalgia Rheumatica
Malaise, fatigue, weight loss
Fever (usually low grade); if high, consider other forms of vasculitis
Elevated ESR and CRP (10-20% may have normal levels at presentation)
Jaw claudication
Visual loss – usually ischaemic optic neuropathy
Gradual onset (1/3 sudden)
Swollen or tender temporal arteries
Sore throat or dysphagia

Figure 1: Hand X-rays can help distinguish between the various arthritides

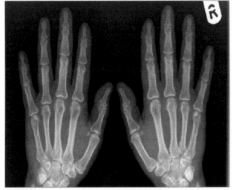

Figure 1a: Normal

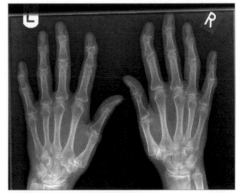

Figure 1b: 'Nodal' Osteoarthritis. Note DIP Changes

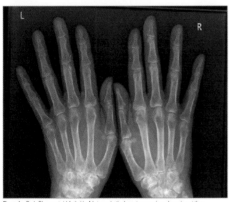

Figure 1c: Early Rheumatoid Arthritis. Note periarticular osteopaenia and erosion at the second MCP bilaterally

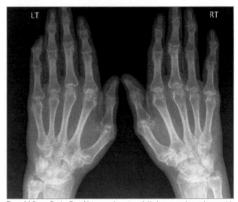

Figure 1d: Severe Erosive Gout. Note secondary osteoarthritis changes, erosions and asymmetric joint involvement

which has led to greatly improved patient outcomes:

1. The recognition that early intervention with disease modifying anti-rheumatic drugs (DMARDs) is significantly better and that some traditional DMARDS like methotrexate are particularly safe and effective in this regard;

2. The development of newer therapies, mainly biologic treatments, including injectable antibodies to tumor necrosis factor alpha, CD-80 costimulatory molecule and CD-20 receptors on B-cells.

These therapeutic advances have been shown not only to halt the inexorable progression of this disease but also to induce remission, something that was rare and exceptional 20 years ago. Studies show today that if treated early up to 50% of persons will go into remission within the first year of therapy and that persons who do can continue a full and active life and

not miss a single day of work due to their illness in the first 5 years of their disease, something that was unthinkable 10 years ago. Those with later onset disease may have milder forms and therapy can be tailored to suit their needs, but similar to younger persons response to early intervention with DMARDs is effective and dramatic and can lead to sustained remissions or minimal progression over many years.

Although there is still debate and research is needed about which is the most effective therapy for this illness, there is general agreement that methotrexate is the initial treatment of choice where there are no contra-indications. When taken weekly at low doses (2.5 - 10mg/week) in those with normal renal function, side-effects are rare. Folic acid supplementation on the non-methotrexate days at doses of 1mg have been shown to reduce the risk of

FEATURES	RA	OA
Primary joints affected	MCP, MTP, PIP, wrist, ankles, other	DIP, CMC, knee, hip
Heberden's nodes	Usually absent	Frequently present
Joint characteristics	Soft, warm, tender	Hard and bony; ± tender
Morning stiffness	Several hours	Several minutes
Change with activity	Improves	Worsens
Extra-articular features	Often present	No
Anaemia	Common	No
Elevated CRP and ESR other	Common (80%)	No (consider presence of diseases if present)
Rheumatoid Factor	Elevated in 80%	Mildly elevated in 5-10%
CCP antibody	Elevated in 80%	Mildly elevated in 5-10%

Note: chronic active rheumatoid arthritis can lead to secondary osteoarthritis.

side-effects in multiple studies. In persons with more active disease or who fail to respond to treatment the dose can be gradually increased to a maximum of 20 - 25mg/week. Side effects are less common when this is performed gradually. Long-term toxicity is rare. However care should be taken to monitor therapy regularly by checking the full blood count, liver function and serum creatinine. Since the medication is renally excreted, caution is advised in older people with mild renal impairment and treatment is contra-indicated in those with moderate-severe renal impairment. Other therapies which can be effective include hydroxychloroquine, salazopyrin, cyclosporin and azathioprine, and a newer agent leflunomide.

Biologic therapies, because they are antibodies, have to be given either by subcutaneous injection or regular infusion. Primarily because they are very expensive, their use is restricted to persons who fail the more traditional therapies already mentioned. These medications in general have an excellent safety profile, although antibodies can form over time which can lead to drug resistance and side effects. Similar to traditional DMARDS they are immuno-modulators and increase the risk of certain infections. Particular care should be taken in this regard since elderly patients are often at increased risk of infections compared to young healthly adults. The general wisdom among experts is that these drugs should not be used on their own, rather in combination with methotrexate, azathioprine or some other DMARD in order to increase their effectiveness, and lower the

risk of drug-induced antibody formation. Detailed guidelines on the management of rheumatoid arthritis have been published by several societies including the American College of Rheumatology, available on line, and several review articles have been published in the New England Journal of Medicine in the past decade. Finally the importance of a multidisciplinary approach to patient management cannot be over-emphasised in all forms of arthritis and expertise from physiotherapists, occupational therapists and clinical nurse specialists to address individual needs and disabilities is invaluable.

Osteoporosis: 'bone with too many holes'

Osteoporosis is the second commonest musculoskeletal disease seen in elderly patients, rivalled only by osteoarthritis. Similar to osteoarthritis, the incidence increases with advancing age, and women are three times more likely to fracture than men. Nearly two million fractures occur annually in the USA and almost 2,000 fractures occur daily throughout Europe. Extrapolating international figures to an Irish population would suggest that approximately 160,000 persons have osteoporosis and approximately 25,000 osteoporotic fractures occur annually. It has been estimated that of the 130,000 falls occurring in elderly Irish people annually, 20% result in an injury. Fractures are associated with significant cost, morbidity and increased mortality. Fracture, in particular hip fracture, represents one of the most serious of such injuries, and accounts for the bulk of the expense. The

TABLE 5	
DIFFERENTIAL DIAGNOSIS OF HIGH AND LOW BONE MINERAL DENSITY	
Low	**High**
Osteoporosis	Osteoarthritis
Osteomalacia	Fracture
Low peak bone mass	Osteosclerosis
Osteolytic lesions	Paget's disease
Transient localised osteoporosis	Osteopetrosis

life-time risk of fracture for a 50 year old Caucasian woman is approximately 40% and approximately 15% for a Caucasian man. The annual risk of fracture for a postmenopausal white woman is greater than her combined risk of stroke, heart attack and breast cancer, yet osteoporosis receives far less attention than any of these diseases.

Osteoporosis can be diagnosed clinically in the presence of a fragility fracture, radiographically by measuring bone mineral density and by histomorphometric analysis of a bone biopsy (rarely used in practice). The presence of a fragility fracture (a fracture sustained by a force ≤ that which is sustained by a fall from a standing position) in men and women over 50 years of age is diagnostic of osteoporosis in the absence of another disease. This point deserves appropriate emphasis since every study that has been published in the last 20 years shows most men and women who suffer a fragility fracture are not evaluated or treated for their underlying osteoporosis. In 1994 the World Health Organisation published criteria by which a post-menopausal white woman could be diagnosed with osteoporosis by measuring bone mineral density at the proximal femur using dual-energy X-ray absorptiometry (DXA). However DXA is a flawed diagnostic test since most people who fracture do not have osteoporosis by these criteria. Nonetheless DXA is used to diagnose low bone mineral density, predict fracture risk, and when available and appropriate to monitor risk and response to therapy. In certain instances such as renal failure, or where there is concern about the diagnosis, a tetracycline labelled bone biopsy can provide more reliable information of the presence or absence of other diseases. Newer technology using micro-magnetic resonance imaging and computerised tomography enables researchers to perform a 'virtual bone biopsy' which will likely be the non-invasive diagnostic test of choice in the future. Similar to other multifactorial

diseases however, the best way to intervene in this disorder is to identify individuals at risk for the outcome, in this case fracture.

There are several important risk factors to consider when deciding whether someone needs to be further assessed with laboratory testing, bone mineral density, or otherwise including:
• Family history
• Advancing age
• Prior fracture
• Low bone mineral density (BMD)
• Increased fall risk or prior falls
• Whether they are taking glucocorticoids
• Low body mass index

Studies have clearly shown that men and women with multiple risk factors for fracture have a much greater risk of fracture than individuals with any single risk factor including low BMD. The single biggest risk factor for predicting fracture risk is a prior fracture, followed by low BMD. Studies from the calcium and vitamin D plus placebo arm of clinical trials of osteoporosis therapies have shown that elderly white women with low BMD have a 1 in 4 risk of fracture in the index year of the study if they have had 2 or more fractures compared to a 1 in 20 risk if they have not had a prior fracture. Extensive lists of diseases, conditions and drugs that are associated with or predispose individuals have been published. At a minimum, patients deemed to have osteoporosis should have some basic additional investigations including a full serum chemistry panel including creatinine, calcium, albumin, phosphorous, alkaline phosphatase and 25-hydroxyvitamin D level, and ideally a full blood count, 24 hour urine calcium and some form of bone mineral density measurement. Additional testing may be helpful if clinically indicated. Disorders of calcium metabolism need to be corrected prior to commencing any of the approved therapies for osteoporosis.

The more effective treatments have been shown to lower future fracture risk by approximately 50%. Ten elderly white women over 65 with 2 or more fractures need to be treated to prevent a single fracture in a single year. Such results clearly show that supplemental calcium and vitamin D is not adequate as sole therapy in individuals at high risk of fracture. The cost of treatment for osteoporosis today represents only a fraction of the economic cost of treating fractures and thus effective fracture prevention therapy would

Treatment	Reduces fracture of			Side effects	Cost	Efficacy in men
	Spine	Hip	Non-spine			
Alendronate	Y	Y	Y	GI Bleed, flu-like symptoms	€€	Y
Calcium plus Vitamin D	Y	Y	Y	Nephrolithiasis, hypercalcaemia, GI distress	€	Y
Estradiol	Y	Y	Y	Breast cancer, cardiovascular disease, thrombophlebitis	€	-
Etidronate	Y	-	-	Osteomalacia, GI distress	€	-
Ibandronate	Y	-	-	GI bleed, flu-like symptoms	€€	
Raloxifene	Y	-	-	Thrombophlebitis, hot flashes, leg cramps	€€	-
Risedronate	Y	Y	Y	GI bleed (?), flu-like symptoms	€€	Y
Strontium Ranelate	Y	Y	Y	GI distress, osteomalacia	€€	-
Teriparatide	Y	-	Y	Headache, leg cramps, hypercalcaemia	€€€€	-
Tibolone	Y	-	Y	Stroke, leg cramps	€€	-
Zoledronate	Y	Y	Y	Hypocalcaemia, flu like symptoms in 10% at first infusion	€€	

Note: GI = gastrointestinal. 'Y' = Yes; '-' = No data; (?) evidence is controversial.

appear more than justifiable. Bisphosphonates represent the greatest breakthrough in the treatment of bone disease in the past century and remain the primary treatment option for patients who have no contra-indications. The number of available effective therapies continues to increase, shown in table 6.

Hip fracture

Epidemiology
Hip fracture is a disease almost exclusively of older people, with over 90% of fractures occurring in patients over the age of fifty years. The annual incidence doubles for each decade after 50 years and is expected to increase two-fold by 2040 due to population ageing. Hip fracture rates are two to three times higher in women, as men sustain fewer falls, have a higher peak bone density, lose less bone during ageing, are less likely to become hypogonadal and die sooner. The risk is two to three times higher in white women than non-white women and approximately one-third of victims will subsequently fracture the other hip. The strongest single risk factor for hip fracture is falling, and the habitus and characteristics of a fall, such as the direction, site of impact and protective response, are important factors influencing this risk in any given fall. Although osteoporosis is a significant risk factor for hip fracture, bone mineral density alone is a poor predictor of fracture for individuals. The World Health Organization has devised a web-based tool to calculate the absolute risk of hip and other fractures that uses age, sex and six clinical risk factors (previous fracture, glucocorticoid use, family history of fracture, current smoking, excessive alcohol consumption and rheumatoid arthritis) as well as bone mineral density (www.shef.ac.uk/FRAX).

Pathology
A hip fracture is a fracture of the proximal femur

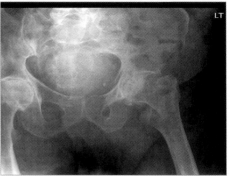

Figure 2: Intertrochanteric Fracture of left hip

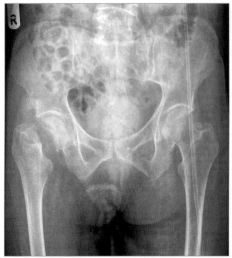

Figure 3: Subcapital fracture of right hip

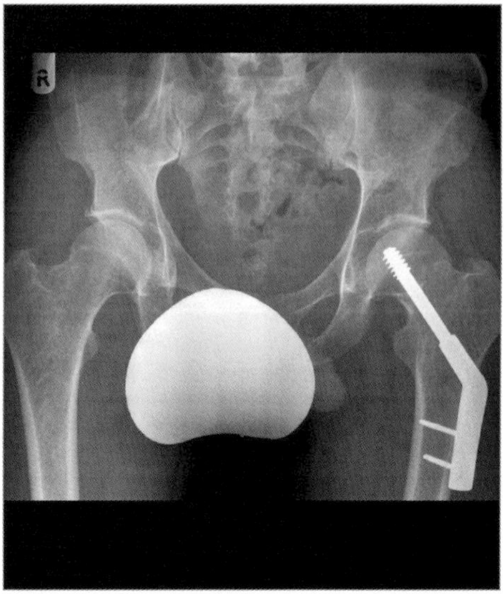

Figure 4. Low subcapital fracture with dynamic hip screw

and injuries are divided into intracapsular and extracapsular categories according to whether or not they occur within the capsule of the hip joint.

Fractures of the femoral neck are intracapsular fractures and occur distal to the femoral head but proximal to the greater and lesser trochanters. Because of the precarious blood supply, fractures of the femoral neck, particularly those that involve marked displacement, can disrupt the blood supply of the femoral head and are consequently associated with an increased incidence of healing complications such as non-union and osteonecrosis of the femoral head.

Extracapsular fractures include intertrochanteric fractures of the well-vascularised metaphyseal region between the greater and lesser trochanters and subtrochanteric fractures that occur just below the lesser trochanter. These fractures do not interfere with the blood supply of the femoral head and are not, therefore, associated with the healing complications that afflict femoral neck fractures. Intertrochanteric fractures occur through the part of the femur that is subjected to the highest mechanical loads and, because of the rich blood supply, often result in significant blood loss of 500ml or more from the fracture itself.

Femoral neck and intertrochanteric fractures occur with almost equal frequency and account for over 90% of hip fractures, with subtrochanteric fractures accounting for the remainder.

Diagnosis

A hip fracture should be suspected in any older adult who falls and is unable to rise or weight bear on the affected side. The physical findings include groin pain which may intensify after striking the heel or when attempting straight leg raising or weight bearing. Displaced fractures are clinically obvious due to shortening and external rotation of the lower limb, but non-displaced fractures may be more subtle. Most hip fractures are easily diagnosed on the basis of clinical findings and standard radiographs that include anteroposterior pelvic views and lateral views of the hip. Some patients, however, report hip or groin pain after a fall and difficulty standing or walking without any fracture being demonstrated using standard radiography. This is an important group in whom a high index of suspicion for hip fracture should be maintained, as the first radiograph will be normal in up to 10% of patients with hip fracture. An anteroposterior view obtained with the hip internally rotated 15-20 degrees facilitates optimal imaging of the femoral neck and may reveal a fracture not evident on a standard anteroposterior view.

If this radiograph is normal and the diagnosis of hip fracture is still likely on the basis of clinical findings, other methods of imaging the hip should be considered such as computed tomography, magnetic resonance imaging and technetium-99m bone scanning. A radionuclide bone scan is generally a sensitive indicator of an unrecognised hip fracture but may be unreliable in older patients in the first two or three days after the event. Computed tomography and magnetic resonance imaging are as accurate as bone scanning in the assessment of occult hip fractures and reliable results may be obtained within 24 hours of incurring the injury. Because of the reliability and low incidence of false negative results, computed tomography and magnetic resonance imaging have become the preferred diagnostic tests.

If a hip fracture has not been demonstrated using the above methodology and the patient has persistent difficulties weight bearing, alternative diagnoses should be considered, including pubic ramus and acetabular fractures, isolated fracture of the greater trochanter and trochanteric bursitis or contusion.

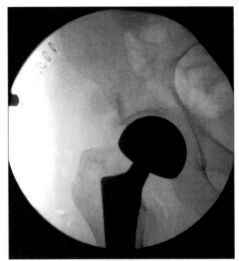

Figure 5: Low subcapital fracture with hip replacement

Treatment

A joint initiative by the British Orthopaedic Association and the British Geriatrics Society (www. boa.ac.uk/site/showpublications.aspx?ID=59) has identified six key care standards for the care of patients with hip fracture: prompt admission to orthopaedic care; early surgery; pressure ulcer prevention; access to acute orthogeriatric medical care; osteoporosis treatment; and falls assessment.

Preoperative care

Early surgery and early mobilisation give patients the best chance of regaining their previous level of function. However, because the occurrence of a hip fracture is often the first indicator of general frailty or an underlying medical problem, surgery poses a substantial increased risk of morbidity or mortality for some patients.

A formal orthogeriatric medical evaluation is essential to identify and treat underlying comorbid conditions and joint medical and orthopaedic care should now be offered to all patients with hip fracture. Electrolyte imbalances, dehydration and volume contraction due to fracture haemorrhage are frequently seen in patients with hip fracture due to delays in presentation and must be corrected prior to surgery. Placement of a urethral catheter will improve patient comfort and aid with the monitoring of fluid resuscitation.

In general, surgery should be performed as soon as the patient is medically stable, within 24 hours if possible. Although a delay to stabilise underlying medical conditions may be beneficial, any deferral must be considered very carefully as early surgical repair reduces the risks of pressure sores, major medical complications, severe pain, prolonged length of stay and mortality at 12 months. Every additional eight hour delay to surgery after the initial 48 hours results, on average, in an extra day in hospital. A recent or concurrent myocardial infarction in a patient with hip fracture is associated with a perioperative mortality rate of approximately 37% within the first three months and surgery in such patients is best delayed. Surgery should also be deferred for patients whose anticoagulation cannot be safely discontinued for 48 - 72 hours perioperatively.

Preoperative skin or skeletal traction was thought to reduce pain and assist with fracture reduction, but studies have failed to confirm any benefit and it is not recommended. Pressure sores are common following hip fracture, with reported incidence rates of 10 - 40%, and affected patients have a greater risk of nosocomial infection and prolonged length of stay. Foam and alternating pressure mattresses substantially reduce the incidence of pressure sore development by up to 80%. Non-ambulatory, institutionalised patients who have minimal discomfort may be candidates for non-operative management, but early mobilisation remains crucial in such patients to help prevent complications associated with prolonged bed rest.

Perioperative care

Regional (spinal) anaesthesia is most commonly used for hip fracture repair due to lower rates of delirium, deep venous thrombosis and mortality at one month postoperatively when compared with general anaesthesia. Adequate hydration is important preoperatively if profound hypotension on induction of anaesthesia is to be avoided in volume depleted patients. Antibiotic prophylaxis has been shown to reduce the rates of deep and superficial wound infections as well as the incidence of urinary and respiratory tract infections in the postoperative period. Single dose regimes with third generation cephalosporins such as ceftriaxone have been shown to be cost effective, but it is unclear if multiple dose regimes confer any added benefit over single dose regimes.

The type of surgical intervention depends on a number of factors, including location of the fracture, displacement, bone quality, the age and overall condition of the patient and the experience of the surgeon involved. Non-displaced fractures of the femoral neck are usually treated by internal fixation with multiple screws. Displaced femoral neck fractures have a non-union and osteonecrosis rate of 30-40% in comparison with a rate of <10% for non-displaced fractures due to interruption of the precarious blood supply to the femoral head. To minimise the risk of these complications, prosthetic replacement of the femoral head by hemiarthroplasty or total hip replacement is the procedure of choice in older patients with displaced femoral neck fractures, but internal fixation may still be considered a reasonable option in younger patients.

Intertrochanteric fractures present the problem of stabilising a fracture in bone that is subjected to high mechanical loads and which is frequently osteoporotic, holding screws and plates poorly. This can be achieved for all but the most unstable of fractures through internal fixation with the aid of a sliding hip screw or similar device. Patients with pre-existing degenerative changes due to rheumatoid arthritis, osteoarthritis or Paget's disease involving a fractured hip generally need a total hip replacement. This is also the preferred surgical intervention for patients who incur pathological hip fractures due to metastatic bone disease.

Postoperative management

Early mobilisation in the postoperative period helps to reduce the risk of many complications associated with prolonged recumbency such as venous thromboembolism, pressure sores, infection and deconditioning. Rehabilitation that encourages weight bearing through walking with assistance should begin on the first postoperative day by initially moving the patient from bed to chair. Progression to walking can usually be accomplished on the first or second postoperative day. Rehabilitation and discharge planning is best achieved through a multidisciplinary team approach, though clear evidence favouring particular rehabilitation strategies is lacking.

Patients with hip fracture are at high risk of venous thromboembolism in the postoperative period, with up to one quarter developing a proximal deep venous thrombosis and mortality rates of up to 7.5% reported from pulmonary embolism in the first 3 months after surgery. Early mobilisation is a critical part of helping to avoid venous thromboembolic complications but the extent of the problem is such that anticoagulation has become an important part of postoperative management. The use of any heparin treatment or a mechanical pumping device significantly reduces risks but, due to ease of administration and supervision and the relatively low risk of haemorrhage, low molecular heparins have become the agents of choice. Aspirin is probably an inadequate measure while warfarin, though probably effective, is unwieldy and the target INR is not clear.

Malnutrition affects approximately half of all patients who suffer hip fracture and is independently associated with increased morbidity and mortality. There is evidence that nutritional supplementation may reduce long-term complications and length of stay and should be offered to all patients with suboptimal nutritional status. Particular attention should be paid to calcium and vitamin D intake and most patients will need appropriate treatment for osteoporosis. The intravenous administration of Zoledronate, a bisphosphonate, to patients specifically recuperating from hip fracture has been shown to reduce the risk of subsequent fractures and mortality.

Prognosis

The occurrence of a hip fracture is a devastating event that is associated with high rates of morbidity and mortality and poor functional, social and emotional outcomes in survivors. The mortality rate in elderly patients with hip fracture is as high as 36% in the first 12 months but is similar to that among age and sex-matched persons thereafter. Mortality rates are higher for institutionalised patients and those with postoperative complications, and increase with age, male sex, and the presence of underlying psychiatric and systemic diseases. Men are two times more likely to die than women in the first two years after a hip fracture, possibly due to a greater comorbidity burden at the time of fracture.

Between 50 - 65% of patients with hip fracture regain their previous level of ambulation, approximately 20% lose the ability to walk entirely and 10 - 15% lose the ability to walk outside the home. To regain functional independence and return home, however, the patient must also recover the ability to perform basic activities of daily living such as feeding, bathing, dressing, toileting and to perform instrumental activities of daily living such as shopping, meal preparation, laundry, housework and using public transport. Up to 75% of patients recover their previous ability to perform basic activities of daily living whereas only 50% regain their ability to perform instrumental activities by one year, with most of the recovery coming in the first six months. Not surprisingly, this markedly influences the number of patients who are discharged to their own home, a major outcome measure in patients with hip fracture. As many as 25% of patients with hip fracture require long-term nursing home care with younger age, ability to walk independently before and soon after the hip fracture, ability to perform activities of daily living and the presence of another person at home being the main predictive factors of a successful home discharge. Attempts to shorten the in-hospital length of stay in patients with hip fracture have consistently resulted in substantial increases in the eventual levels of dependency and overall care costs.

Hip fracture frequently results in significant psychological symptoms, most commonly depression and loss of self-esteem as patients struggle with pain, physical limitations and lifestyle and cosmetic changes. The high morbidity and dependency associated with hip fracture can challenge interpersonal relationships and social roles for patients and carers.

The crystal arthropathies
Crystal deposition disorders are commonly seen in elderly patients. Unlike rheumatoid and osteoarthritis, patients tend to present with an acutely swollen, red and tender joint. Sometimes in chronic untreated disease, the symptoms can be polyarticular in nature, occasionally mimicking a rheumatoid like pattern. Acutely these represent the most painful arthritides, making ambulation, sleep or footwear impossible. Treatment produces rapid resolution of symptoms but can be problematic, particularly in elderly persons where side effects are more common, and where comorbidities and other medications need to be taken into consideration when prescribing therapy.

The commonest forms of these arthropathies in the elderly result from the deposition of the following crystals in or around the joints:
• Uric acid (gout)
• Calcium pyrophosphate (CPPD disease) and
• Calcium hydroxyapatite disease ('Milwaukee shoulder')

Gout is the most common inflammatory arthritis in men over 40 years of age, and very rare in premenopausal women. It manifests as acute or chronic arthritis, tophaceous depositions and nephrolithiasis. The male to female ratio is 4:1. The main causes of hyperuricaemia and risk factors for gout are shown in table 7. Although the risk for developing gout increases with increasing hyperuricaemia, approximately 10% of gout patients have a normal uric acid level, and many persons with marked hyperuricaemia never develop gout. Acute attacks can be precipitated by acute raising or lowering of the serum uric acid level in predisposed individuals, and thus the diagnosis should be considered very likely in hospitalised patients where large fluxes in vascular fluid occur such as congestive heart failure, sepsis and surgery. Thus although measurement of uric acid can help predict risk and monitor therapy it cannot diagnose gout. Although a history of podagra suggests gout, it is not specific for gout. Other disorders such as infection, pseudogout and osteoarthritis can mimic podagra. A definite diagnosis of gout can be made by identifying classic negatively birefringent (appear yellow when they lie parallel to the y-axis of the red compensator) needle shaped crystals on microscopic examination of fresh joint fluid using a polarising microscope, demonstration that the tophaceous material is indeed uric acid crystals, the presence of classic 'bite erosions' with an 'overhanging

TABLE 7		
RISK FACTORS FOR GOUT		
PRIMARY GOUT	Male gender	
	Family history	
	Genetic disorders	
	Advancing age	
	Obesity	
URIC ACID OVER PRODUCTION	Cell lysis-tumour lysis syndrome, myeloproliferative disease, haemolytic anaemia, psoriasis, trauma, obesity, drugs: alcohol, cytotoxics, warfarin	
URIC ACID UNDER EXCRETION	Renal failure	
	Drugs including alcohol, low dose salicylates, diuretics, laxatives, cyclosporin, levodopa, ethambutol, pyrazinamide	

It can be very difficult to differentiate an infectious arthritis from crystalline arthopathy as the clinical picture and synovial fluid leukocyte count is often very similar, so care should be taken to send synovial fluid for routine culture and staining when aspiration is obtained. This is particularly true for hospitalised patients since infections appear more likely to affect damaged or inflamed joints than healthy ones.

Once a diagnosis has been made, analgesia as appropriate is the treatment of choice. In the absence of infection, intra-articular injection of corticosteroids is preferable for monoarthritis than systemic therapy in terms of safety and efficacy. Colchicine can be used effectively at doses of 0.5mg 2 - 3 times daily. Hourly dosing is not indicated and can result in severe diarrhoea and death from bone marrow suppression. Chronic colchicine has advantages over NSAIDs in that it does not increase the risk of GI bleeding, cardiovascular disease or renal failure. However care needs to be taken in persons with renal insufficiency and the dose adjusted accordingly. Allopurinol provides definitive treatment for preventing gout but persons may take several months to reach a flare-free nadir. The dose can be increased to normalise the uric acid level understanding that changes in serum uric acid levels can precipitate flares. Thus colchicine 0.5mg once or twice daily is usually co-prescribed for the first six to twelve months of therapy. Allopurinol is indicated only for tophaceous gout, erosive gout, severe gout ($\geq$ 2 attacks per year or polyarticular disease) or nephrolithiasis. It has no proven benefit for other forms of crystal arthritis.

edge' on radiographs, or the predominance of uric acid in the formal analysis of a kidney stone. The acute attack occurs in the big toe in 60 - 70%. Some 70% will have a recurrent attack within 2 years. If untreated the pattern of monoarticular disease changes to polyarticular with shorter periods of remissions and joint damage. Elderly people with primary nodal OA, on diuretics are more likely to have polyarticular gout.

Pseudogout as its name suggests is the great gout mimicker. This disorder is associated with several other metabolic diseases including haemochromatosis, hyperparathyroidism and hyperthyroidism. Unlike gout crystals, the crystals of pseudogout are classically positively birefringent (appear pale blue when they lie parallel to the y-axis of the red compensator) rectangular or rod shaped crystals on microscopic examination of fresh joint fluid. Chronic CPPD disease results in chondrocalcinosis, which is diagnostic if seen on radiographs. Hydroxyapatite crystals can produce a bloody effusion, occur mainly in the shoulder joint and although harder to see on microscopy at times, may produce severe joint damage. Definite diagnosis is made by identification of the crystals on microscopy following Alizarin red staining, something that is not available in many hospitals.

Summary

Musculoskeletal disorders are common in elderly persons. Many are clearly linked to advancing age. Diagnosis and management can be difficult but a systematic approach will easily identify the majority of cases. Management can be difficult, especially in elderly patients where the presence of other diseases, medications and their propensity to side effects and toxicity can be challenging. When diagnosis remains doubtful or management complicated, consultation with appropriate specialty services should be sought. Similar to other diseases a multidisciplinary and multifaceted approach to management can greatly improve disease outcomes and patients lives.

Suggested further reading
- *Ad Hoc Committee on clinical guidelines for initial evaluation of adult patient with acute muscloskeletal*

symptoms. *Arthritis Rheum* 1996, 39: 1-8.

- Altman RD, Hochberg MC, Moskowitz RW et al. Recommendations for the Medical Management of Osteoarthrits of the Hip and Knee. *Arthritis and Rheumatism*. 2000; 43: 1905-15.

- Antman EM, Bennett JS, Daugherty A, et al. Use of nonsteroidal antiinflammatory drugs: an update for clinicians: a scientific statement from the American Heart Association. *Circulation* 2007; 115: 1634-1642.

- Chapuy MC, Arlot ME, Duboeuf F. Vitamin D3 and calcium to prevent hip fractures in elderly women. *N Engl J Med* 1992; 327: 1637-42.

- Choy EHS, Panayi GS Cytokine Pathways and Joint Inflammation in Rheumatoid Arthritis. *N Engl J Med* 2001; 344: 907-916.

- Clegg DO, Reda DJ, Harris CL, et al. Glucosamine, chondroitin sulfate, and the two in combination for painful knee osteoarthritis. *N Engl J Med.* 2006; 354: 795-808.

- Cummings SR, Nevitt MC, Browner WS. Risk factors for Hip fracture in White Women. *N Engl J Med* 1995; 332: 767-73.

- Ebeling PR. Osteoporosis in Men. *N Engl J Med* 2008; 358: 1474-1482.

- Felson DT. Osteoarthritis of the knee. *New England J Medicine* 2006; 354: 841-848.

- Genta MS, Gabay C. *N Engl J Med* 2006; 354; 2.

- Hunder GG. The early History of Giant Cell Arteritis and Polymyalgia Rheumatica: First Descriptions to 1970. *Mayo Clin Proc.* 2006; 81: 1071-1083.

- Hunder GG, Valente RM. Giant Cell Arteritis: Clinical Aspects: 425-4442. In Inflammatory Diseases of Blood Vessels. Hoffman GS, Weyand CM eds. Marcel Dekker, Inc. New York.

- Jordan KM, Arden NK, Doherty M et al. EULAR Recommendations 2003: an evidence based approach to the management of knee osteoarthritis: Report of a Task Force of the Standing Committee for International Clinical Studies Including Therapeutic Trials (ESCISIT). *Ann Rheum Dis* 2003; 62: 1145-55.

- Kanis JA, Melton LJ, Christiansen C, et al. The diagnosis of osteoporosis. *J Bone Min Res* 1994; 8: 1137-1141.

- Kirkley A, Birmingham TB, Litchfield RB et al. A Randomized Trial of Arthroscopic Surgery for Osteoarthritis of the Knee. *N Engl J Med* 2008; 359: 1097-107.

- Lane NE. Osteoarthritis of the Hip. *New England J Medicine* 2007; 357: 1413-21.

- Lindsay R, Silverman SL, Cooper C et al. Risk of new verterbral fracture in the year following a fracture. *JAMA* 2001; 285: 320-3.

- Loh GH, LaValley M, McAlindon T, Felson DT. Intra-articular hyaluronic acid in treatment of knee osteoarthritis: a meta-analysis. *JAMA.* Dec. 2003: 3115-21.

- Lonner JH. A 57-year-old man with osteoarthritis of the knee. *JAMA* 2003; 289: 1016-25.

- McGettigan P, Henry D. Cardiovascular risk and inhibition of cyclooxygenase: a systematic review of the observational studies of selective and nonselective inhibitors of cyclooxygenase 2. *JAMA* 2006; 296: 1633-44.

- Moseley JB, O'Malley K, Petersen NJ, et al. A controlled trial of arthroscopic surgery for osteoarthritis of the knee. *N Engl J Med* 2002; 347: 81-8.

- NIH Consensus Development panel. Osteoporosis prevention, diagnosis and management. *JAMA* 2001; 285: 785-95.

- NOF's 2008 Clinician's Guide to Prevention and Treatment of osteoporosis. Available at: http://www.nof. org/professionals/Clinicians_Guide.htm.

- O'Dell JR. Therapeutic Strategies for Rheumatoid Arthritis *N Engl J Med* 2004; 350: 2591-2602.

- Olsen NJ, Stein CM. New Drugs for Rheumatoid Arthritis. *N Engl J Med* 2004; 350: 2167-2179.

- Raynauld JP, Buckwald-Wright C, Ward R, et al. Safety and efficacy of long-term intraarticular steroid injections in osteoarthritis of the knee: a randomized, double-blind, placebo-controlled trial. *Arthritis & Rheumatism* 2003; 48(2): 370-7.

- Rosen CJ. Postmenopausal Osteoporosis. *N Engl J Med* 2005; 353: 595-603.

- Saag KG, Teng GG, Patkar NM et al. American College of Rheumatology 2008 Recommendations for the use of Nonbiologic and Biologic Disease-Modifying Antirheumatic drugs in Rheumatoid Arthritis. *Arthritis & Rheumatism* 2008; 59: 762-84.

- Salvarani C, Cantini F, Boiardi L, Hunder GG. Polymyalgia Rheumatica and Giant Cell Arteritis. *N Engl J Med* 2002; 347: 261-271.

- Terkeltaub RA. Gout. *N Engl J Med* 2003;349:1647-55.

- Turkcapar N. Late onset rheumatoid arthritis: clinical and laboratory comparisons with younger onset patients. *Arch Gerontol Geriatr* 2006: 42(2): 225-31.

- Wainwright SA, Marshall LM, Ensrud et al. Hip fracture in women without osteoporosis. *JCEM* 2005; 90: 2787-2793.

- Zhang W, Doherty M, Arden N et al. EULAR evidence based recommendations for the management of hip osteoarthritis: report of a task force of the EULAR Standing Committee for International Clinical Studies Including Therapeutics (ESCISIT). *Ann Rheum Dis.* 2005;64: 669-81.

- Zhang Y, Xu L, Nevitt MC, et al. Lower prevalence of

hand osteoarthritis among Chinese subjects in Beijing compared with white subjects in the United States: the Beijing Osteoarthritis Study. Arthritis Rheum 2003; 48: 1034-40.

Case Study 1

A 66 year old lady was referred by her GP for further evaluation. On questioning the patient denies pain in her knees; however she does describe morning 'stiffness' for several minutes which has become progressive over several years. She has difficulty rising from a chair, going up and down stairs, and getting up from the floor after bending down to do chores. The discomfort worsens with prolonged activities but is relieved with short periods of rest and paracetamol.

Her most likely diagnosis is osteoarthritis. The next best step in her evaluation at this point is physical examination and standing radiographs of both knees. The patient's examination reveals normal range of movement of her knees and hips, moderate crepitus in both knees and small medial osteophytes bilaterally. There is no effusion, redness or marked tenderness in either knee. X-ray of both knees is shown in figure 6.

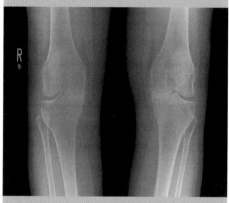

Figure 6: Standing antero-posterior radiographs of both knees

The best treatment options for this patient at this time are reassurance, explanation, paracetamol and isometric knee exercises.

Case Study 2

A 62 year old male presents to clinic with weight loss, anorexia, generalised pain and depression. He is accompanied by his wife. On further questioning he was well several months earlier and, though retired, active and physically well. His symptoms appear to affect mainly his shoulders, back, neck, hips and thighs. Although he says he has pain all the time, he does feel a bit better after several hours. The diagnosis is likely to be polymyalgia rheumatica. Physical examination reveals a flattened affect, restricted movement of the neck, back, shoulders, hips and knees and some diffuse musculoskeletal tenderness. There are no rashes, nodules or adenopathy. ESR is mildly elevated at 60mm/hr. Corticosteroid therapy results in a marked resolution of his symptoms. The patient is then lost to follow-up.

A decade later you are asked to do a pre-op assessment on a 72 year old gentleman for repair of a hip fracture. You note a pulsatile abdominal mass and bilateral renal artery bruits. A diagnosis of giant cell arteritis is confirmed by temporal artery biopsy and the disease is complicated by an abdominal aortic aneurysm.

Case Study 3

A 66 year old lady was referred by her GP with pain in both knees, shoulders, back and hips for further evaluation. She has a prior history of polymyalgia rheumatica and has been treated with various doses of oral corticosteroids for the past 2 years. Although her symptoms improve with corticosteroids, she has been unable to taper off and was referred to you for further evaluation. Examination shows slight puffiness of her hands, restricted movement of her shoulders, elbows, knees and ankles. She has morning stiffness for a couple of hours daily.

Her most likely diagnosis is rheumatoid arthritis. X-rays of her hands and feet which show some peri-articular osteopaenia and juxta-articular erosions. Her ESR and CRP are raised and rheumatoid factor is positive. Appropriate first line therapy would be methotrexate 10mg once weekly with folic acid supplementation.

Case Study 4

A 70 year old woman is lifting her shopping out of her car one day she suddenly experiences low back pain. The pain increases in intensity such that she makes an urgent appointment to see you. You note she is walking with a stooped posture. An x-ray of her spine is shown in Figure 7.

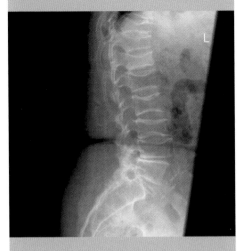

Figure 7: Lateral lumbar spine X-ray of elderly lady with back pain

Her diagnosis is osteoporosis with compression fractures. Her FBC and bone profile are normal and 25OH vitamin D level is 25 mmol/l (NR>50). Initial treatment should include vitamin D supplements and a bisphosphonate.

📂 Case Study 5

A 75 years old male, 3 days after left hip replacement surgery developed acute congestive heart failure. He is commenced on diuretic therapy and he recovers well. His medications prior to admission are not available and due to his delirium he is unable to give a cogent history. Two days later he has of severe pain in his right knee. Examination reveals a swollen, red and very tender knee, he is reluctant to let you examine him and he cannot flex his knee.

His most likely diagnosis is gout. Aspiration of his knee reveals negatively birefringent crystals and he is commenced on colchicine therapy with good effect.

Data Interpretation

Question 1

A 75 year old lady complains of early morning stiffness in both knees. She has crepitus in both knees with mild swelling of her right knee.

a. What is the likely diagnosis?
b. What is the next best diagnostic test?
c. Describe the appropriate initial management

Question 2

A 65 year old lady has pain in her shoulders and both hands and examination reveals swelling of the joints in both hands.

a. What is the likely diagnosis?
b. Name 3 tests which would be of diagnostic help
c. What is the first line therapy?

Question 3

An 80 year old woman bends down and feels a sudden, severe pain in her lower back. She is on treatment for COPD for 10 years.

a. What is the diagnosis?
b. What are the essential tests as part of her initial assessment?
c. What is the first line treatment?

Best of five questions

Question 1

A 70 year old woman falls and fractures her hip. She is admitted to hospital and has surgery. The correct management on day 1 post surgery is:

a. Bed rest and analgesia
b. Hoist transfer to chair but no mobilisation
c. Avoid analgesia
d. Analgesia, physiotherapy with active mobilisation
e. Passive movements of affected limb within limits of pain

Question 2

A 68 year old woman with uncontrolled hypertension is commenced on a thiazide diuretic and 3 days later develops severe pain in her left knee and right foot which is swollen and exquisitely tender. What is the most appropriate first line treatment?

a.   Splinting of the joint
b.   Paracetamol
c.   Indomethacin
d.   Diclofenac
e.   Colchicine

Question 3

An 85 year old lady with known osteoarthritis develops a sudden painful right shoulder. Her radiograph demonstrates chondrocalcinosis. The next appropriate treatment is?

a.   Arthrocentesis and injection of the shoulder with corticosteroid
b.   Indomethacin
c.   Colchicine
d.   Paracetamol
e.   Collar and cuff

Answers are on page 311

Falls and syncope

B Carey

Epidemiology of falls

Definitions and classifications

Falls in older people are a major public health concern in terms of morbidity, mortality and costs to health and social services. The definitions and classifications used for falls are contentious and, to a large extent, affect the discussion regarding the occurrence, prevalence, and time and place of falls. Tinetti defined a fall in 1988 as 'an event which results in a person coming to rest unintentionally on the ground or other lower level, not as a result of a major intrinsic event (such as a stroke) or overwhelming hazard'. Although rather cumbersome, this definition has served the medical community well since then and most authorities agree that falls resulting from violence, road accidents and acute major events such as stroke should be excluded. Other definitions exist and it is important to note that even small alterations in the definition of a fall can alter the main message of research studies.

Falls have been classified in a variety of ways including:
- Explained or unexplained eg. caused by a simple slip or by an undetermined medical event such as syncope
- Intrinsic or extrinsic eg. where some event or condition affects postural control or where an environmental factor is the main precipitant
- Injurious or non-injurious

In practice, as the majority of falls are multifactorial in aetiology, such classifications are often unhelpful due to a large overlap between them.

Fallers have also been classified in a variety of ways. A faller, as opposed to a non-faller, is usually defined as someone who has fallen at least once during a particular time period and a recurrent faller is often defined as someone who falls more than once during that time as compared with a 'once-only faller'. Some evidence exists, however, to suggest that 'once-only fallers' are characteristically more closely related to non-fallers than recurrent fallers. This may prove to be a significant point as there is evidence to suggest that 'once-only fallers' may experience more significant injuries after a fall than recurrent fallers.

Incidence and occurrence

Studies that have attempted to estimate the annual incidence of falls have been plagued by a number of difficulties. In addition to the problems associated with definition and classification outlined above, it is now recognised that retrospective studies underestimate the incidence of falls by up to one-third, depending on the time period of recall. The frequency of data collection and method used (eg. postal questionnaire, telephone interview, face-to-face interview, interview of witnesses) may also affect the incidence.

Notwithstanding these difficulties, it is clear that between 29 - 35% of people older than 65 years living in the community can be expected to fall each year and this incidence rises with age, probably due to increased co-morbidity. Up to 15% of 'healthy' older people and over half of all institutionalised patients will also fall annually. Previous fallers have a two-thirds chance of falling again within one year and approximately half of all fallers do so repeatedly, emphasising the fact that a history of a prior fall is an important risk factor for future falls.

Of those who fall, up to two-thirds fall in their normal residence, usually in the most frequently used rooms such as the bedroom, kitchen and dining room. People under 75 years of age are more likely to fall outdoors. Most falls occur during the day with only 20% occurring at night, while cold weather increases the incidence of falls and fractures in women.

Risk factors

The many risk factors for falling are listed in Table 1 according to whether the risk is intrinsically related to the patient or an extrinsic factor. Perhaps even more important than recognising risk factors for falling is to appreciate the interaction and probable synergism between multiple factors. Many studies have demonstrated that the risk of falling increases

TABLE I
RISK FACTORS FOR FALLING

Intrinsic risk factors
History of falls
Muscle weakness
Gait abnormality
Balance deficit
Visual impairment
Arthritis
Cognitive dysfunction
Depression
Impaired activities of daily living
Age >80 years
Urinary incontinence
Cardiovascular abnormalities
Stroke

Extrinsic risk factors
Environmental factors eg. clutter, poor lighting, loose mats, lack of bathroom aids etc
Use of assistive device
Polypharmacy
Medications
    psychotropics
    hypnotics / anxiolytics
    antihypertensives
    antiarrhythmics
    digoxin
    diuretics
    anticonvulsants
    anticholinergics
    caffeine

markedly as the number of risk factors increases. For example, Tinetti reported an increase in the fall risk in community-dwelling elderly persons from 27% in those with no or one risk factor to 78% in those with four or more risk factors.

Impact

Falling is associated with considerable morbidity and mortality. Accidental injuries are the fifth leading cause of death in older adults after cardiovascular, neoplastic, cerebrovascular and pulmonary causes. Falls are responsible for two-thirds of deaths resulting from accidental injuries and 75% of deaths due to falls occur in the 13% of the population over 65 years of age. Approximately half of all falls lead to some degree of injury, with major injuries occurring in 10% after a fall. Up to 1% of falls in older people result in hip fracture which is associated with substantial morbidity and mortality.

As well as resulting in physical injury, falls can also have huge social and psychological consequences. Recurrent falls are a common reason for the admission of previously independent older people to long-stay institutions. In addition, the loss of self confidence to walk safely often results in self-imposed functional limitations. Up to 80% of women would rather be dead than experience loss of independence and quality of life as a result of a bad hip fracture.

Falls assessment

Many trials have confirmed that the detection of a history of falls and the subsequent implementation of a falls-related assessment and intervention strategy significantly reduces the likelihood of future falls. Due to the absence of prospectively collated evidence, however, it is not clear who should undergo a falls assessment, how often they should be assessed and what the assessment should entail. A number of screening tools exist, but most have either been poorly validated or validated in selected populations only.

Most authorities agree, however, that all patients presenting with recurrent falls or a single, unexplained fall with a significant injury warrant formal assessment. In addition, recent guidelines have suggested that all older persons under the care of a health professional should be asked at least once a year about falls. All those who report a single fall should be observed as they perform the 'get up and go test', in which the patient is asked to stand up from a chair without using their arms, walk a few metres and return. This test is easy to perform and can be incorporated into short clinical consultations. Further evaluation is needed for those who have difficulty or demonstrate unsteadiness.

A formal falls assessment should ideally be performed by a dedicated multidisciplinary team including a physician, physiotherapist and occupational therapist. Although 'one-stop' falls assessment clinics have become popular, the occupational therapy assessment is best performed in the patient's own home where a proper appraisal of the environment can be undertaken. The medical assessment should include an assessment of the history and circumstances of any fall, medications, acute and chronic medical problems, mobility levels, vision, gait and balance and an examination of neurological and cardiovascular function. Laboratory investigations may help to identify treatable abnormalities and should include a full blood count, serum urea and electrolytes, creatinine, glucose, vitamin B_{12} and an assessment of thyroid function. Neuroimaging is only helpful in the presence of a head injury or if new, focal deficits are detected during neurological examination. Electroencephalography is rarely helpful and is only indicated if there is a high clinical suspicion of a seizure disorder. The usefulness of cardiovascular investigations is discussed below.

Interventions
Multifactorial risk assessment by a multidisciplinary team followed by targeting of interventions to an individual's risk factors is regarded as the best method of reducing falls. In general, trials with higher intensity interventions have shown the greatest risk reductions but evaluation of the success of individual intervention strategies is difficult due to inconsistent trial design.

In community dwelling older adults, reducing the dosages and total number of medications to 4 or fewer has been shown to significantly reduce the risk of falling. In particular, the tapering and discontinuation of psychotropic medications may reduce the rate of falling by up to 40%. Older people with recurrent falls should be offered long-term exercise and balance training, including Tai Chi C'uan and muscle strengthening programs, though the optimal type, duration and intensity of exercise for falls prevention remains unclear. In addition, advice should be given on the appropriate use of assistive devices such as canes, Zimmer frames and bed alarms.

Medical assessment followed by specific intervention for underlying medical problems, including cardiovascular problems and orthostatic hypotension, has been shown to be beneficial. First cataract surgery reduces the risks of falling and fractures as well as improving visual function and general health status. Despite the significant relationship between visual acuity, falls and fractures, evidence for intervention in patients with visual problems other than cataract is patchy.

Standardised assessment of home environmental hazards by an occupational therapist with specific recommendations and follow up after hospital discharge may reduce falls by as much as 20%. The commonest useful modifications include the removal of rugs, the use of non-slip bathmats, the use of lighting at night, changing to more appropriate footwear and the installation of stair and bathroom rails.

Evidence for interventions in the acute hospital setting is very sparse, but it is clear that ward design can influence fall rates. Wards in which most beds are visible from the nurses' station have significantly lower fall rates than wards where few beds are visible. No evidence exists to suggest that the use of restraints or indeed, that the removal of restraints, affects the overall fall risk. Bedrails have not been shown to affect fall or total injury rates and may even contribute to an increase in the number of serious injuries.

All intervention strategies should include the education of patients and carers regarding the multifactorial nature of most falls and about the presence of, and recommended interventions for, specific risk factors. Persons at risk for falling who live alone or who spend large amounts of time alone should be taught what to do if they fall and cannot get up. In addition, they should have a personal emergency-response system or at least a telephone that is accessible from the floor. Hip protectors do not reduce the risk of falling but may reduce the risk of hip fracture following a fall in high risk individuals. As such, hip protectors may be considered as a prophylactic measure for high risk groups, though poor compliance due to bulkiness, discomfort, incontinence, difficulty of application and expense limits their effectiveness. Finally, there is solid evidence that appropriate treatment of coexisting osteoporosis and vitamin D deficiency significantly reduces fracture risk.

Syncope
Syncope, defined as transient loss of consciousness and postural tone with spontaneous recovery, has been recognised as a clinical entity for thousands of years. Crucifixion is the only method of execution in history that relies on the induction of recurrent syncope to induce death. Syncope is common, comprising up to 3% of accident and emergency attendances and as many as 6% of hospital admissions. It is more common in older people, particularly after 70 years, and up to one-third of the population will experience a syncopal episode at least once during their lifetime. Syncope can be dangerous, disabling and difficult to diagnose and recurrent episodes can have huge physical,

NEURALLY MEDIATED SYNDROMES
Vasovagal syncope
Carotid sinus syndrome
Orthostatic hypotension
Postprandial hypotension
Situational syncope - swallow, cough, sneeze, micturition, defecation, valsalva, diving

CARDIAC
Arrhythmias
Bradyarrhythmias
    sinus node disease
    bifascicular / second / third degree heart block
    pacemaker malfunction
Tachyarrhythmias
    ventricular fibrillation
    ventricular tachycardia
    torsades de pointes
    Brugada syndrome
    long QT syndrome
    supraventricular (atrial fibrillation / flutter / tachycardia)
    junctional (Wolff-Parkinson-White, Lown-Ganong-Levine)

Structural abnormalities
Aortic stenosis
Hypertrophic obstructive cardiomyopathy
Aortic dissection
Cardiac tamponade
Atrial myxoma
Coronary spasm

MISCELLANEOUS
Pulmonary embolism
Subclavian steal syndrome
'Cerebral' syncope
Transient ischaemic attack
Migraine
Iatrogenic

causes and miscellaneous causes. Neurally mediated syndromes are common and generally have a benign prognosis, while cardiac syncope is less common but more alarming due to the much poorer prognosis. Although the advent of head-up tilt testing has greatly improved the diagnostic yield, many centres still report up to one-third of syncope presentations as unexplained despite extensive investigations.

Presentation

Irrespective of the aetiology of syncope, the final pathophysiological pathway is common to all causes. Progressive systemic hypotension (figure 1) eventually results in a failure of cerebral autoregulation, a fall in cerebral flow and cerebral hypoxia which ultimately causes loss of consciousness and postural tone. Syncope allows adoption of the supine position which facilitates a recovery in blood pressure, cerebral blood flow and consciousness. During syncope, as well as being unconscious, patients are usually pale and have a thready or absent pulse, a presentation often initially indistinguishable from sudden cardiac death.

Syncope itself is usually preceded by a prodromal period lasting from seconds to minutes which consists of a wide variety of presyncopal symptoms including dizziness, light-headedness, palpitations, dyspnoea, chest pain, vertigo, sweating, nausea, diplopia, tinnitus, hallucinations, anxiety and many others. Most patients learn to recognise presyncopal symptoms and take evasive action by sitting or lying down, thereby aborting progression of hypotension and avoiding syncope. The prodrome, however, may be absent or attenuated in older people and patients with cardiac abnormalties, thereby removing the opportunity to take evasive action and increasing the risk of sustaining significant injuries. The post syncopal period is variable in duration, generally lasting seconds or minutes, and is characterised by symptoms similar to those during presyncope. More prolonged recovery periods following episodes of loss of consciousness are more suggestive of generalised seizures than syncope.

Neurally mediated syndromes

Vasovagal syncope

Considerable overlap exists between the various neurally mediated disorders with two or more diagnoses commonly co-existing. Vasovagal syncope is by far the commonest cause of syncope, affecting

psychological and social consequences similar to those resulting from chronic disabling illnesses such as rheumatoid arthritis.

The causes of syncope are extensive in number but can be conveniently classified into three categories (table 2), namely, neurally mediated syndromes, cardiac

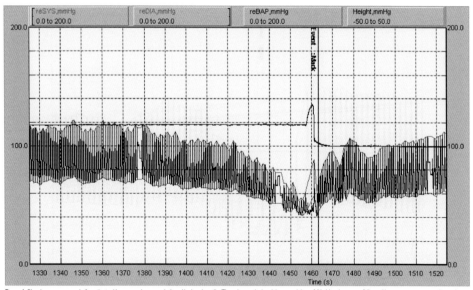

| reSYS,mmHg 0.0 to 200.0 | reDIA,mmHg 0.0 to 200.0 | reBAP,mmHg 0.0 to 200.0 | Height,mmHg -50.0 to 50.0 |

Figure 1: Blood pressure record of a patient with vasovagal syncope induced by head-up tilt. There is a gradual and then precipitous fall in blood pressure followed by a recovery on returning to the supine position

all age groups with an equal sex incidence. A family history is present in about a third of patients. Events usually occur in the standing position, but may occur while sitting and, less commonly, lying. Vasovagal syncope often has identifiable precipitating factors such as pain, emotional trauma, prolonged standing, warm environments, venesection and medications with hypotensive effects. Progressive hypotension (figure 1) prior to vasovagal syncope may be exacerbated by a concurrent bradycardia (vagal effect) but episodes without bradycardia are at least as common.

A suggestive clinical history of presyncopal symptoms, pallor, collapse, brief loss of consciousness, thready or impalpable pulse, and relatively rapid recovery is enough to make the diagnosis of vasovagal syncope in uncomplicated cases. Eye-witness accounts are particularly invaluable and should be actively sought, especially in view of the fact that up to one-third of patients who lose consciousness deny having done so.

Cases with more obscure presentations can be confirmed by head-up tilt testing (figure 2) which helps to precipitate episodes of vasovagal syncope in a controlled environment by encouraging venous pooling in both lower limbs and reducing cardiac

venous return. Patients undergo non-invasive continuous monitoring of heart rate and blood pressure and are tilted head-up, usually to an angle of 70°. Symptom reproduction during the test in association with the classic haemodynamic profile (figure 1), with or without a bradycardia, confirms the diagnosis. Although head-up tilt testing has improved the diagnostic yield in patients with unexplained syncope from 50% to 75 - 100%, it is complicated by

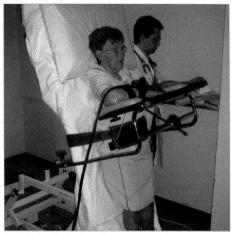

Figure 2: A patient undergoing a head-up tilt test

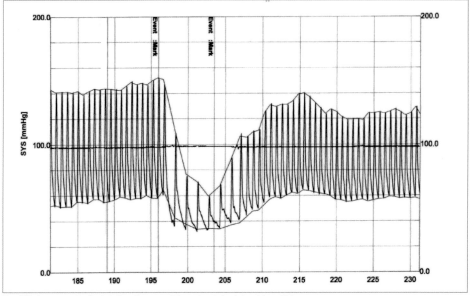

Figure 3: Blood pressure recording of a patient with vasodepressor carotid sinus syndrome before, during and after carotid sinus massage

relatively high false negative and false positive rates of approximately 10% which often make the test difficult to interpret. Patients who do not experience vasovagal episodes in the first 30-40 minutes of head-up tilt testing often undergo added pharmacological or physical stressors to accentuate lower limb venous pooling. Such added stressors include intravenous nitrate and isoproterenol infusions, sublingual nitrate administration and lower body negative pressure. Although syncopal episodes may be expedited by such manoeuvres, this is at the expense of much higher false positive rates which render interpretation of results even more difficult.

Carotid sinus syndrome

Carotid sinus syndrome is a disease of older people, being rare under the age of 50 years, and is associated with a substantial increase in morbidity, but not mortality. It is the commonest cause of 'drop attacks' (syncopal episodes with no warning and recovery within seconds) and accounts for up to one-third of unexplained non-accidental falls in older people. Symptoms are classically precipitated by manoeuvres that mechanically stimulate the carotid sinus, such as head turning and shaving, and may also result from straining, prolonged standing and pain but clear precipitating factors are often lacking. Amnesia for loss of consciousness is particularly common,

emphasising the importance of a collateral history from witnesses. Males are more commonly affected and the majority have cardiovascular co-morbidity in the form of ischaemic heart disease, cerebrovascular disease or hypertension.

A diagnosis of carotid sinus syndrome is confirmed by reproducing symptoms in the presence of carotid sinus hypersensitivity demonstrated by carotid sinus massage. Carotid hypersensitivity responses are defined as follows:
• Vasodepressor - a fall in systolic blood pressure of ≥50mmHg (figure 3)
• Cardioinhibitory - a ≥ 3s period of asystole (figure 4),
• Mixed vasodepressor and cardiohibitory

Carotid sinus massage is performed for five seconds longitudinally over the point of maximal carotid impulse, with one minute between stimuli. Massage is performed bilaterally (not simultaneously) in the supine position, but, if negative, must be repeated in the head-up tilt position as approximately 30% of patients with the syndrome exhibit positive findings in the head-up position only. Heart rate responses occur almost immediately on stimulation but the blood pressure fall takes approximately 18 seconds to reach its nadir.

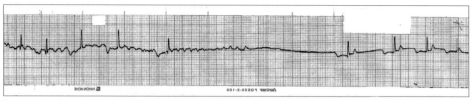

Figure 4: ECG tracing of a patient with cardioinhibitory carotid sinus syndrome demonstrating a 5.6 second R-R interval in response to carotid sinus massage

Carotid sinus massage is a relatively safe procedure with a low risk of complications (<1%) if patients with carotid bruits, recent myocardial infarction, recent cerebral ischaemia and previous ventricular tachyarrhythmias are excluded. The test, however, is associated with a significant stroke risk of 1:1000 and written informed consent should be obtained in advance. In addition, recent evidence suggests that hypersensitive responses to carotid sinus massage may be present in as many as 39% of healthy older people with no history of syncope, dizziness or falls. Whether this population is at increased risk of syncope or falls in the future is unclear, but evidently, hypersensitive responses to carotid sinus massage without symptom reproduction must be interpreted with great caution.

Orthostatic hypotension

Orthostatic hypotension is defined as a reduction in systolic blood pressure of at least 20mmHg or in diastolic blood pressure of at least 10mmHg within 3 minutes of standing or head-up tilt. It is common, being present in up to 30% of asymptomatic healthy elderly people living at home and over half of older people living in care facilities, and is probably under-diagnosed in both settings. The prevalence of orthostatic hypotension increases with age and is associated with increased morbidity and mortality, due in part to the increased incidence of falls and vascular death, especially stroke.

Orthostatic hypotension is poorly reproducible and the lack of a blood pressure fall in the presence of suggestive symptoms, therefore, warrants further investigation in view of the numerous factors that may influence the condition, including drug use, speed of postural change, prolonged recumbency, warm environment and food and alcohol ingestion. Symptoms of syncope and presyncope occur on postural change, but correlate poorly with measured blood pressure changes. The reasons for this are unclear, but co-existing impaired cerebral autoregulation may play a role. Supine hypertension

is common in patients with orthostatic hypotension, affecting over half of all patients in some series.

Orthostatic hypotension in older people is usually due to failure of the autonomic nervous system with impairment of the sympathetic vasoconstrictor system and absent or suboptimal compensatory heart rate increases on standing. Failure of the autonomic nervous system may originate centrally, due to degenerative neurological illnesses such as Parkinson's disease, multi-system atrophy, dementia with Lewy bodies and pure autonomic failure, or peripherally, due to illnesses such as diabetes mellitus, amyloidosis, vitamin B_{12} deficiency, inflammatory neuropathies, neurotoxins, porphyria, familial dysautonomia and human immunodeficiency virus. Medications with hypotensive effects, particularly antihypertensives and antidepressants, are frequently implicated and dehydration and haemorrhage should be considered, particularly in acutely ill patients. Entities such as Addison's disease and phaeochromocytoma are uncommon causes but treatable and should be considered.

Other neurally mediated syndromes

Postprandial hypotension may be exacerbated by posture change, but is a distinct entity that differs from orthostatic hypotension. It is defined as a fall in systolic blood pressure >20mmHg, or an absolute systolic blood pressure <90mmHg when pre-prandial systolic blood pressure was >100mmHg, within two hours of the start of a meal. The prevalence of postprandial hypotension is unknown, but it may be more common than orthostatic hypotension, being present in up to one-half of patients with unexplained syncope. Prevalence studies are complicated by the fact that mild, meal-induced decreases in blood pressure are common in healthy older people. Postprandial hypotension occurs in both sitting and supine positions, can be found at all meal times and is associated with symptoms similar to those produced by orthostatic hypotension. The causes are unclear, but the size and nutrient content of meals affect the magnitude of the decrease in postprandial blood pressure, with carbohydrates and, more specifically, simple carbohydrates such as glucose being particularly implicated.

Syncope may also be precipitated by a wide variety of everyday physiological manoeuvres such as micturition, swallowing, coughing, sneezing, defaecation and diving. Syncope in such cases is usually precipitated by hypotension due to a vagally induced profound bradycardia, though vasodepression in the absence of cardioinhibition has also been described. The occurrence of syncope in such settings should alert one to the possibility of an underlying pathology in the relevant organ, for example, oesophageal cancer in swallow syncope.

Management of neurally mediated syncope

Once a diagnosis of syncope or presyncope of neural origin is confirmed, patients can be reassured regarding the relatively benign nature of the diagnosis. Many patients with vasovagal syncope experience a progressive amelioration of symptoms over time, even without intervention. The majority of patients with neurally mediated syncope syndromes need no treatment other than reassurance and education regarding avoidance of precipitating factors and how to take evasive action should presyncopal symptoms occur. Patients should be encouraged to increase their daily intake of fluid and salt and should be educated regarding physical counter-manoeuvres, such as leg crossing, stooping, squatting and tensing of the muscles of the legs, abdomen and buttocks, which may help to maintain blood pressure during daily activities. Physical exercise should be encouraged as it helps to avoid deconditioning, which exacerbates orthostatic intolerance, and has been shown to improve outcomes in patients with vasovagal syncope and orthostatic hypotension. Rapid ingestion of 0.5 litres of cold tap water over 3 - 4 minutes has been shown to significantly elevate systemic blood pressure and may aid recovery. Patients with orthostatic hypotension should be advised to get from a supine position to a standing position gradually and to raise the head of the bed by 10 - 20 degrees. Custom-fitted elastic stockings and abdominal binders can be tried in orthostatic hypotension but tend to be poorly tolerated by patients. Advice should be given to avoid physiological manoeuvres that reduce venous return to the heart by raising intrathoracic pressure, such as straining and coughing. In this regard, older patients with orthostatic hypotension should be specifically advised to be cautious when standing from a toilet seat.

Discontinuation of medications with hypotensive effects (eg. antihypertensives, antidepressants, antipsychotics, anticholinergics) may improve matters, but if episodes of syncope continue to affect quality of life, further pharmacological intervention may be considered. Due to the relapsing and remitting nature of the neurally mediated syndromes, however, it is often difficult to know whether improvement in symptoms has been spontaneous or due to the introduction of a particular medication.

Fludrocortisone attenuates hypotension during presyncope by promoting salt and water retention and enhancing sensitivity of blood vessels to circulating catecholamines. It has proven benefit in patients with orthostatic hypotension, vasovagal syncope and vasodepressor carotid sinus syndrome and is usually started at a dose of 0.05mg, increasing up to 0.3mg as necessary. Older patients who fail to tolerate fludrocortisone due to the development of oedema may respond to midodrine, a peripheral, selective, direct α1-adrenoreceptor agonist, which has been shown to be of benefit in orthostatic hypotension, vasovagal syncope and vasodepressor carotid sinus syndrome. An initial dose of 2.5mg two or three times daily can be increased to 10mg three times daily as necessary. Combinations of fludrocortisone and midodrine may prove effective, though formal evidence is lacking. Supine hypertension often limits the use of both agents, particularly in patients with carotid sinus syndrome and orthostatic hypotension.

Patients with vasovagal syncope who do not respond to the above measures may show a response to beta-blockers such as propranolol and metoprolol, or serotonin reuptake inhibitors such as paroxetine and fluoxetine, though the evidence that they are much better than placebo is sparse. Tilt training programs have shown promise in patients with resistant vasovagal syncope but are time consuming and compliance is variable. Desmopressin is a vasopressin analogue that encourages volume expansion and reduces nocturnal diuresis and may be beneficial in patients with orthostatic hypotension. It can be administered orally, sublingually, intranasally, subcutaneously or intramuscularly but fluid and electrolyte status should be monitored carefully due

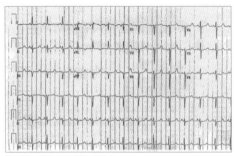

Figure 5: Long QT syndrome (QTc = 510ms)

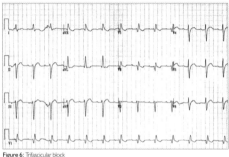

Figure 6: Trifascicular block

to the risk of hyponatraemia and water intoxication. Erythropoeitin increases standing blood pressure and improves orthostatic tolerance in patients with orthostatic hypotension and anaemia, particularly normochromic, normocytic anaemias associated with autonomic failure. Other agents used in the treatment of orthostatic hypotension such as pyridostigmine, ephedrine, pseudoephedrine, dihydroergotamine, clonidine, cyclooxygenase inhibitors, indomethacin, metoclopramide, domperidone and potassium supplements are of less certain value.

The long term effects of elevating systemic blood pressure with pressor agents in patients with neurally mediated syncope are unknown but caution is advised as increased hypertensive end-organ damage exacerbating cerebrovascular disease, nephropathy and cardiomyopathy is a potential concern.

Patients with documented bradycardias as the cause of their syncope syndromes may benefit from the insertion of cardiac pacemakers. Cardioinhibitory and mixed subtypes of carotid sinus syndrome may be treated with permanent cardiac pacing which reduces the risk of falls, syncope and injuries by two-thirds. Dual chamber demand pacing is best tolerated and results in less hypotension during pacing than single lead ventricular pacemakers. Intervention is generally recommended for patients with a history of two or more symptomatic episodes. In view of the high injury rate associated with symptomatic episodes, however, intervention should also be considered in individuals with a solitary severe event. A significant number of paced patients may continue to experience residual presyncopal symptoms despite pacing, possibly as a result of an untreated vasodepressor component. Permanent pacemakers with rate hysteresis may benefit some patients with a profound bradycardia during

vasovagal syncope but this remains a controversial area and is fortunately rarely necessary.

Cardiac syncope

In marked contrast with the generally benign prognosis associated with neurally mediated syncope, the prognosis in patients with syncope attributable to a cardiac cause is very guarded, with mortality rates of greater than 10% and up to 30% reported at 6 and 12 months respectively. A diagnosis of cardiac syncope doubles the risk of death from any cause and increases the risk of fatal and nonfatal cardiovascular events. Patients with no cause identified for syncope carry an intermediate risk, probably due to undiagnosed cardiac syncope in this group.

The challenge in managing older patients who present with syncope, therefore, is to identify those who are high risk for sudden death. Syncope on exercise, in the supine position, without warning and with convulsive elements have been found to be the most predictive clinical features of a cardiac cause of syncope. Unlike the neurally mediated syndromes, identifiable trigger factors are uncommon. The presence of suspected or definite heart disease doubles the probability of a diagnosis of cardiac syncope at presentation from 39% to 79%. The presence of any cardiac abnormalities on physical examination, therefore, such as atrial fibrillation, murmurs or signs of congestive cardiac failure should raise the possibility of a cardiac cause of syncope.

A chest radiograph displaying an enlarged cardiothoracic ratio or a 12-lead ECG demonstrating abnormalities such as electrical left ventricular hypertrophy, second or third degree heart block, bifascicular block or a prolonged QT interval (figure 5) should also raise suspicion. Patients with syncope and bifascicular or trifascicular block (figure 6) are

TABLE 3
DRUGS THAT MAY PROLONG THE QT INTERVAL

Antiarrhythmic drugs
  Amiodarone
  Sotalol
  Flecainide
  Disopyramide
  Quinidine
  Procainamide

Antihistamines
  Terfenadine
  Astemizole

Antibiotics
  Erythromycin
  Clarithromycin
  Ciprofloxacin
  Levofloxacin

Gastrointestinal motility agents
  Cisapride
  Domperidone

Antidepressants
  Tricyclics
  Serotonin reuptake inhibitors

Antipsychotic drugs
  Haloperidol
  Chlorpromazine
  Clozapine
  Quetiapine
  Risperidone
  Thioridazine
  Droperidol

listed in table 3. Older patients presenting with syncope and a prolonged QT interval in the presence of such drugs should be suspected of having a ventricular arrhythmia as the cause of syncope and offending drugs should be discontinued immediately.

Transient ventricular tachyacardia and bradyarrhythmias are the most common cardiac causes of syncope and usually occur in the presence of structural heart disease. The risk of ventricular arrhythmias and sudden death increases with the severity of left ventricular dysfunction. Echocardiography should be used, therefore, to assess left ventricular function in all syncopal patients with a previous history or current evidence of ischaemic heart disease and cardiac failure. In addition to allowing assessment of the severity of left ventricular dysfunction, echocardiography will detect cardiac structural abnormalities such as aortic stenosis or hypertrophic obstructive cardiomyopathy in 5-10% of unselected cases of syncope. Patients with an ejection fraction of <30% should be considered for the insertion of an implantable cardioverter-defibrillator. Syncopal patients with ischaemic heart disease and less severe left ventricular dysfunction ought to be considered for electrophysiological testing as those with inducible ventricular tachycardia have a prognosis similar to those who present with spontaneous sustained ventricular arrhythmias. Such patients should also be considered candidates for an implantable cardioverter-defibrillator. Outside of these parameters, the role of electrophysiological testing in unexplained syncope is unclear.

Holter monitoring over 24 hours yields a diagnosis in up to 18% of patients with unexplained syncope or pre-syncope and excludes the diagnosis in a further 15%. Extending the period of monitoring to 72 hours does not, however, increase the yield for arrhythmias associated with symptoms. External ambulatory loop electrocardiography may be performed for 30 days or more and is most useful in patients with palpitations, but a high degree of patient compliance and cooperation is essential. Exercise stress testing is generally unhelpful for diagnostic purposes with a yield likely to be <1%. Where all these investigations are normal and a high index of suspicion remains for arrhythmia-induced syncope in the face of uncertainty regarding the presence of organic heart disease, implantable loop

at increased risk of developing complete heart block and sudden death and should undergo evaluation of the need for empirical permanent pacemaker insertion. The Brugada syndrome (characterised by ST segment elevation in the anterior leads), right ventricular dysplasia (characterised by T wave inversion in the anterior leads), and congenital forms of the long QT syndrome are pathologies of younger people and rarely present with syncope in later life. The QT interval may, however, be prolonged by electrolyte disturbances such as hypokalaemia, hypomagnesaemia and hypocalcaemia and a large number of drugs, the most common of which are recorders may reveal treatable arrhythmias, usually bradycardias, in as many as 20% of patients.

Differential diagnosis of syncope
The initial presentation of syncope with collapse, loss of consciousness, pallor and pulselessness is very similar to the presentation of sudden cardiac death, and its occurrence can often lead to understandable alarm among witnesses. Most 'successful' cardiopulmonary resuscitations in the community without defibrillation are of patients with syncope.

In patients who lose consciousness and spontaneously recover, however, the main diagnostic dilemma is between syncope and a generalised seizure. Investigations such as CT/MRI scans of brain and EEGs are generally unhelpful being, more often than not, normal in both clinical conditions. Clinical features of cerebral hypoxia such as limb jerking and incontinence may occur during syncope as well as generalised seizures and should not be used to discriminate between the conditions. Physical injuries can also occur in both conditions, but lateral tongue biting is highly suggestive of a seizure. The nature and duration of the postictal period, however, is probably the best discriminating feature. Recovery following syncope is generally complete within minutes and sometimes even seconds and is characterised by symptoms similar to those during presyncope. Recovery following a seizure, however, is usually much more delayed, often taking many hours. Confusion and drowsiness are prominent features and patients may sleep for several hours. Diagnostic difficulties arise in cases where the recovery period is of interim duration with mixed clinical features and misdiagnoses are unfortunately quite common. Up to one-third of patients diagnosed as having treatment-resistant epilepsy have abnormalities during head-up tilt testing, suggesting the alternative diagnosis of recurrent syncope.

Transient ischaemic attack (TIA) seems to be quite an abused term and is unfortunately frequently applied to patients with 'funny turns' of varying aetiologies. A clinical event involving loss of consciousness is almost never due to a transient ischaemic attack and almost always due to syncope or seizure.

Syncope is a common presenting complaint of pulmonary embolism in older people with evidence that up to 30% of older patients may present in this manner.

Patients with panic attacks experience many symptoms that also occur during presyncope such as dizziness, palpitations, chest pain and dyspnoea and may hyperventilate as well as experience a feeling of panic. A diagnosis of recurrent presyncope should be considered in patients diagnosed with panic attacks who subsequently develop episodes of loss of consciousness or who appear otherwise psychiatrically normal.

Episodes of loss of consciousness may be psychogenic in origin, but this is fortunately unusual. In such patients, injuries are exceptional and recovery is usually very rapid. Episodes may be precipitated by stressful events and it may be possible to distract patients during episodes. A psychogenic origin should be suspected in patients who appear to gain rewards when events occur or who have pre-existing behavioural problems.

Syncope and driving
The ability to drive a motor vehicle is a very significant contributing factor to the quality of life of older people. It is not surprising, therefore, that many patients with syncope are more concerned with their continued ability to drive rather than their own overall prognosis. In most jurisdictions, patients have a legal duty to inform the licencing authorities about any condition likely to affect their ability to drive. In addition, failure to notify their insurance company may also affect the validity of their insurance. It is the doctor's responsibility to advise patients when they should cease driving and when to inform relevant authorities. In addition, doctors have ethical and moral obligations to directly inform authorities where there is evidence that an individual continues to drive despite advice to the contrary.

Although the law varies from one jurisdiction to another, the following recommendations may be considered reasonable. Patients with simple episodes of vasovagal syncope are not usually restricted from driving, as long as the episodes are uncomplicated, have identifiable precipitating factors, are associated with prodromal symptoms and are unlikely to occur while sitting or lying. Patients who have syncopal episodes that are unexplained and without a prodrome can be advised to resume driving 4 weeks after the event if they are deemed to have a low risk of recurrence. Factors that suggest a high risk of recurrence include clinical evidence of structural heart disease, more than one episode in the previous six months and events that cause injury or occur while driving, sitting or lying. Such patients may be allowed to drive again 4 weeks after the event if the cause has been identified and treated. If no cause has been identified in patients at high risk of recurrence and there are no epileptiform features, the licence should be revoked for a period of six months. In patients where the event cannot be clearly differentiated from a seizure, the licence should be revoked for a period of 12 months. Those with cough syncope must not drive until the liability to attacks has been successfully controlled.

There is evidence that the adherence of syncopal patients to driving recommendations is very poor, even when they remember the advice. It is important, therefore, that any counselling regarding driving should be convincing and repeated at subsequent visits.

Suggested further reading

- American Geriatrics Society, British Geriatrics Society, and American Academy of Orthopaedic Surgeons Panel on Falls Prevention.
- Guideline for the prevention of falls in older persons. Journal of the American Geriatrics Society. 2001; 49: 664–672.
- British Orthopaedic Association. The care of patients with fragility fracture. www.boa.ac.uk/site/showpublications.aspx?ID=59
- Caird FI, Andrews GR, Kennedy RD. Effect of posture on blood pressure in the elderly. British Heart Journal. 1973; 35: 527–530.
- Carey BJ, Potter JF. Cardiovascular causes of falls. Age & Ageing. 2001; 30-S4: 19-24.
- MC, Arlot ME, Delmas PD, Meunier PJ. Effect of calcium and cholecalciferol treatment for three years on hip fractures in elderly women. BMJ 1994; 308: 1081-2
- Close J. Ellis M, Hopper R et al. Prevention of falls in the elderly trial (PROFET): A randomised controlled trial. Lancet 1999; 353: 93-97.
- FRAX World Health Organization fracture risk assessment tool. www.shef.ac.uk/FRAX
- Gillespie LD, Gillespie WJ, Robertson MC, Lamb SE, Cumming RG, Rowe BH. Interventions for preventing falls in elderly people. Cochrane Database of Systematic Reviews 2003, Issue 3 Art. No. CD000340. DOI:10.1002/14651858.CD000340
- Kenny RA (editor). Syncope in the Older Patient. Chapman & Hall. 1996
- Kenny RA, Richardson DA, Steen N, Bexton RS, Shaw FE, Bond J. Carotid sinus syndrome: a modifiable risk factor for nonaccidental falls in older adults (Safe Pace). Journal of the American College of Cardiology. 2001; 38: 1491-1496.
- Leipzig RM, Cumming RG, Tinetti ME. Drugs and falls in older people: A systematic review and meta-analysis: I. Psychotropic drugs. J Am Geriatr Soc 1999; 47: 30-39. 33
- Linzer M, Yang EH, Estes NAM, Wang P, Vorperian VR, Kapoor WN. Clinical guidline: Diagnosing syncope. Parts I & II. Annals of Internal Medicine 1997; 126&127: 989-996&76–86
- Lord SR, McClean D, Stathers G. Physiological factors associated with injurious falls in older people living in the community. Gerontology 1992: 38: 338-46.
- Mathias CJ, Kimber JR. Treatment of postural hypotension. Journal of Neurology, Neurosurgery & Psychiatry. 1998; 65: 285-289.
- Mathias S, Nayak US, Isaac B. Balance in elderly patient: The "get-up and go" test. Arch Phys Med Rehabil 1986;67: 387-389.
- McIntosh SJ, Lawson J, Kenny RA. Clinical characteristics of vasodepressor, cardioinhibitory and mixed carotid sinus syndrome in the elderly. American Journal of Medicine. 1993; 95: 203-208.
- Sutton R, Petersen M, Brignole M, Raviele A, Menozzi C, Giani P. Proposed classification for tilt induced vasovagal syncope. European Journal of Cardiac Pacing & Electrophysiology. 1992; 3: 180–183.
- Tinetti ME, Baker DI, McAvay G et al. A multifactorial intervention to reduce the risk of falling among elderly people living in the community. N Engl J Med 1994; 331: 821–827.
- Tinetti ME, Speechley M, Ginter SF. Risk factors for falls among elderly persons living in the community. N Eng J Med 1988; 319; 1701-7.
- Tinetti ME, Speechley M. Prevention of falls among the elderly. N Eng J Med 1989; 320: 1055-9.
- Wolf SL, Barnhart HX, Kutner NG et al. Reducing frailty and falls in older persons: an investigation of Tai Chi and computerised balance training. J Am Geriatr Soc 1996; 44: 489.

Case Study 1

A 75 year old widow with a history of rheumatoid arthritis and a left mastectomy for breast adenocarcinoma suffered an intertrochanteric fracture of her right hip after slipping while getting out of the bath. She lives alone and was on the floor for 36 hours before being found by a neighbour and brought to the Accident & Emergency department.

This patient needs a formal medical opinion to assess her medical condition prior to any planned surgery. Dehydration and electrolyte imbalance due to prolonged incapacitation prior to being discovered will need to be corrected and attention should be paid to any potential underlying pressure sores, rhabdomyolysis, respiratory infections and cardiac and cerebrovascular conditions. Once stable, surgery should be considered without delay for the hip fracture. In view of her history of breast carcinoma, the possibility of a pathological fracture should be considered. If the fracture is a result of metastatic bone disease or rheumatoid arthritis has caused degeneration of the hip joint, a total hip replacement should be the procedure of choice. Early postoperative rehabilitation should be undertaken. Formal bone mineral densitometry should be considered. If she is taking oral corticosteroids for rheumatoid arthritis, they should be discontinued if possible, especially if her rheumatoid arthritis is inactive, to help prevent corticosteroid induced osteoporosis. Calcium and vitamin D supplementation should be considered as well as the introduction of a bisphosphonate for fracture prophylaxis. Hormone replacement therapy is contraindicated in view of her previous breast carcinoma. As a high risk candidate for future falls and fractures, hip protectors should also be considered. After discharge, a home hazard assessment and modification by an occupational therapist, especially of the bathroom, would be beneficial. If, as is likely, balance or gait abnormalities are detected, a progressive program of balance and gait training and muscle strengthening may be helpful. A personal alarm should be provided.

Case Study 2

A 68 year old male with longstanding hypertension and glaucoma fell in the street without warning and suffered a fracture of nasal bones. He denied loss of consciousness but had two similar episodes in the previous 2 years after getting out of bed to urinate which resulted in a head laceration on each occasion. He is an avid golfer and, apart from being overweight and having a sitting casual blood pressure measurement of 175/95mmHg, physical examination was unremarkable.

A collateral history from an eye-witness to the most recent fall is important in this case as the history regarding loss of consciousness may be unreliable. The history of falls after getting out of bed should lead to a high index of suspicion for orthostatic hypotension and erect and supine blood pressure measurements should be performed, repeatedly if necessary. In addition, the presentation on this occasion is suggestive of a drop attack and, due to the facts that carotid sinus syndrome is the commonest cause of drop attacks and that there is an overlap between orthostatic hypotension and carotid sinus syndrome, a head-up tilt test with erect and supine carotid sinus massage should be organised to exclude carotid sinus syndrome. If significant cardioinhibition is discovered on tilt testing, any medications used to treat hypertension or glaucoma with cardioinhibitory effects (eg. β-blockers) should be discontinued and the tilt test repeated. If significant cardioinhibition persists, a permanent dual chamber pacemaker should be considered. If orthostatic hypotension or vasodepressor carotid sinus syndrome are found, postural advice should be given. Pharmacological interventions for these diagnoses are limited due to coexisting hypertension and higher than ideal systemic blood pressure levels may have to be tolerated to reduce the risks posed by significant vasodepression. Exercise should be encouraged to help induce weight loss, lower systemic blood pressure and improve orthostatic tolerance. If tilt testing does not reveal an abnormality, Holter monitoring and the insertion of an implantable loop recorder should be considered. As the history is very suggestive of carotid sinus syndrome and the tilt test is notoriously irreproducible, a repeat tilt test with carotid sinus massage may be an option. A formal visual assessment is indicated in view of the occurrence of falls at night and history of glaucoma and a post discharge visit by an occupational therapist to assess and modify home hazards, especially in the bedroom and bathroom, may be helpful. The cause of the patient's nocturia (e.g. prostatism, cardiac failure, diabetes mellitus) should be ascertained and treated where possible. If it cannot be eliminated or improved, the provision of a bedside commode may help. In view of the high future fall risk, bone mineral density testing should be considered, but osteoporosis is unlikely in view of his sex, body mass index and regular exercise. He should be advised not to drive until he has been event-free for 12 months or unless a diagnosis and definitive intervention have been made (eg dual chamber pacemaker insertion for cardioinhibitory carotid sinus syndrome).

📂 Case Study 3

An 82 year old woman with dementia who has been living in a residential home for the past 3 years has fallen twice in the last three months without suffering injury, but denies ever having fallen. She has a history of congestive cardiac failure, osteoarthritis of both knees, depression and staff at the residential home report increasing difficulties in the last 6 months due to aggression and nocturnal wandering.

A collateral history from workers at the residential home who may have witnessed the falls is very important and, in view of her high future fall risk, formal bone mineral densitometry should be considered. As she is institutionalised and probably 'housebound', calcium and vitamin D supplementation should be commenced. Hip protectors should also be considered. The fact that her falls are temporally related to her new onset behavioural difficulties raises the possibility that the introduction of antipsychotic medications in an attempt to control behaviour may be contributing to the fall risk. The possibility of polypharmacy in such a patient is high with a likely treatment regime consisting of an antidepressant, diuretic, angiotensin converting enzyme inhibitor, antiplatelet agent, hypnotic, analgesics and antipsychotics. A reduction in medications, especially antipsychotics and hypnotics, may markedly reduce the fall risk. Potential cardiovascular contributing factors such as orthostatic hypotension should be considered and a visit by an occupational therapist to the residential home with targeted recommendations may be helpful. In view of her cognitive dysfunction, balance training is probably not an option due to likely difficulties in participation and retention of information.

Data Interpretation

Question 1

An 80 year old man with a history of angina and hypertension presented with a hip fracture but was unsure of how he fell. He reported one other fall two weeks previously and is also unsure of how he fell on that occasion but is adamant that he did not lose consciousness. The figure below represents a non-invasive beat-to-beat tracing of the patients blood pressure before, during and after right sided carotid sinus massage commencing at 294 seconds and ending at 299 seconds.

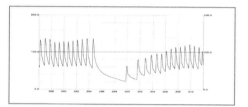

a.   Describe the two main abnormalities.
b.   What is the diagnosis?
c.   What are the two most important aspects of management?

Question 2

A 74 year old woman complains of a tremor and dizziness when getting out of bed and has fallen on 3 occasions in the bathroom when getting off the toilet, suffering a colles fracture on one occasion. Her husband reports that she has slowed up in the last 12 months and that it now takes her a long time to dress herself. The below represents a non-invasive beat-to-beat record of her blood pressure before and after standing at 683 seconds.

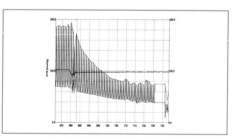

a)   What is the cause of her dizziness?

b) Is there any potential underlying cause in this case?

c) Name the two most relevant interventions for her dizziness.

Question 3

A 78 year old man with a history of a myocardial infarction presents with recurrent drop attacks and palpitations. Below is his ECG recording before, during and after right carotid sinus massage.

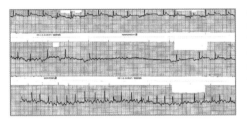

a. What cause is suggested by the above recording for the drop attacks?

b. Are there any other more sinister potential causes for the drop attacks in this case?

c. What complication has arisen from the performance of carotid sinus massage in this case?

d. What is the most significant complication associated with this procedure?

Best of five questions

Question 1

Dual chamber pacemakers may be of benefit in patients with the following diagnoses

a. Cardioinhibitory carotid sinus syndrome

b. Mixed carotid sinus syndrome

c. Sick sinus syndrome

d. All of the above

e. None of the above

Question 2

The most important intervention for a patient with symptomatic orthostatic hypotension is

a. Postural related advice

b. Elastic stockings

c. Fludrocortisone

d. Midodrine

e. Fludrocortisone & midodrine combined

Question 3

The test most likely to reveal a diagnosis in a patient with a drop attack is

a. Electrocardiogram

b. Holter monitor (24 hour ECG) examination

c. Echocardiogram

d. Carotid sinus massage

e. Electroencephalogram

Question 4

An 82 year old man with a history of hypertension and glaucoma collapsed to the ground and lost consciousness while attending Church. A nurse who witnessed the event reported that he looked deathly pale and could not feel a pulse. In addition, she noticed some jerking of the left upper limb lasting about 10 seconds. She commenced cardiopulmonary resuscitation and he regained consciousness within 2 minutes, though was initially drowsy, confused and dysarthric. He was taken outside and given a drink of water and after a further 10 minutes regained his colour and was once again talking clearly and coherently. After another 30 minutes he reported that he was once again "feeling fine" and walked home with his wife. What is the most likely diagnosis?

a. Vasovagal syncope

b. Transient ischaemic attack

c. Vertebrobasilar insufficiency

d. Generalised seizure

e. Cardiac arrhythmia

Question 5

A 78 year old woman with a history of hypertension, myocardial infarction and congestive cardiac failure with an ejection fraction of 22% has had recurrent syncopal episodes without warning resulting in bilateral colles fractures. The most important intervention is likely to be

a. Postural related advice

b. Medication reduction

c. Hip protectors

d. Dual chamber pacemaker

e. Implantable cardioverter defibrillator

Question 6

The following interventions are commonly used to reduce the risk of falling

1. Falls clinics

2. Tai Chi

3. Home hazard assessment and modification

4. Pacemaker insertion for fallers with cardioinhibitory carotid sinus syndrome

5. Bed rails

There is good evidence to support

a. All of the listed interventions

b.   None of the listed interventions
c.   1,2 and 4
d.   2,3 and 4
e.   1,4 and 5

Answers are on page 311

Endocrine and metabolic disorders

EC Mulkerrin, M Bell, G Flaherty, T O'Brien

Introduction

The ageing kidney has a reduced ability to respond to physiologic and pathologic stresses. Renal blood flow decreases from 1200 ml/min at age 30 years to 600 ml/min at age 80. The glomerular filtration rate (GFR), as indexed by the creatinine clearance, is stable until age 40 and then declines linearly at an average rate of about 8 ml/min/1.73 m^2/decade in about two-thirds of older persons without renal disease. This decline often occurs without influencing blood urea and creatinine levels and can only be identified by accurate measurement of the GFR. Lower renin levels in older persons result in 30-50% reductions in plasma aldosterone levels and contribute to the increased risk of hyperkalaemia in various clinical settings. The tendency toward hyperkalaemia is enhanced by acidosis because the ageing kidney is slow to correct an increase in acid load. Ageing is associated with impaired glomerular filtration of sodium and water and diminished renal tubular conservation of sodium. With age, total body water decreases because of an increase in fat and a decrease in lean body mass, so that the margin of error for maintaining normal electrolyte balance when water losses occur during acute illness is reduced. Furthermore, older patients frequently suffer from co-morbid conditions, such as hypertension and heart disease, which may be additive to the effects of ageing, thereby amplifying these abnormalities. This section addresses the principal electrolyte abnormalities found in older patients in clinical practice from a problem based perspective.

Disturbances in potassium metabolism

Hyperkalaemia

Hyperkalaemia is less common but more dangerous than hypokalaemia. A reduction of the resting membrane potential in hyperkalaemia will lead, if uncorrected, to muscle weakness and ultimately death from cardiac arrhythmias. Hyperkalaemia must be distinguished from pseudohyperkalaemia due to haemolysis of the blood sample, or the release of potassium from white blood cells or platelets in patients with marked leukocytosis or thrombocytosis. Hyperkalaemia is also associated with acidosis due to accumulation of inorganic acids, hyperglycaemia (in the presence of insulin deficiency), moderately heavy exercise, digitalis intoxication, tumour lysis syndrome, acute intravascular haemolysis, hyperkalaemic familial periodic paralysis, and excessive consumption of apple juice.

In an older patient, hyperkalaemia due to excessive oral intake of potassium may occur after overdose with slow-release potassium preparations. Parenteral infusion of potassium may cause dangerous hyperkalaemia if rates of infusion exceed 40 mmol/h or concentrations exceed 40 mmol/l in the presence of renal insufficiency. Older patients with impaired renal function who are transfused with whole blood are also at risk of hyperkalaemia. Since the kidneys normally excrete potassium loads rapidly, sustained hyperkalaemia usually implies diminished renal potassium excretion, a common concomitant of ageing. Hyperkalaemia is to be expected in cases of acute renal failure, especially when this is associated with gastrointestinal bleeding, severe sepsis, major burns, rhabdomyolysis or myonecrosis. Hyperkalaemia is rarely a problem in patients with chronic renal failure until the GFR falls below 15 to 20 ml/min. Hyperkalaemia due to impaired renal excretion of potassium may also be a feature of any cause of renal tubular acidosis.

Potassium-sparing diuretics may cause severe hyperkalaemia, even in older patients with normal renal function (case study 1). The reduction in angiotensin II concentrations induced by angiotensin-converting enzyme (ACE) inhibitors may cause elevation of plasma potassium but severe hyperkalaemia (> 6 mmol/l) is only likely when these agents are given to patients with a creatinine clearance less than 20 ml/min. The majority of older patients who develop hyperkalaemia on ACE inhibitors have chronic renal failure and diabetes. Inhibition of prostaglandin synthetase by non-steroidal anti-inflammatory drugs serves to reduce GFR and may

TABLE I
CAUSES OF HYPERKALAEMIA IN OLDER PATIENTS

Pseudohyperkalaemia
- Tourniquet method of drawing blood
- Haemolysis of drawn blood
- Increased white blood cell or platelet count

True hyperkalaemia
- Redistribution
  - Acidosis
  - Insulin deficiency
  - Adrenal insufficiency
  - Hepatic cirrhosis
  - Drugs
- Digitalis intoxication
- Alpha-adrenergic agonists
- Decreased excretion
  - Chronic renal failure
  - Potassium-sparing diuretics
  - Deficiency of adrenal steroids
  - Addison's disease
  - Hypoaldosteronism
- Drugs
  - Heparin
  - Angiotensin-converting enzyme inhibitors
  - Non steroidal anti-inflammatory drugs
  - Cyclosporine
- Inhibition of tubular secretion
  - Spironolactone
  - Triamterene
  - Amiloride
- Increased input
  - Endogenous input
  - Haemolysis
  - Rhabdomyolysis
- Exogenous input
  - Salt substitute
  - Potassium penicillin

elevated blood urea. The commonest cause of chronic hyperkalaemia in the absence of severe renal failure is probably hyporeninaemic hypoaldosteronism. The association of this disorder with old age, diabetes and renal disease reflects the decreasing activity of the renin-angiotensin system with age, reduced sensitivity of renal stretch receptors with increased rigidity of arteriolar walls, insulin deficiency and autonomic neuropathy. Moreover it has been shown that older subjects have lower basal levels of plasma aldosterone and a blunted aldosterone response to potassium infusion.

Although flaccid paralysis occasionally occurs, hyperkalaemia is usually asymptomatic until cardiac toxicity supervenes. Concentrations over 6.5 mmol/l with ECG changes and levels exceeding 7 mmol/l constitute a medical emergency. ECG changes, in order of severity, include tall, tented T-waves, diminished or absent P-waves, widening of the QRS complex, slurring of the ST segment, and a sinusoidal pre-cardiac arrest pattern. In an emergency an intravenous infusion of dextrose and insulin must be administered. This may need to be repeated, as its duration of action is 2 to 4 hours. Intravenous sodium bicarbonate achieves a similar shift of potassium from extracellular to intracellular fluid. Intravenous calcium gluconate reduces the serum potassium concentration and antagonises the deleterious effects of hyperkalaemia on the heart. The beneficial effects of calcium gluconate are evident within 2 minutes of infusion but last less than 1 hour. In less urgent cases potassium should be strictly excluded from the diet and a cation-exchange resin such as calcium resonium administered. This has a slower onset of action and its effects last 4 to 6 hours. In cases of intractable hyperkalaemia, especially in the setting of oliguric acute renal failure, haemodialysis must be promptly instituted.

Hypokalaemia

Hypokalaemia is also commonly seen in older patients and it is usually associated with a deficit in total body potassium. The resultant hyperpolarisation across excitable membranes may be apparent clinically as muscle weakness, paralysis and ultimately death from cardiac arrhythmias. Hypokalaemia potentiates the toxicity of digitalis since both reduce the excitability of the myocardial cell membrane. The need for potassium supplements in older patients on long-term digoxin therapy, especially if they are also taking potassium-losing diuretics, should always be considered. Hypokalaemia may

cause hyperkalaemia, especially in older patients with chronic renal failure. These effects are more likely to occur when two or more agents are co-prescribed to an older patient, particularly in the presence of coexisting disease. Malignant hyperthermia is associated with hyperkalaemia and is precipitated by inhaled anaesthetics in patients with an inherited increase in skeletal muscle calcium concentration.

The adrenal insufficiency of Addison's disease is associated with hyperkalaemia, hyponatraemia, and produce changes in the ECG, including ST segment depression, flattening of the T-waves and prominent U waves. These changes correlate poorly, however, with the development of significant arrhythmias. In addition to impairment of skeletal muscle function, hypokalaemia also reduces intestinal smooth muscle activity with occasional paralytic ileus. Hypokalaemia may increase production of renal prostaglandins thereby inhibiting the activation of adenyl cyclase by antidiuretic hormone particularly in older patients. The consequent failure of the kidneys to concentrate urine normally is an example of nephrogenic diabetes insipidus and is characterised by polyuria and polydipsia. Potassium deficiency also causes a metabolic alkalosis through its tendency to promote retention of sodium and bicarbonate.

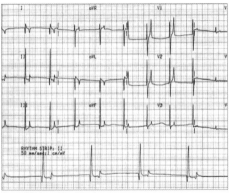
Figure 1: ECG changes in hyperkalaemia

There is more potassium in liquid stools than in gastric and upper intestinal secretions, so that any condition in which stool volumes are high may cause hypokalaemia. This is particularly pertinent to older, frail patients with diminished total body potassium. The hypokalaemia of vomiting is largely due to a renal potassium leak, secondary to the associated hypochloraemic alkalosis. Diarrhoea-associated hypokalaemia is usually accompanied by loss of bicarbonate, with a resultant metabolic acidosis. A colorectal villous adenoma may cause profound hypokalaemia, as may chronic laxative abuse, a common problem among older patients.

All diuretics, other than those acting directly on the distal tubule, tend to increase urinary potassium excretion. About 20% of patients receiving thiazide diuretics develop hypokalaemia. If hypokalaemia occurs, it is usually observed early in the course of treatment. Supplemental potassium is often required in patients who are prone to cardiac arrhythmias and in patients with severe liver disease in whom hypokalaemia may precipitate hepatic encephalopathy. In older hypertensive patients with unexplained hypokalaemia, primary hyperaldosteronism especially that associated with adrenal adenoma may cause renal potassium wasting. However, hypokalaemia in such patients is much more likely to be iatrogenic. Secondary hyperaldosteronism with hypokalaemia may complicate renal artery stenosis, congestive cardiac failure, cirrhosis and nephrotic syndrome treated with diuretic agents. Cushing's syndrome may cause renal depletion of potassium, especially if associated with adrenal cortical carcinoma or ectopic ACTH production. Excessive consumption of liquorice may cause hypokalaemia by inhibiting renal 11-ß-hydroxysteroid dehydrogenase. Renal potassium wasting and hypokalaemia may complicate acute myeloid, monocytic, and myelomonocytic leukaemias. Rarer causes of hypokalaemia include Bartter's syndrome, Liddle's syndrome and the autosomal dominant hypokalaemic periodic paralysis.

Correction of the underlying cause may suffice when hypokalaemia is minimal. In patients with myocardial disease, it is reasonable to treat all levels of hypokalaemia. In otherwise healthy subjects, most physicians will treat patients in whom potassium concentrations are consistently below 3 mmol/l with oral potassium. Indications for rapid parenteral infusion of potassium include hypokalaemic cardiac arrhythmias, paralysis and hypokalaemic diabetic ketoacidosis. Care must be taken to monitor plasma potassium levels closely in all patients receiving supplemental potassium. Hypokalaemia should be corrected very carefully in older patients with renal insufficiency using prescriptions, which expire within a limited timeframe eg. 2 days.

Disturbances in sodium metabolism

Hypernatraemia
Hypernatraemia is less commonly observed in hospital practice than hyponatraemia. Hypernatraemia is generally the result of water losses that exceed sodium losses in conjunction with inadequate water intake. The prevalence of hypernatraemia is about 1% in older hospitalised patients and in residents of long term care facilities. Precipitating factors include the inability to obtain water for themselves due to infirmity, impaired thirst,

TABLE 2
DISORDERS AND DRUGS ASSOCIATED WITH THE SYNDROME OF INAPPROPRIATE SECRETION OF ANTIDIURETIC HORMONE IN OLDER PATIENTS

Carcinomas	Pulmonary Disorders	Central Nervous System Disorders	Drugs
Bronchogenic carcinom	Viral pneumonia	Encephalitis (viral or bacterial)	ADH analogue
Carcinoma of the duodenum	Bacterial pneumonia	Meningitis (viral, bacterial, tuberculous, and fungal)	Chlorpropamide
Carcinoma of the pancreas	Pulmonary abscess	Head trauma	Carbamazepine
Carcinoma of the ureter	Tuberculosis	Brain tumours	Haloperidol
Lymphoma	Aspergillosis	Guillain-Barré syndrome	Amitriptyline
Mesothelioma	Positive pressure breathing	Subarachnoid haemorrhage	Thioridazine
Carcinoma of the bladder		Cerebellar and cerebral atrophy	NSAIDS
Prostatic carcinoma		Hydrocephalus	Diuretics
		Shy-Drager syndrome	SSRIs
		Delirium tremens	PPIs
		Cerebrovascular accident (cerebral thrombosis or haemorrhage)	
		Acute psychosis	

impaired renal concentrating ability and increased insensible losses due to fever and/or tachypnoea. Iatrogenic factors account for the increased frequency of hypernatraemia in older patients receiving nasogastric or gastrostomy tube feedings or parenteral nutrition. Hypernatraemia is also common in older patients with cirrhosis, in whom therapy for encephalopathy with lactulose produces osmotic diarrhoea and replacement of water losses is inadequate. Hypernatraemia may also occur in the setting of cardiopulmonary resuscitation, as a result of excessive administration of hypertonic sodium bicarbonate solutions. In hyperosmolar non-ketotic hyperglycaemia there is marked hyperglycaemia, hyperosmolality, and absence of ketosis, usually associated with combined sodium and water depletion. Correcting the serum sodium for the serum glucose level can alleviate water depletion.

Cranial diabetes insipidus most often results from hypophysectomy or head trauma. It may also occur in association with pituitary infarction due to cerebral oedema from acute hyponatraemia, intracranial tumours or infiltrative disorders such as sarcoidosis. Nephrogenic diabetes insipidus may be congenital and is usually acquired from the use of drugs such as amphotericin B and lithium carbonate. It may also result from impairment of the renal concentrating mechanism by parenchymal disease or electrolyte abnormalities such as hypokalaemia and hypercalcaemia.

The major clinical feature of hypernatraemia resulting from water deficit is central nervous system dysfunction secondary to brain cell shrinkage. Confusion, neuromuscular excitability, seizures or coma may result. Hyperviscosity may increase the likelihood of cerebral infarction in predisposed older patients. The mortality rate is about 40% in the older hospitalised patient and is highest in patients with a rapid onset of hypernatraemia and in those with serum sodium concentrations >160 mmol/l. The initial treatment of hypernatraemia involves water replacement, which can be accomplished orally in the conscious patient without GI disturbance. Otherwise, patients may respond to intravenous infusion of 5% dextrose. In cases of severe volume disturbances, 0.9% NaCl may be required before using hypotonic 0.45% NaCl. Since over-rapid correction may lead to cerebral oedema, the serum sodium concentration should be lowered by no more than 2 mmol/l/h. In cranial diabetes insipidus, administration of vasopressin prevents renal water loss. In nephrogenic diabetes insipidus, administration of a thiazide diuretic along with sodium restriction reduces free water loss.

Hyponatraemia

Hyponatraemia is the commonest electrolyte

disturbance in older patients and is a common contributor to delirium. The clinician must be aware of the possibility of spurious hyponatraemia in patients with hyperlipidaemia or hyperproteinaemia. Pseudohyponatraemia may also occur in the setting of severe hyperglycaemia, where high blood glucose concentrations draw intracellular water into the extracellular space.

In all hyponatraemic states there is an excess of extracellular water relative to the total sodium content of the extracellular compartment. In hypovolaemic hyponatraemia the total extracellular sodium level is lower than normal, resulting in extracellular hypovolaemia. Sodium losses can be incurred through persistent vomiting and/or diarrhoea, extensive skin burns and excessive prolonged sweating. The healthy kidney will conserve sodium so that urinary sodium concentrations will be <10mmol/l. Renal sodium loss accounts for the hyponatraemia of renal diseases such as analgesic nephropathy, chronic pyelonephritis and polycystic kidney disease. A similar mechanism partially explains the hyponatraemia of mineralocorticoid deficiency in Addison's disease or overdiuresis. Hyponatraemia is associated with the use of serotonergic antidepressants in older patients.

Normovolaemic hyponatraemia is usually due to the syndrome of inappropriate antidiuretic hormone release (SIADH) or inappropriate administration of intravenous hypotonic solutions and rarely to prolonged severe hypothyroidism. To diagnose SIADH, there must be plasma hypo-osmolality proportional to the hyponatraemia (i.e., dilutional hyponatraemia). Urine osmolality must be greater than plasma osmolality and renal sodium excretion should be persistently >50mmol/l. In addition, hypovolaemia and oedema must be absent. Disorders associated with SIADH (Table 2) include neoplasms, especially oat cell carcinoma of the bronchus; pneumonia (the commonest cause in older patients); subdural haematoma; cytotoxic agents and carbamazepine.

Hypervolaemic hyponatraemia in older patients is commonly seen in severe heart failure, but also in decompensated cirrhosis and the nephrotic syndrome. In these conditions there is a reduced GFR and increased proximal tubular reabsorption of sodium. Renal afferent arteriolar perfusion is diminished, leading to increased circulating levels of angiotensin II, which contributes to thirst stimulation and release of ADH which promotes water retention. Chronic mild hyponatraemia is often asymptomatic but a rapid fall from normal values can cause convulsions. Clinical features of mild hyponatraemia include anorexia, nausea, headache and lethargy. Moderate hyponatraemia may be associated with personality change, muscle cramps, confusion and ataxia. Severe hyponatraemia causes drowsiness, hyporeflexia and convulsions and may progress to coma and death.

Treatment of the underlying cause of hyponatraemia frequently corrects the serum sodium concentration. Infusion of normal saline is usually sufficient in hypovolaemic hyponatraemia. Addisonian crisis demands prompt hydrocortisone as well as intravenous saline. Identification and successful treatment of the underlying cause of SIADH will usually correct the hyponatraemia. If specific treatment of the hyponatraemia is required, this usually takes the form of fluid restriction to 500 ml/24h. If this fails, partial nephrogenic diabetes insipidus may be induced with demeclocycline but maximal effect may take two weeks to achieve. Over-rapid correction of profound hyponatraemia can result in central pontine myelinolysis with quadriparesis, respiratory arrest, pseudobulbar palsy, mutism and fits. In the management of severe hyponatraemia, most authorities agree that the plasma sodium concentration should not rise by more than 10 to 12 mmol/24h. When the fall in plasma sodium is known to have occurred within 12 to 24 hours it is safer to correct plasma sodium more quickly than if the hyponatraemia is more chronic.

Disturbances in calcium metabolism

Hypercalcaemia

The most common cause of hypercalcaemia in older hospitalised patients is malignant disease. Tumours of the breast, lung, kidney, head and neck are particularly associated with bone metastases and hypercalcaemia. The most common mechanism by which hypercalcaemia arises in malignancy is the widespread bone destruction induced by metastases. Tumours may secrete parathyroid hormone-related peptide (PTH-rP) which causes a generalised increase in bone resorption and an increased tubular reabsorption of calcium. Many solid tumours, including squamous cell carcinoma of the lung and oesophagus secrete PTH-rP and specific assays are available.

Primary hyperparathyroidism is the most common cause of hypercalcaemia in the general population.

Often the patients are older females who are found to have a single parathyroid adenoma. Up to 10% of cases are due to hyperplasia of two or more glands or parathyroid carcinoma. Primary hyperparathyroidism is a component of the autosomal dominant multiple endocrine neoplasias – types I and II. Familial hypocalciuric hypercalcaemia is transmitted as an autosomal dominant trait and is characterised by persistent hypercalcaemia, hypocalciuria and hypermagnesaemia. Unlike primary hyperparathyroidism, the hypercalcaemia is usually asymptomatic, renal function is normal and nephrolithiasis is unusual. The fractional excretion of calcium is <1%, whereas it is almost invariably elevated in primary hyperparathyroidism. Affected patients have a mutation in the calcium-sensing receptor causing a reduction in its activity. Serum PTH levels are normal and parathyroidectomy is not indicated. Secondary hyperparathyroidism occurs in the setting of hypocalcaemia caused by renal insufficiency, intestinal malabsorption and inadequate dietary intake. When secondary hyperparathyroidism has been present for some time, sensitivity of the parathyroid glands to calcium may be diminished so that hypersecretion of PTH may continue in the face of normocalcaemia or even hypercalcaemia (i.e., tertiary hyperparathyroidism).

Vitamin D in pharmacological doses produces excessive bone resorption as well as increased intestinal calcium absorption and hypercalciuria. In the milk-alkali syndrome, excessive amounts of calcium and absorbable alkali are ingested resulting in hypercalcaemia. This uncommon disorder may become more prevalent in older patients as the use of calcium preparations increases in efforts to prevent osteoporosis. Likewise, latent primary hyperparathyroidism may be unmasked by calcium and vitamin D replacement in older subjects with undiagnosed osteomalacia. Immobilisation may lead to a rapid increase in bone resorption and hypercalcaemia, especially in the presence of renal insufficiency or Paget's disease of bone. Sarcoidosis is associated with hypercalcaemia in about 20% of patients. It appears to result from the unregulated conversion of 25-hydroxycholecalciferol to 1,25-dihydroxycholecalciferol due to the expression of 1-α-hydroxylase in mononuclear cells within sarcoid granulomas. Hypercalcaemia may also occur in Addison's disease and thyrotoxicosis.

Many older patients with mild hypercalcaemia are asymptomatic and the condition is discovered incidentally. Symptoms include anorexia, constipation, nausea and vomiting and abdominal pain. Impairment of the renal concentrating mechanism leads to nephrogenic diabetes insipidus. Severe hypercalcaemia is associated with emotional lability, confusion, stupor and coma. There may be prominent skeletal muscle weakness. Hypercalciuria with urolithiasis is common. Less frequent is nephrocalcinosis causing reversible acute renal failure or irreversible renal damage. Peptic ulcers and acute pancreatitis may be associated with hyperparathyroidism. The Q-T interval on the ECG is shortened in severe hypercalcaemia. Severe hyperparathyroidism often leads to subperiosteal resorption of bone in the appendicular skeleton and to osteitis fibrosa cystica.

Hypercalcaemia that is neither symptomatic nor progressive requires treatment only of any underlying disorder. Patients with serum calcium concentrations >3 mmol/l are usually dehydrated and the extracellular fluid volume must be restored with intravenous saline. Care should be taken in older patients with impaired cardiac or renal function. Loop diuretics increase urinary calcium excretion but the use of diuretics without adequate volume expansion may aggravate hypercalcaemia. Thiazide diuretics should be avoided since these increase renal tubular reabsorption of calcium. Calcitonin may induce a decrease in serum calcium but this may be of short duration. Bisphosphonates induce a slower but more sustained response. When indicated, intravenous administration of large volumes of fluid over at least 4 hours is recommended because of the nephrotoxicity of precipitated calcium bisphosphonate. The efficacy of corticosteroids in the acute management of hypercalcaemia is doubtful except in patients with myeloma, lymphoma, vitamin D intoxication and sarcoidosis.

Hypocalcaemia

Hypocalcaemia is an infrequent laboratory finding in older patients. It is usually asymptomatic but any clinical manifestations are primarily neurologic. Slowly developing hypocalcaemia may produce diffuse encephalopathy and should enter the differential diagnosis in the older patient with unexplained dementia, depression or psychosis. Cataracts may develop after prolonged hypocalcaemia and papilloedema occasionally exists. Severe hypocalcaemia may cause generalised

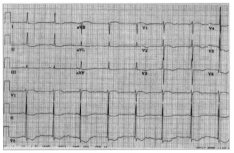
Figure 2: Prolonged QT in a patient with hypocalcaemia

TABLE 3	
PRESENTING FEATURES OF TYPE 1 DIABETES	
Osmotic symptoms	**Associated symptoms**
Thirst	Muscular cramps
Polyuria	Blurred vision
Nocturia	Fungal or bacterial infection
	(oro-genital and cutaneous)
	Fatigue
	Weight loss

seizures. The most characteristic clinical feature is tetany, resulting from severe hypocalcaemia or a reduction in the ionised fraction of serum calcium without marked hypocalcaemia; e.g., in the setting of respiratory or metabolic alkalosis. Tetany gives rise to perioral paraesthesiae, carpopedal spasm, generalised muscle aches, laryngospasm and spasm of the muscles of facial expression. Chvostek and Trousseau's signs may be positive. The ECG typically shows a prolonged Q-T interval.

Hypoparathyroidism causing hypocalcaemia usually complicates the inadvertent removal of or damage to several parathyroid glands during thyroidectomy. Clinical tetany usually begins about 24 to 48 hours postoperatively but may be delayed for months. Pseudohypoparathyroidism is characterised, not by deficiency of PTH, but by target organ unresponsiveness to its action. These patients also commonly have shortened metacarpals, obesity and heterotopic calcification and can survive to old age. Vitamin D deficiency, due to inadequate dietary intake, decreased exposure to sunlight, hepatobiliary disease or malabsorption, may be associated with osteomalacia in older patients. In these patients serum phosphate is mildly reduced, and alkaline phosphatase is elevated. Prolonged therapy with phenytoin may also cause vitamin D deficiency and hypocalcaemia by increasing the turnover of vitamin D into inactive compounds. Chronic renal failure may produce hypocalcaemia due to diminished formation of 1,25-dihydroxycholecalciferol coupled with hyperphosphataemia. Serum magnesium must be measured and corrected if low in every patient being investigated for hypocalcaemia. Metastatic prostate cancer may cause hypocalcaemia by increasing osteoblastic activity in older patients. Acute pancreatitis, although sometimes the result of hypercalcaemia, may itself cause hypocalcaemia when calcium is chelated by lipolytic products. Although high levels of calcitonin

might be expected to cause hypocalcaemia, it is rare in patients with medullary carcinoma of the thyroid. Septic shock is associated with hypocalcaemia through unknown mechanisms.

Acute hypocalcaemia is treated initially with an intravenous infusion of calcium gluconate. Infusions of calcium salts are hazardous in older patients receiving digitalis and should be given slowly with telemetric monitoring. In the postoperative patient with transient hypoparathyroidism after thyroidectomy, oral calcium supplements may be sufficient to prevent hypocalcaemia. Hypocalcaemia may be severe in the so-called hungry bone state that develops following subtotal parathyroidectomy in patients with chronic renal failure due to rapid uptake of calcium into bones. In the chronic hypocalcaemia of hypoparathyroidism or renal failure, calcium usually is given orally with one alpha hydroxylated cholecalciferol. Treatment of hypocalcaemia in patients with renal failure must be combined with dietary phosphorus restriction and phosphate-binding agents such as aluminium hydroxide.

Diabetes mellitus

Diabetes Mellitus is a chronic, debilitating disease and is costly in terms of both human suffering and health care expenditure. It is a metabolic disease characterised by hyperglycaemia resulting from defects in insulin secretion, insulin action or both. Type 2 diabetes, is particularly common in older patients. There is a gradual increase in blood glucose levels with normal ageing and so the prevalence of diabetes also rises; in many western countries 10-20% of those aged 65 or above have diabetes. About 85% of diabetic patients in developed countries will have type 2 diabetes; the remainder have type 1. Type 2 diabetes has become epidemic in the past several decades owing to the advancing age of the population,

TABLE 4	
PRESENTING FEATURES OF TYPE 2 DIABETES	
• Classical symptoms (see Table 3)	50%
• Infections – usually skin, urinary tract or perineal	15%
• Complications- usually retinopathy or macrovascular disease	5%
• Incidental finding	30%

a substantially increased prevalence of obesity and decreased physical activity. The prevalence of type 2 diabetes is predicted to increase to 216 million cases worldwide in 2010, from 99 million in 1994.

Clinical classification:
In 1997 the American Diabetes Association (ADA) classified diabetes into two types based on aetiology rather than therapy. They also introduced the new category of impaired fasting glucose:

• Type I diabetes
(Previously 'insulin-dependent diabetes')
Absolute insulin deficiency, where insulin treatment is necessary for survival.

Type 1 diabetes is caused by autoimmune destruction of the beta-cells in the pancreas, resulting in no insulin production. Ten percent of those diagnosed with diabetes over the age of 65 are insulin dependent.

• Type 2 diabetes
(Previously 'noninsulin-dependent diabetes')
Insulin resistance or relative insulin deficiency, where lifestyle changes or oral therapy may achieve control of blood glucose levels, although insulin may also be used to improve control.

Type 2 diabetes occurs more often in older people who are obese and live sedentary lifestyles. It is believed that up to 50% of people with type 2 diabetes remain undiagnosed and the majority of these are in the older population.

• Impaired glucose tolerance
This represents an intermediate category between normality and diabetes.
Patients with impaired glucose tolerance are not at risk of developing microvascular complications

of diabetes. However, they are at increased risk of developing type 2 diabetes and macrovascular disease. The diagnosis of impaired glucose tolerance relies on glucose tolerance testing. A proportion of individuals who have impaired glucose tolerance diagnosed by an oral glucose tolerance test (OGTT) may revert to normal glucose tolerance on retesting or after implementing diet and lifestyle changes. Intervention studies including the Diabetes Prevention Programme (DPP) and the Study To Prevent Non-Insulin-Dependent Diabetes Mellitus (STOP-NIDDM) have shown that diet and exercise, metformin and acarbose can prevent or delay the development of type 2 diabetes in subjects with IGT.

Establishing the diagnosis
The ADA uses the following criteria for the diagnosis of diabetes:
• Fasting plasma glucose >7.0mmol/l; no calorific intake for previous 8 hours
• Random plasma glucose>11.1mmol/l in association with symptoms of hyperglycaemia
• Plasma glucose level of >11.1mmol/l two hours after a glucose load of 75g (an oral glucose tolerance test)

The diagnosis should be confirmed by repeat testing on a different day unless there is overt metabolic decompensation. Because of the economic implications of the widespread use of the OGTT in testing for diabetes, its use is reserved mainly for research studies and for defining impaired glucose tolerance particularly in relation to pregnancy. The WHO, Diabetes UK and the Diabetic Federation of Ireland have accepted the diagnostic criteria outlined by the ADA. However, there remains some concern that basing the diagnosis on a fasting glucose will still miss some patients who would have had a blood glucose level of greater than 11.1mmol/l 2 hours after a glucose load of 75g. These patients may be at particularly high risk of macrovascular disease. It has therefore been suggested that those people with impaired fasting glucose (defined as a glucose level of 6.1-7.0mmol/l) should have an OGTT performed. It is suggested that as a minimum all patients over 45 years should have a fasting glucose performed at 3 yearly intervals and an OGTT thereafter if necessary.

The insulin resistance syndrome
It has been recognised for many years that diabetes is an important and independent risk factor for large vessel disease, particularly cardiovascular

disease. This association is particularly strong in type 2 diabetes, which is also associated with a number of other cardiovascular risk factors including hypertension, dyslipidaemia and obesity. This cluster of risk factors has a number of synonyms: 'syndrome x', 'Reaven's syndrome' and the 'metabolic syndrome'. The key features include:

• Insulin resistance (eventually low insulin levels)
• Glucose intolerance or diabetes mellitus
• Dyslipidaemia
• Obesity
• Essential hypertension

Environmental factors such as physical inactivity and possibly cigarette smoking may exacerbate insulin resistance. There is considerable epidemiological and experimental evidence that the insulin resistance syndrome confers an increased risk of cardiovascular disease. It is felt that the effects are synergistic rather than simply additive. Treatment of the insulin resistance syndrome with diet, exercise and weight loss may prevent progression to diabetes and heart disease.

Vascular complications of diabetes
Diabetes is associated with long term vascular complications at the macrovascular and microvascular levels. Although these two classes of complications have been defined separately, the vascular damage caused by diabetes often develops concurrently and affects several systems, resulting in severe disability and reduced life expectancy. The average delay of four to seven years in diagnosing type 2 diabetes translates into approximately 20% of patients having some evidence of diabetic complications at the time of diagnosis.

Macrovascular complications
• Ischaemic heart disease
• Cerebrovascular disease
• Peripheral vascular disease

Microvascular complications
• Nephropathy
• Retinopathy
• Neuropathy

Diabetes and hypertension
Hypertension is up to three times as prevalent in diabetics as in non-diabetics. The prevalence of hypertension increases with age. Hypertension in diabetes accelerates the progression of microvascular

and macrovascular complications. In those with type 1 disease hypertension becomes established with the development of diabetic nephropathy. A sustained rise in BP within the normal range and a disturbance in the diurnal changes in BP may be early features of nephropathy. Hypertension causes progression of the nephropathy and thus a further rise in BP. The hypertension associated with type 2 diabetes is multifactorial. It is often associated with the metabolic syndrome and its development is similar to that in non-diabetic patients. Obesity is an important contributor to the prevalence of hypertension in type 2 diabetes but other factors include sodium retention and activation of the renin-angiotensin system. As with type 1 patients the development of nephropathy further contributes to the development of hypertension and the progression of microvascular and macrovascular complications.

Isolated systolic hypertension (ISH), which may result from decreased arterial elasticity, is most commonly seen in older patients but occurs about 20 years earlier in diabetic patients. Hypertension should be treated early and aggressively to reduce the development of diabetic complications. Multiple clinical trials have been done in this area to determine optimum blood pressure targets and best therapies to use. These include the following:
• The blood pressure control arm of the UK Prospective Diabetes Study Group (UKPDS)
• The Hypertension Optimal Treatment (HOT) trial
• The Captopril Prevention Project (CAPPP)
The above studies and many others have lead to guidelines for the treatment of hypertension in diabetic patients. The ADA and the WHO endorse these guidelines. The target BP levels for diabetic patients are as follows:
<130/85 mmHg (normoalbuminuria)
<130/80 mmHg (abnormal albumin excretion)

Less ambitious goals for the older patient may be acceptable if they experience troublesome side effects on antihypertensive medication, particularly postural hypotension. If postural hypotension is suspected twenty-four hour blood pressure monitoring should be performed to confirm this. Meanwhile the target systolic blood pressure level in ISH is 160-140mmHg.

An ACE inhibitor is recommended for the treatment of hypertension in the following groups:

TABLE 5
SUGGESTED ANTIHYPERTENSIVE TREATMENT IN OLDER DIABETIC PATIENTS

DRUGS AND POSSIBLE INDICATION	AVOID WITH CONCURRENT
ACE Inhibitors - first line if tolerated	Renal artery stenosis
	Aortic stenosis
Angiotensin receptor blockers - if ACE not tolerated	
β Blockers - especially if history of MI	Asthma or COPD
	Obesity
± Diuretic - use low dose in older patients	
± Calcium channel blockers	Sick sinus syndrome
± Alpha blockers	Postural hypotension

- Type 1 and Type 2 diabetic patients with abnormal albumin excretion
- Type 1 normotensive patients with abnormal albumin excretion

Guidelines for the treatment of normotensive type 2 diabetics with normoalbuminuria are less clear but there is some evidence that these patients also benefit from the addition of an ACE inhibitor providing there are no contraindications to their use. Analysis of the outcomes in the diabetic subgroup of the Heart Outcomes Prevention Evaluation (HOPE) trial showed that these patients with one other cardiovascular risk factor who were commenced on an ACE inhibitor had a reduction in the incidence of all cause mortality and morbidity. In addition, an ACE inhibitor reduced the development of diabetic complications and overt nephropathy. Although drug selection is important and several factors should be considered when choosing drugs the attained blood

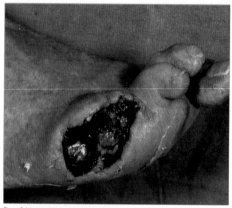

Figure 3: Neuropathic ulcer in diabetic patient

pressure level appears to be more important than the drugs used. In the UKPDS it was found that multiple drug therapies (three or more agents) were required in the tight blood pressure control group.

Long term follow up of patients over more than 10 years after enrolment in the UKPDS study, recently confirmed that the benefit of tight control of blood pressure fails to endure over that period. This absence of a 'legacy effect' contrasts with the persistence of reduction of poor outcomes over many years in those who had tight glycaemic control during the same study.

Diabetes and dyslipidaemia
Patients with well-controlled type 1 diabetes do not have abnormal lipid profiles. The lipid profile becomes abnormal with poor control and with the development of nephropathy. Type 2 diabetes is associated with the characteristic dyslipidaemia of elevated very low-density lipoprotein (VLDL) and low-density lipoprotein (LDL) and reduced high-density lipoprotein (HDL). This lipid profile is associated with obesity and may precede diabetes. Poorly controlled diabetes may lead to hypertriglyceridaemia. However, even in the presence of normoglycaemia, hypertriglyceridaemia is more common in type 2 diabetics and is associated with insulin resistance. Diabetics without symptomatic atherosclerotic disease experience a similar rate of major cardiovascular events to nondiabetics with pre-existing coronary disease. This together with recent results from clinical trials of lipid modifying drugs has lead to an increased awareness of the importance of detecting and treating dyslipidaemia. It is apparent that cholesterol lowering may not only prevent coronary events but may also reduce

TABLE 6		
ADA CLINICAL PRACTICE GUIDELINES		
Biochemical Index	**Normal**	**Goal**
Preprandial glucose (mmol/l)	<6.1	4.4 – 6.7
Bedtime glucose	<6.7	5.6 – 7.8
HbAIC %	<6	<7

ischaemic symptoms and episodes. Although no large randomised placebo controlled trials have primarily addressed the role of lipid lowering in diabetics, several of the major recent studies have included diabetic subjects including The Scandinavian Simvastatin Survival Study (4S), The Cholesterol and Recurrent Events Study (CARE) and The Heart Protection Study (HPS).

Dyslipidaemia and the older patient
Data from the Framingham study suggest that average annual rates of a first major CHD event increases from 5/1000 men at age 35-44 years to 59/1000 age 85-94 years. Studies suggest that treating patients with dyslipidaemia over 65 years of age is effective in reducing CHD and death. All studies when analysed showed that older people in particular benefited from statin therapy. The PROSPER study looked specifically at the benefits of pravastatin in an older population with, or at high risk of developing cardiovascular disease or stroke. It showed a 24% reduction in mortality from CHD in the treated group. The 4S and CARE studies also suggest that a mortality rate benefit is achieved within 12 – 18 months of commencing a statin and that endothelial function and symptoms may be improved within 6 months. This clearly opposes the argument that older patients may not live long enough to benefit from cholesterol treatment. Assuming that there are no other significant co-morbidities all patients should be considered for treatment, independent of age.

Therapeutic targets in diabetic dyslipidaemia
The treatment of dyslipidaemia in diabetics often involves diet, weight-reduction, increased exercise and improved glycaemic control. The question then arises as to which diabetic patients should be on lipid lowering agents. The HPS would suggest that all patients with diabetes irrespective of cholesterol levels should be on a statin. If, after maximising statin therapy and controlling diabetes, the triglyceride level remains high then the addition of a fibrate should be

TABLE 7		
CAUSES OF HYPOTHYROIDISM		
Goitre present	**TSH**	**Free T4**
Chronic thyroiditis (Hashimoto's thyroiditis)	↑	↓
Goitre absent		
Following radioiodine or surgery for hyperthyroidism	↑	↓
Atrophic thyroiditis	↑	↓
Drug induced eg: amiodarone or lithium	↑	↓
Pituitary failure	↓	↓
Hypothalamic causes	↓	↓
→tumour		
→infection		
→infiltration eg. sarcoid		

considered. The clinical practice recommendations of the ADA published in 1999 state that the target levels should be as follows:
- LDL cholesterol ≤ 2.6mmol/l
- Triglyceride < 2.0mmol/l
- HDL cholesterol > 0.9 mmol/l in men and >1.15 mmol/l in women

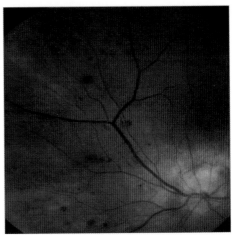

Figure 4: Diabetic retinopathy

Microvascular complications
Diabetic microangiopathy is a specific disease of the small blood vessels, clinically apparent in the kidneys,

eyes and peripheral nerves. The microvascular complications of diabetes account for a high incidence of morbidity and in the case of nephropathy, mortality. Risk factors for diabetic microangiopathy include poor metabolic control, hypertension and duration of diabetes.

Diabetic nephropathy

This is the commonest cause of end-stage renal failure worldwide and it occurs in patients with type 1 or type 2 diabetes. The earliest feature of diabetic nephropathy is microalbuminuria. Screening should occur annually. Results from the Diabetes Control and Complications Trial (DCCT) and the UKPDS have shown that intensive glycaemic control can allay the onset and delay the progression of nephropathy in type 1 and type 2 diabetic patients respectively. Blood pressure control may be one of the most important factors in protecting the kidney against progressive renal disease in diabetes. ACE inhibitors appear to have a renoprotective effect that is additional to their antihypertensive action.

Diabetic retinopathy

This is the commonest cause of blindness among adults aged 20-74. The prevalence of retinopathy is strongly related to the duration of diabetes. The results of the DCCT and the UKPDS showed that good glycaemic control reduces the risk of development and progression of diabetic retinopathy. Proteinuria and high BP are also risk factors. Data from the ELUCID study suggest that ACE inhibitors may also prevent the development and progression of retinopathy in patients with type 1 diabetes, irrespective of BP. Patients should be screened annually for the presence of retinopathy. Laser photocoagulation is the mainstay of treatment for sight-threatening diabetic retinopathy.

Diabetic neuropathy

The diabetic neuropathies are diverse disorders of nerve function associated with diabetes. Approximately 60-70% of patients with diabetes have some form of diabetic neuropathy. The major complication of diabetic neuropathy is foot ulceration. The diabetic neuropathic foot may develop callouses and ulcers, which are painless. If they become infected amputation of the foot or leg may be necessary. The DCCT and the UKPDS demonstrated a reduction in the progression of clinical neuropathy in those individuals with tight glycaemic control. The mainstay of treatment for patients with significant neuropathy is education to reduce the risk of foot ulceration and symptomatic relief.

Management of diabetes

The aims of treatment are firstly, to save life and to alleviate symptoms and secondly, to achieve the best possible control of diabetes with blood glucose concentrations as near normal as possible to minimise long term complications. In the older patient the aims of management will depend on the individual. A healthy 70-year-old lady has a life expectancy of at least 12 years and therefore should be treated aggressively to avoid complications. However, in a patient whose life expectancy is likely to be much less the aims of treatment might be to alleviate symptoms and to prevent acute complications with the minimum of unwanted effects from treatment. As in all other age groups standard treatment goals need to be set for the older patient. These may be modified if there are co-morbidities or risks of treatment side-effects. Results from the DCCT in type 1 diabetic patients and the UKPDS in type 2 diabetic patients showed that improved glycaemic control significantly reduced the risk of microvascular complications. Tight diabetic control, however, was associated with up to a three-fold increase in the incidence of hypoglycaemic episodes. In 1999 the ADA published clinical practice recommendations as shown in Table 6.

In type 1 diabetes insulin is necessary for survival. Subcutaneous insulin is administered usually in one of two regimens depending on patient's lifestyle and ability and willingness to self inject.

• A Multiple Daily Injection Programme: Here, short acting insulin is given preprandially with a long-acting insulin at night
• A Twice Daily Regimen: This involves injecting a mixture of short and long acting insulin twice daily

Traditionally the treatment of type 2 diabetes has been a step wise approach commencing with dietary and lifestyle changes followed by oral agents. Insulin therapy despite being the most effective and durable hypoglycaemic intervention available has generally been saved until last. All diabetic patients should be advised on a diabetic diet. This differs little from a normal healthy diet that is recommended to the general population. Those who are overweight (BMI >25) should be advised on a hypocaloric diet. Plasma glucose levels fall with hypocaloric diets, before weight loss occurs, and levels can decline into the near normal range with a weight loss of even 2.3 to 4.5kg. Patients should also be advised to increase their activity levels. For type 2 diabetic patients who are unable to change their lifestyle through weight loss and increased activity and for those who make these lifestyle changes but continue to have blood glucose levels above the target range oral agents should be added. When choosing an oral agent in the diabetic patient any co-existing comorbidity must be considered. In particular for an older population the following should be remembered:

- Cerebrovascular and cardiovascular disease are common
- Polypharmacy is often necessary and therefore carries the risk of drug interactions
- Impaired renal and hepatic function may increase the risk of adverse events with antidiabetic medication

The sulphonylureas and the biguanide, metformin are the oldest and most commonly used classes of oral hypoglycaemic drugs.

Metformin

Its main action is to decrease hepatic glucose output and to improve insulin sensitivity. In appropriately selected older patients, particularly those who are overweight, it is the oral agent of first choice, as it does not carry the same risk of weight gain or hypoglycaemia as other agents. About 10% of patients cannot tolerate the drug because of GI side effects. It is contraindicated in patients with moderate to severe renal impairment because of the risk of developing lactic acidosis. It is also contraindicated in liver and heart failure.

Sulphonylureas

These act by stimulating insulin secretion. There must be some pancreatic β-cells functioning for sulphonylureas to act. The shorter acting second-generation drugs such as gliclazide should be used in older patients to minimise the risk of hypoglycaemia. The once daily preparations may aid compliance. Side effects include weight gain. Hypoglycaemia especially with the shorter acting agents is rare but has a high case-fatality rate. Chlorpropamide and glibenclamide are associated with a high risk of hypoglycaemia and should not be used in older patients. Other oral hypoglycaemic agents have become available in the past few years, but currently play a supporting role in older patients. They include:

- Glucosidase inhibitors eg. acarbose

Inhibit the absorption of carbohydrates in the small intestine. They are associated with a high risk of GI disturbance

- Thiazolidinediones eg. rosiglitazone

Increase peripheral glucose uptake and act as insulin sensitisers in adipose tissues, liver and muscle cells. Avoid in heart failure, IHD, PAD

- Prandial glucose regulators eg. nateglanide

Act on β-cell surface to transiently stimulate insulin release

- Incretin mimetic drugs eg. exanatide

Increase insulin secretion, suppress glucagon secretion and slow gastric emptying

Combination therapy

Control may not be achieved with monotherapy alone and as diabetes is a progressive disease with worsening of metabolic control likely over time, combination therapy often needs to be used. The principle behind combination therapy is to use drugs with different mechanisms of action, such as:

- A sulphonylurea and metformin
- A sulphonylurea and a thiazolidinedione
- Metformin and a thiazolidinedione
- Metformin and insulin

Insulin therapy becomes necessary in a significant proportion of older type 2 diabetic patients. Insulin therapy should not be denied to older patients and many may derive a feeling of wellbeing from better control of their diabetes. A trial of insulin therapy may therefore be warranted if drug failure occurs. Most patients with type 2 diabetes will be started on one of the following regimens:

- Once daily insulin
- Once daily insulin with an oral hypoglycaemic agent, usually metformin
- Twice daily mixed insulin

A few patients will opt for a Multiple Daily Injection Programme for flexibility. The most common regime for successful insulin therapy involves the use of a sufficiently large dose of insulin, typical range 0.6 to 1.0U per kilogram of body weight per day, to achieve or approach normoglycaemia, rather than any specific pattern of insulin administration. Guidelines have been issued by the American Geriatrics Society (AGS) for the management

TABLE 8
SYSTEMIC FEATURES OF HYPOTHYROIDISM IN OLDER PATIENTS

Nervous system	• Cerebellar dysfunction which may lead to ataxia and falls
	• Sensorineural deafness
	• Rarely reversible dementia
	• Paradoxical hyperactivity of myxoedematous madness
Cardiovascular	• Heart block and arrhythmias
	• Hypertension (hypotensive in severe hypothyroidism)
	• Angina and myocardial ischaemia, which may improve with thyroxine replacement, however, initiation of treatment in these patients must be done very cautiously.

TABLE 9		
CAUSES OF THYROTOXICOSIS		
	TSH	**Free T4**
Graves Disease	↓	↑
Toxic Adenoma	↓	↑
Subacute (De Quervain's) thyroiditis	↓	↑
Drug induced thyroiditis (amiodarone)	↓	↑
Over-treatment with thyroid hormone	↓	↑

of diabetes in older patients. These include, specifically, a recommendation for screening for six geriatric 'syndromes' which are more prevalent in older diabetic patients. They include polypharmacy, depression, cognitive impairment, urinary incontinence, injurious falls and neuropathic pain.

New ADA guidelines and European guidelines have recently been published regarding management of diabetes mellitus in older patients. These emphasise the potential role of incretin mimetic agents such as exenatide, a synthetic form of exendin-4. Of significance in these guidelines is the fact that rimonabant, a cannabinoid receptor antagonist used for adjunctive management of obesity has been withdrawn from the market due to unacceptable side effects. Details relating to these guidelines can be accessed using the reference at the end of this chapter.

Thyroid disease

The normal thyroid weighs between 15 and 25g. It comprises of a midline isthmus lying just below the cricoid cartilage and has two lateral lobes that extend upward over the lower half of the thyroid cartilage. Thyroid hormone abnormalities are usually due to a problem with the thyroid gland itself. Primary abnormalities of thyroid stimulating hormone (TSH) and thyroid releasing hormone (TRH) are very rare. The levels of thyroid hormones in the body are tightly controlled by the negative feedback mechanisms involved in the hypothalamic – pituitary - thyroid axis. The thyroid gland produces mainly T4, which is much less active than T3. Over 80% of T3 is formed from the peripheral conversion of T4. In the blood T4 and T3 are mainly bound to proteins. Only the free hormone is active. The widespread availability of precise measurements of thyroid hormone levels and TSH in blood has transformed the determination of thyroid status.

Hypothyroidism
Hypothyroidism may affect every organ system in the body. In its extreme form it is clinically obvious; however, the signs may be subtle and go undiagnosed for years.

Older hypothyroid patients may occasionally develop myxoedema coma, which can be precipitated by cold exposure, trauma, infection and administration of centrally acting depressants such as sedatives. The neurological and cardiovascular systems of the older patient may be more susceptible to the effects of hypothyroidism and specific symptoms are summarised in Table 8.

Hyperthyroidism.
Hyperthyroidism refers to those conditions where hyperfunction of the thyroid gland leads to thyrotoxicosis. Thyrotoxicosis refers to the clinical and biochemical findings that result when tissues are exposed to excess thyroid hormone. Age plays a major role in determining the clinical picture of thyrotoxicosis. Atypical presentations occur more frequently in older patients. Anorexia is very common and older patients often lack eye signs or goitre.

The antithyroid drugs namely, carbimazole and propylthiouracil are well tolerated, however 1– 5%

of patients may present with allergic type reactions; rash, fever and arthralgia. If a patient develops these side effects on one drug, it is worth trying them on a second agent. The rare but serious side effect of agranulocytosis occurs in 0.1- 0.5% of patients. Because of cross reactivity of this reaction, one drug should never be substituted for the other.

Treatment of thyrotoxicosis in older patients

Patients are initially commenced on anti-thyroid drugs with or without the addition of a beta- blocker for early symptomatic relief. Beta-blockers are avoided in asthma or possibly in heart failure. Subacute thyroiditis does not require treatment with antithyroid drugs. Most cases of thyrotoxicosis will require more definitive treatment. The options are either surgery or radioiodine therapy.

Surgery is usually reserved for the following older patients:
• those in whom a rapid control in symptoms is desired
• those with severe Grave's opthalmopathy
• those with large goitres which are causing local compressive symptoms

Most older patients requiring definitive treatment of their hyperthyroidism should have radioiodine therapy. The following should be remembered about radio-iodine therapy:
• The thyrotoxicosis may not be controlled for months following treatment
• Some patients need more than one treatment
• Those with Grave's disease must not have active opthalmopathy as this may be acutely worsened by radioiodine therapy

Suggested further reading

• Ahuja TS, Freeman Jr D, Mahnken JD, et al. Predictors of the development of hyperkalemia in patients using angiotensin-converting enzyme inhibitors. Am J Nephrol 2000; 20(4): 268-72.
• American Diabetes Association. Clinical Practice Recommendations. Diabetes Care 1999; 22(Suppl 1): S1-S114.
• Baylis PH. Water and electrolyte metabolism. In Weatherall DJ, Ledingham JGG, Warrell DA, eds, Oxford Textbook of Medicine, 3rd ed., Vol. 3, Section 20.2, pp. 3116-35. Oxford University Press 1996.
• Biswas K, Mulkerrin EC. Potassium homoeostasis in the elderly. Q J Med 1997; 90: 487-92.
• Bushinsky DA, Monk RD. Electrolyte quintet – Calcium. Lancet 1998; 352: 306-11.
• California Healthcare Foundation/AGS Panel on Improving Care for Elders with Diabetes. Guidelines for Improving the Care of the Older Person with Diabetes Mellitus. J Am Ger Soc 2003; 5(suppl): S265-S280.
• Castelli WP, Garrison RJ, Wilson PW, Abbott RD, Kalousdian S, Kannel WB. Incidence of coronary heart disease and lipoprotein cholesterol levels. The Framingham Study. JAMA 1986; 256: 2835-8.
• Chiasson JL, Josse RG, Gomis R et al. Acarbose for prevention of type 2 diabetes mellitus: the STOP-NIDDM randomised trial. Lancet 2002; 359: 2072-77.
• Colbert D. Fluid and electrolyte balance. In Colbert D, Fundamentals of Clinical Physiology, Cambridge: Prentice Hall International (UK) Ltd., 1993.
• Curb JD, Pressel SL, Cutler JA et al. Effects of diuretic-based antihypertensive treatment on cardiovascular disease risk in older diabetic patients with isolated systolic hypertension. Systolic Hypertension in the Elderly Program Co-operative Research Group. JAMA 1996; 276: 1886-97.
• DAIS Investigators. Effect of fenofibrate on progression of coronary-artery disease in type 2 diabetes: the Diabetes Atherosclerosis Intervention Study, a randomised study. Lancet 2001; 357: 905-10.
• Diabetes Control and Complications Trial Research Group. The effect of intensive treatment of diabetes on the development and progression of long-term complications in insulin-dependent diabetes mellitus. N Engl J Med 1993; 329: 977-86.
• Diabetes Control and Complications Trial Research Group. Effect of intensive diabetes management on macrovascular events and risk factors in the Diabetes Control and Complications Trial. Am J Cardiol 1995; 75; 894-903.
• Diabetes Prevention Program Research Group. Reduction in the incidence of type 2 diabetes with lifestyle intervention or metformin. N Engl J Med 2002; 346: 393-403.
• Epstein M. Aging and the kidney. J Am Soc Nephrol 1996; 7(8): 1106-22.
• Erkelens DW, Insulin resistance syndrome and type 2 diabetes mellitus. Am J Cardiol, 2001; 88(suppl): 38j-42j.
• Estacio RO, Jeffers BW, Gifford N, Schrier RW. Effect of blood pressure control on diabetic microvascular complications in patients with hypertension and type 2 diabetes. Diabetes Care 2000; 23(suppl. 2): B54-64.
• EUCLID Study Group. Effect of lisinopril on progression of retinopathy in normotensive people with type 1 diabetes. Lancet 1998; 351: 28-31.
• Fonseca V, Rosenstock J, Patwardhan R, Salzman A. Effect of metformin and rosiglitazone combination

therapy in patients with type 2 diabetes mellitus; a randomised controlled trial. JAMA 2000; 283: 1695-702.

• Goldberg RB, Mellies MJ, Sacks FM et al. Cardiovascular events and their reduction with pravaststin in diabetic and glucose-intolerant myocardial infarction survivors with average cholesterol levels: subgroup analyses in the cholesterol and recurrent events (CARE) TRIAL. The Care Investigators. Circulation 1998; 98: 2513-9.

• Grover SA, Coupal L, Zowall H, Dorais M. Cost-effectiveness of treating hyperlipidaemia in the presence of diabetes: who should be treated? Circulation 2000; 102: 722-7.

• Haffner SM, Alexander CM, Cook TJ et al. Reduced coronary events in simvastatin-treated patients with coronary heart disease and diabetes or impaired fasting glucose levels: subgroup analyses in the Scandinavian Simvastatin Survival Study. Arch Intern Med 1985; 313: 1557-63.

• Halperin ML, Kamel KS. Electrolyte quintet - Potassium. Lancet 1998; 352:135-40.

• Hansson L, Zanchetti A, Carruthers SG et al. Effects of blood pressure lowering and low-dose aspirin in patients with hypertension: principal results of the Hypertension Optimal Treatment (HOT) randomised trial. HOT Study Group. Lancet 1998; 351: 1755-62.

• Hansson L et al. Effect of angiotensin-converting-enzyme inhibition compared with conventional therapy on cardiovascular morbidity and mortality in hypertension: the Captopril Prevention Project (CAPPP) randomised trial. CAPPP Study Group. Lancet 1999; 353: 611-16.

• Heart Outcomes Prevention Evaluation (HOPE) Study Investigators. Effects of ramipril on cardiovascular and microvascular outcomes in people with diabetes mellitus: results or the HOPE study and MICRO-HOPE substudy. Lancet 1999; 355: 253-9.

• Heart Protection Study Collaborative Group. MRC/BHF Heart Protection Study of cholesterol lowering with simvastatin in 20536 high-risk individuals: a randomised placebo-controlled trial. Lancet 2002; 360: 7-22.

• Kannel WB, McGee DL. Diabetes and cardiovascular disease. The Framingham Study. JAMA 1979; 241; 2035-8.

• Kumar S, Berl T. Electrolyte quintet - Sodium. Lancet 1998; 352: 220-28.

• Li CL, Pan CY, Lu JM et al. Effect of metformin on patients with impaired glucose tolerance. Diabetes Med 1999; 16: 477-81.

• Maury E, Lemant J, Dussaule J, et al. Case report: A reversible paralysis. Lancet 2002; 360: 1160.

• Movig KL, Leufkens HG, Lenderink AW, et al. Serotonergic antidepressants associated with an increased risk for hyponatraemia in the elderly. Eur J Clin Pharmacol 2002; 58(2): 143-8.

• Mulkerrin E, Epstein FH, Clark BA. Aldosterone responses to hyperkalemia in healthy elderly humans. J Am Soc Nephrol 1995; 6(5): 1459-62.

• Nathan DM. Initial Management of Glycemia in Type 2 Diabetes Mellitus. N Engl J Med 2002; 347: 1342-48.

• National Cholesterol Education Program. Executive Summary of the Third Report of the NCEP Expert Panel on Detection, Evaluation and Treatment of High Blood Cholesterol in Adults (Adult Treatment Panel III). JAMA 2001; 285: 2486-2497.

• Palevsky PM. Hypernatremia. Semin Nephrol 1998; 18(1): 20-30.

• Sowinski KM, Mueller BA. Hyperkalaemia and apple juice. Lancet 2001; 358: 841-2.

• Tuomilehto J, Lindstrom J, Eriksson JG et al. Prevention of type 2 diabetes mellitus by changes in lifestyle among subjects with impaired glucose tolerance. N Engl J Med 2001; 1343-50.

• UK Prospective Diabetes Study (UKPDS) Group. Effect of intensive blood-glucose control with metformin on complications in overweight patients with type 2 diabetes. (UKPDS 33) Lancet 1998b; 352: 837-53.

• UK Prospective Diabetes Study Group. Tight blood pressure control and risk of macrovascular and microvascular complications in type 2 diabetes: UKPDS 38. BMJ 1998c; 317; 703-13.

• UK Prospective Diabetes Study Group. Efficacy of atenolol and captopril in reducing risk of macrovascular and microvascular complications in type 2 diabetes: UKPDS 39. BMJ 1998d; 317:713-20.

• Rury R. Holman, Sanjoy K. Paul, M. Angelyn Bethel, David R. Matthews,., and H. Andrew W. Neil. 10 – year follow – up of intensive glucose control in type 2 diabetes. N Engl J Med 2008; 359: 1577-89.

• Rury R. Holman, Sanjoy K. Paul, M. Angelyn Bethel, David R. Matthews. Long-term follow up after tight control of blood pressure in Type 2 diabetes. N Engl J Med 2008; 359: 1565-76.

• McGreevy C, Horan J, Jones D, Biswas K, O'Meara YM, Mulkerrin EC. A study of tubular potassium secretory capacity in older patients with hyperkalaemia. J Nutr Health Ageing. 2008 Feb; 12(2): 152-5.

• Nathan DM, Buse JB, Davidson MB, Ferrannini E, Holman RR, Sherwin R, Zinman B. Diabetologia. 2008 October 22nd. Medical management of hyperglycaemia in type 2 diabetes mellitus: a consensus algorithm for the initiation and adjustment of therapy: A consensus statement from the American Diabetes Association and the European Association for the Study of Diabetes.

Case Study 1

A 78 year old lady is seen at the GP surgery complaining of generalised weakness. Past medical history included late onset asthma, hypertension and venous insufficiency. Medications are prednisolone, frusemide/amiloride combination and theophylline. Bloods: sodium 128mmol/l, potassium 5.9mmol/l, urea 14mmol/l, creatinine 126umol/l.

The most likely cause is iatrogenic due to diuretic therapy, the hyponatraemia and hyperkalaemia being secondary to amiloride. The raised urea, with relatively normal creatinine are due to dehydration secondary to the loop diuretic. A less likely cause of similar biochemistry would be Addison's disease.

Case Study 2

An 80 year old man was seen in the accident and emergency department with a 2-day history of increased confusion. He had been generally well until he had an accidental fall with bruising on his shoulder and leg two weeks previously. Bloods: sodium 123mmol/l, potassium 3.1mmol/l, urea 2.0mmol/l, creatinine 57umol/l and glucose 6.2mmol/l.

This is likely to be a dilutional hyponatraemia secondary to SIADH. A CT brain scan is urgently indicated as a likely underlying cause is chronic subdural haematoma subsequent to his recent fall. Confirmation of SIADH by urine and serum osmolalities and urine sodium estimation would be appropriate and a search for other causes would be necessary if CT scan was negative.

Case Study 3

After an overnight fast, an asymptomatic 70 year old gentleman has a plasma glucose level of 8.2mmol/l on initial evaluation and 7.9mmol/l on re-evaluation. Other than a steady weight gain over the previous 10 years, despite attempts at weight loss, and dyslipidaemia, his medical history is unremarkable. He is 175cm tall and weighs 95kg with a body-mass index of 31.2, and his BP is 145/89mmHg. His physical examination is notable only for abdominal obesity and absent ankle reflexes. The result of a fasting lipid profile is as follow: cholesterol 5.5mmol/l, LDL 3.0mmol/l, HDL 0.7mmol/l, triglycerides 2.8mmol/l.

This gentleman has newly diagnosed type 2 diabetes with associated dyslipidaemia. He is overweight and hypertensive. The absent ankle reflex may suggest peripheral neuropathy raising the possibility that he has had diabetes undiagnosed for some time. The fact that he has previously tried in vain to lose weight would warrant thyroid function tests to outrule associated hypothyroidism. The gentleman should be commenced on a diet (low calorie and low fat) and encouraged to increase his physical activity. He should be educated about diabetes and its complications and encouraged to monitor his blood sugars regularly. He should be assessed for evidence of end organ damage including microalbuminuria, fundoscopy, detailed history for evidence of cardiac ischaemia and peripheral vascular disease. He should be commenced on aspirin and possibly an ACE inhibitor if there are no contra-indications. Based on the HPS data, statin therapy should be added independent of his cholesterol and LDL levels. If, after three months of diet and exercise, his glycosylated haemoglobin (HbA1C) values are not less than 7%, he should be commenced on an oral hypoglycaemic agent. Metformin should be considered as first line here, since it is less likely to cause weight gain. If after a further three-month period he fails to reach treatment goals a sulphonylurea or thiazolidinedione should be added. Thereafter if his goals are not achieved insulin therapy should be commenced if feasible.

Case Study 4

An 82 year old gentleman with a history of type 2 diabetes for 15 years presents with an ulcer on the sole of his left foot. His examination shows an infected ulcer, 1cm in diameter under the head of the first metatarsal, he has loss of sensation to light touch, vibration and pinprick in a glove and stocking distribution. His feet are cold, the foot pulses are not palpable and he has loss of hair growth on the lower legs. His blood pressure is 125/72, he has proteinuria and fundoscopy shows evidence of background diabetic retinopathy. His usual medications are as follows: metformin 1g bd, gliclazide 120mg od, aspirin 75mg od. His HbA1C is 9%.

This man has an infected neuropathic ulcer on the sole of his foot with evidence of peripheral vascular disease. He should have an x-ray of his foot to ensure that there is no evidence of osteomyelitis. He should be commenced on appropriate empirical antibiotic therapy and kept on bed rest to allow ulcer healing. The degree of his peripheral vascular disease should be assessed and treated as appropriate. His diabetes is not controlled and he has evidence of established mircovascular and macrovascular complications. He should be considered for insulin therapy to improve his glycaemic control. A once daily nocturnal injection of insulin glargine in combination with his usual dose of metformin may achieve good glycaemic control. He should be commenced on a statin and an ACE inhibitor providing he has no contraindication to either. He should be given foot care advice and followed up regularly by a podiatrist.

Case Study 5

A 68 year old lady presented to her GP with increasing myalgia and fatigue. On examination she was overweight with a myxoedematous facies with thickened and coarse facial features, periorbital puffiness and pallor. Her skin was dry and cold with a yellowish tint from hypercarotenaemia. Her movements were slow and her daughter reported that recently she has been forgetful. There was thinning of her hair, which was dry and brittle. She had no palpable goitre. The relaxation phase of her ankle jerk was slow and multiphasic. Baseline investigations were as follows:

↑ TSH/↓ T4
Dyslipidaemia→ elevated total cholesterol and triglyceride level.
Normochromic anaemia
Mildly elevated creatinine kinase level
ECG showed sinus bradycardia with low volume complexes

The diagnosis is primary atrophic hypothyroidism – a common autoimmune disease, which is associated with other autoimmune diseases. The treatment is thyroxine replacement therapy. It is usual to commence with a low dose in older patients to avoid precipitating angina in patients with pre-existing heart disease eg: 25-50μg/day for 2-4 weeks. The dose is thereafter adjusted according to the TSH level. The patient represented 3 weeks later with worsening of her myalgia. This is not uncommon as myalgia may occasionally worsen transiently when thyroid hormone replacement is begun in older patients. The patient should be encouraged to continue with therapy.

Case Study 6

An asymptomatic 65 year old gentleman had routine blood tests done and his results included the following; an elevated TSH of 8.5mU/l with normal free T4 and T3 levels.

This gentleman has subclinical hypothyroidism. The risk of progression from subclinical hypothyroidism to frank hypothyroidism is 2%, however if thyroid autoantibodies are positive this risk increases. Therefore, patients with subclinical hypothyroidism should have thyroid antibodies checked. If these are positive or TSH > 10 treatment with thyroxine should be commenced.

Case Study 7

An 82 year old lady presents with increasing dyspnoea and decreasing mobility over a six-week period. She has anorexia and marked weight loss. On examination, her movements are very slow and she has a flat affect. She has bilateral temporalis muscle wasting and a bilateral ptosis. Palpation of her neck reveals a small diffuse non tender goitre. She has uncontrolled atrial fibrillation and evidence of heart failure.

This patient is suffering from apathetic thyrotoxicosis. The diagnosis is confirmed with biochemical testing and the patient responds to treatment with anti-thyroid drugs. Beta-blockers are avoided because of the co-existing heart failure. Apathetic thyrotoxicosis is the presentation most removed from the classical picture and because of the associated inertia and cachexia other diagnoses including malignancy and hypothyroidism may be considered.

Case Study 8

A 68 year-old lady presented with palpitations. She was thin, had sweaty palms and a fine tremor. She had a sinus tachycardia and appeared uncomfortable at rest. She had exophthalmos and lid lag and she had a small diffuse goitre with a bruit.

Here, the diagnosis is Grave's disease with uncontrolled thyrotoxicosis. This lady was commenced on carbimazole and propranolol was added for symptomatic relief. Eight days later, she represents with a maculopapular, pruritic rash. She was felt to be allergic to carbimazole and commenced on propylthiouracil instead.

Data Interpretation

Question 1

A 66-year-old previously well female attends her GP complaining of lethargy. No abnormalities are detected on physical examination. The following abnormal laboratory investigations are documented:

Plasma Calcium	2.96 mmol/l
Plasma Albumin	32 mmol/l
24-hour urinary calcium	2.1 mmol/l (normal range 1.25-3.75 nmol/l)

a. Calculate the corrected calcium concentration.
b. What is the most likely diagnosis?
c. How should the patient be managed?

Question 2

A 68-year-old male is referred by his GP for management of intractable hypertension. One year ago he was commenced on a calcium channel blocker, and since then a beta-blocker and ACE inhibitor have been added to his antihypertensive drug regime. He is compliant with his medications. His blood pressure remains elevated at 190/100 mmHg. Fundoscopy reveals grade III hypertensive retinopathy. The apex beat is displaced. No other abnormalities are detected. The following investigations are obtained:

Sodium	149 mmol/l
Potassium	2.9 mmol/l
Bicarbonate	32 mmol/l
Urea	4.2 mmol/l
Urinalysis	No proteinuria

a. List 3 further investigations.
b. What is the most likely cause for the patient's hypertension?
c. What is the most likely pathogenesis of the underlying condition?

Question 3

A 62 year old male complains of a dry cough, an 8 kg weight loss, loss of appetite and intermittent abdominal pain. His blood pressure is 120/82 mmHg lying and 102/76 mmHg standing. There is digital clubbing. The following laboratory results are obtained:

Sodium	126 mmol/l
Potassium	6.2 mmol/l

Glucose	3.2 mmol/l
Urea	13.8 mmol/l
Calcium	2.82 mmol/l
Albumin	30 mmol/l

a. List 3 appropriate investigations.
b. What is the most likely unifying diagnosis?
c. What treatment is indicated for this patient?

Best of five questions

Question 1

Recognised features of the sick euthyroid syndrome include each of the following except:
a. Low total T3
b. Elevated TSH
c. No p roven benefit from thyroxine replacement
d. Normal TSH
e. Low total T4

Question 2

A 72 year old man presents with confusion and weakness. The plasma sodium is 124 mmol/l. Which one of the following findings makes the diagnosis of SIADH most likely?
a. Plasma osmolality 300 mOsm/kg
b. Urine osmolality 80 mOsm/kg
c. Urine sodium 50mmol/l
d. Elevated JVP
e. Elevated urea and creatinine

Question 3

A 78 year old male with a 14-year history of poorly controlled type 2 diabetes is found in a comatose state. The plasma glucose is 42 mmol/l and the serum osmolality is 382 mOsm/kg. Appropriate initial steps in the management of this patient include each of the following except:
a. 1L of 0.9% NaCl over the first hour
b. Central venous monitoring
c. Intravenous broad-spectrum antibiotics
d. Subcutaneous low molecular weight heparin
e. 6 units of intravenous insulin per hour

Answers are available on page 311

Anaemia and weight loss

M O'Connor, C O'Sullivan

Introduction

From the physician's perspective, the demographic curve strongly argues that medical practice in the future will entail a great deal of Geriatric Medicine. Older patients pose a challenge in that disease presentation and illness behaviour differ significantly from that seen in younger patients. Non-specific symptoms and signs are often the only evidence of serious illness. However there are certain syndromes that are more common in older people such as cognitive impairment, falls, incontinence and immobility. In addition older patients may present with a 'failure to thrive' syndrome characterised by weight loss, reduced vitality, fatigue and anaemia. This symptom complex poses difficult diagnostic challenges due to its vague nature. However a systematic assessment will frequently yield an underlying aetiology.

Weight loss in older patients

Unintentional weight loss in the elderly patient can be difficult to evaluate and is associated with increased morbidity and mortality. Regulation of food intake changes with increasing age leading to what has been called a 'physiologic anorexia of ageing.' The amount of circulating cholecystokinin, a satiating hormone, increases in the circulation as we grow older. Other substances are also thought to increase satiety including cytokines, cachectin, interleukin-1 and interleukin-6. Loss of lean body mass is also common with increasing age. Furthermore advancing age is associated with a decrease in the basal metabolic rate as well as changes in the senses of taste and smell. By the age of 65 years, approximately 50% of Americans have lost teeth and resultant chewing problems can affect food intake. Weight loss is the result of decreased energy intake, increased energy expenditure or loss of energy in the urine or stools. It is not always a patient's chief complaint but is a feature of many different disorders and should always be asked about. Weight loss may be involuntary or voluntary. Involuntary weight loss, where appetite can either be increased or decreased, is nearly always a sign of a serious medical or psychiatric illness and should be thoroughly investigated. Voluntary weight loss may not be a matter of concern in an overweight patient who is dieting but can otherwise be a manifestation of psychiatric illness. Involuntary weight loss and being underweight are both important predictors of increased morbidity and mortality in older patients. Significant involuntary weight loss can be defined as follows;

- >5% weight loss in one month
- >7.5% weight loss in 3 months
- >10% weight loss in 6 months

A prospective study of community-dwelling men over 65 years showed that a documented weight loss of >4% was the single best predictor of death within 2 years. In the same study, mortality rates were 28% in those with weight loss versus 11% in the control group. A similar study in older patients with involuntary weight loss, followed up after discharge from hospital, found a two-fold increase in mortality at one year. Correcting the progressive decline in weight by identifying and treating the cause has not been shown to improve survival but may significantly impact on quality of life and functional status in this age group. The approach to management should consist of a careful attempt to identify the cause of weight loss with targeted aggressive treatment. Failure to find a cause for weight loss is generally associated with a poorer prognosis.

Causes of involuntary weight loss in older patients

It is useful when determining a cause for weight loss to consider changes in appetite. However poor dentition, poverty and social isolation may also be significant factors in older individuals. There are many causes of weight loss and anorexia but only a few of weight loss with an increased appetite, (Table 1).

Assessment of weight loss

The assessment of patients with involuntary weight loss should include history, examination, neuropsychological assessment as well as a basic laboratory work up. Key features that should be elucidated from the history should include the

TABLE I
MAJOR CAUSES OF WEIGHT LOSS

INVOLUNTARY WEIGHT LOSS WITH INCREASED APPETITE
Hyperthyroidism
Uncontrolled diabetes mellitus
Malabsorption syndrome

INVOLUNTARY WEIGHT LOSS WITH REDUCED APPETITE
Medical Disorders
Malignancy
Endocrinopathies
Chronic illness including chronic renal failure
Chronic obstructive pulmonary disease
Gastrointestinal disorders
Chronic infections
Tuberculosis

Psychiatric Disorders
Depression
Dementia

Drugs
Selective serotonin reuptake inhibitors
Opiates
Anti-cholinergics
Metformin
Non-steroidal anti-inflammatory drugs
Anti-neoplastic drugs

The Mini Nutritional Assessment (MNA) is an 18-item tool used to assess nutritional risk; it includes anthropometric measurements (body mass index, mid-arm and calf circumferences and weight loss), a dietary questionnaire (number of meals consumed, food and fluid intakes and feeding autonomy), global assessment (lifestyle, medication, and mobility) and self-assessment (self-perception of health and nutrition). The MNA was designed and validated to rapidly assess the nutritional status of frail older persons so that nutritional intervention may be facilitated. The estimated time required to administer the MNA is 10 min. A scoring algorithm assigns subjects to well-nourished, at-risk and malnourished categories. Copies of the assessment can be viewed or downloaded at http://www.mna-elderly.com/

Although unexplained weight loss in the elderly can have a myriad causes, an undirected or 'shotgun' approach to laboratory tests and other diagnostic studies is rarely fruitful. However initial targeted studies can determine the cause in many patients. The findings of the history and physical examination guide the initial diagnostic assessment. Some diagnostic modalities, such as CT scanning, have particularly low yields. In one series, CT scanning provided no new information beyond confirming one cancer that was already suspected. In the same series, diagnostic yields were highest for faecal occult blood testing (18%), sigmoidoscopy (18%), thyroid function testing for both hyperthyroidism and hypothyroidism (24%), upper endoscopy (40%) and upper gastrointestinal series (44%). Further evaluation and investigation should be guided by history, examination and initial investigations (Table 2).

Anaemia in older patients

Anaemia is one of the most common medical problems of older people. It occurs when the quantity of circulating erythrocytes falls below normal. It has been suggested that an age-related decline in haematological parameters occurs and therefore that haematological norms should be lowered for older patients. Conversely other authors suggest that while anaemia is prevalent, it should not be regarded as a normal aspect of ageing and advise against establishing lower haematological norms for older people. The World Health Organisation criteria for anaemia are a haemoglobin below 13g/dl for men and 12g/dl for women. Based upon these criteria, cross-sectional studies have shown a very high prevalence of anaemia in older patients, particularly

arrangements for meal preparations, drug therapy, presence of upper or lower gastrointestinal symptoms, recent respiratory symptoms, cigarette pack years and night sweats. Examination should focus on oral and dental examination, swallow assessment, abdominal examination, digital rectal examination as well as routine examination of other systems. A Mini Mental State Examination and Geriatric Depression Score are appropriate in selected patients. Evaluation of urine for protein and blood is often forgotten. Laboratory work up should include full blood count, haematinics, ESR, thyroid, liver and renal function as well as bone chemistry and glucose. A chest x-ray is mandatory in smokers and patients with respiratory symptoms. Further evaluation should include nutritional assessments and measurements of Body Mass Index (weight (kg)/height (m^2)):
• <20 severe under-nutrition
• <22 mild-moderate under-nutrition

TABLE 2
FURTHER EVALUATION OF INVOLUNTARY WEIGHT LOSS

Indications	Investigation
Upper GI Symptoms	Gastroscopy and duodenal biopsy
Lower GI symptoms	Barium enema and colonoscopy and biopsy
	Coeliac antibodies if radiology negative
Headache and raised ESR	Temporal artery biopsy
Bone pain	Plain x-rays
	Bone scan
	PSA in males
	MR Imaging of abnormal area
Iron deficiency anaemia	Gastroscopy and colonoscopy
Normochromic anaemia	Bone marrow
	Myeloma screen
Abnormal chest x-ray	Sputum culture and cytology
	Bronchoscopy, CT thorax and mantoux
Abnormal renal function	Urine microscopy
	Urine cytology
	Renal tract imaging
	Autoimmune screen
High inflammatory markers	Autoimmune screen
Possible chronic infection	Blood cultures
	Serology

among older men. Surveys of the prevalence of anaemia have shown an incidence ranging from 8-40% for men and 10 - 22% for women, (Table 3). The high prevalence of mild anaemia among men and the relative frequency at which no obvious aetiology can be identified suggests that an appropriate cut-off point may be 12g/dl. This could result in the avoidance of intensive and at times, invasive investigations but the possibility of missing an underlying disease process in a patient population at risk is enhanced. A careful and targeted history and physical should be performed prior to further investigations.

Presentation and initial assessment of anaemia

Anaemia in older patients generally presents in a similar manner as in younger adults. However there may also be more subtle symptoms and signs. The older patient may present with weakness, lethargy, falls, syncope, worsening ischaemic chest pain, exertional dyspnoea or worsening confusion. The history may give useful clues as to the likely aetiology. Careful attention must be paid to the presence of upper or lower gastro-intestinal symptoms, significant involuntary weight loss,

TABLE 3
AGE AND GENDER-STRATIFIED PREVALENCE OF ANAEMIA IN OLDER COMMUNITY DWELLERS

	Men			Women	
(Age yrs)	n	% Anaemic (Hb < 13g/dl)		n	% Anaemic (Hb < 12g/dl)
71 - 74	452	8.6		630	8.6
75 - 79	484	13.0		867	12.0
80 - 84	268	18.3		590	13.7
85 - 89	143	26.6		303	16.2
>90	59	40.7		150	20.7

TABLE 4
CLASSIFICATION OF ANAEMIA IN THE OLDER PATIENT

HYPOPROLIFERATIVE	INEFFECTIVE HAEMOPOIESIS	HAEMOLYSIS
Intrinsic marrow lesion	**Megaloblastic**	**Immunologic**
Aplastic anaemia	Vitamin B$_{12}$ deficiency	Idiopathic
Red blood cell aplasia	Folate deficiency	Secondary
Marrow fibrosis		• Drugs
Tumour infiltration		• Lymphoma
		• Vasculitis
Erythropoietin lack	**Microcytic/normocytic**	**Intrinsic**
Renal disease	Thalassaemia	Metabolic
Nutritional	Myelodysplastic syndrome	Haemoglobinopathy
Sideroblastic		
Iron deficient erythropoiesi		**Extrinsic**
Iron deficiency anaemia		Mechanical
Anaemia of chronic disease		Drugs

night sweats, haemoptysis, haematuria and rheumatological symptoms. Examination should be detailed and specifically look for presence or absence of lymphadenopathy, hepatomegaly, splenomegaly and iliac fossa masses. In addition it is important to check for signs of polymyalgia and temporal arteritis as they may present in a subtle manner. A detailed respiratory examination may reveal signs such as tracheal deviation or a subtle pleural effusion. A digital rectal examination including a test for occult blood is mandatory in all anaemic patients as is urinalysis. The Full Blood Count (FBC) and blood film will give the most useful indication as to the likely aetiology.

All patients should have an Erythrocyte Sedimentation Rate (ESR), electrolytes, renal function, liver function, bone chemistry, haematinics and thyroid function performed. In addition patients should have a chest x-ray.

Classification of anaemias

Anaemia is traditionally classified according to the red cell mean cell volume (MCV). Although this classification is useful an alternative is to consider the basis for the anaemia. Broadly speaking anaemia in older patients can be considered in the three following categories as summarised shown in Table 4.
• Hypoproliferative; decreased red blood cell production
• Ineffective haemopoiesis
• Haemolytic; red blood cell destruction

Excluding acute blood loss as a cause of anaemia studies have identified iron deficiency and the anaemia of chronic disease as the commonest causes in older patients. Other causes, though rarer are relevant due to their higher predilection for affecting older individuals. These include folate and vitamin B$_{12}$ deficiency as well as multiple myeloma.

Iron deficiency anaemia

Iron deficiency is the commonest cause of anaemia worldwide and is frequently seen in general practice. The anaemia of iron deficiency is caused by defective synthesis of haemoglobin, resulting in red cells that are smaller than normal (microcytic) and contain reduced amounts of haemoglobin (hypochromic). Iron has a pivotal role in many metabolic processes and the average adult has 3 - 5g of iron, of which two thirds is in the oxygen-carrying molecule

TABLE 5
DAILY DIETARY IRON REQUIREMENTS

Male	1mg
Adolescence	2 - 3mgs
Female of reproductive age	2 - 3mgs
Pregnancy	3 - 4mgs
Older male and female	1mg

TABLE 6
COMMON CAUSES OF IRON DEFICIENCY IN OLDER PATIENTS

Gastrointestinal blood loss	Peptic ulcer disease
	Oesophagitis
	Gastic cancer
	Oesophageal varices
	Angiodysplasia
	Colorectal cancer
	Inflammatory bowel disease
	Haemorrhoids
Malabsorption	Coeliac disease
	Post gastrectomy
	Bacterial overgrowth
Genitourinary loss	Transitional cell cancer
	Renal cell cancer
	Endometrial cancer
Dietary	Depression
	Neglect
	Vegans

loss, most commonly from the gastro-intestinal tract, frequently as a result of non-steroidal anti-inflammatory drug and steroid usage or because of occult cancer, ulcers, polyps or angiodysplasia. More rarely neoplasms of the genito-urinary tract, bleeding disorders or chronic intravascular haemolysis may cause iron deficiency as shown in Table 6.

Confirming the diagnosis of iron deficiency
The laboratory diagnosis of iron deficiency may be suggested by a reduced serum ferritin concentration which should be less than 50mg/l, in association with transferrin saturation below 15%. The peripheral blood smear usually contains hypochromic and microcytic red blood cells. The blood findings in iron deficiency anaemia may be altered in older patients with anaemia of chronic disease where normal or high serum ferritin is the norm. When both conditions coexist, the only definitive test may be a bone marrow examination after which iron deficiency is diagnosed with certainty by lack of bone marrow iron stores, (Table 7).

Investigation of patients with iron deficiency anaemia
The investigation of patients with iron deficiency anaemia should focus on identifying the source of blood loss. Stool should be examined for evidence of occult blood. Further investigation, including colonoscopy and oesophagogastroduodenoscopy with duodenal biopsy may also identify upper or lower gastrointestinal bleeding sources. Concomitant lesions of both the upper and lower gastrointestinal tract are rare, such that detection of the likely source of blood loss during the initial examination may obviate the need for further investigations. However one must be cautious about attributing significant iron deficiency anaemia to trivial lesion such as gastritis or reflux oesophagitis without fully investigating the lower gastrointestinal tract. Symptoms related to a specific site in the gastrointestinal tract usually predict disease in the corresponding part of the bowel. The positive predictive value of lower GI symptoms associated with iron deficiency anaemia and positive faecal occult blood is very high; 86% for detecting lesions. CT colonography may be an alternative to colonoscopy and barium enema in frail older patients. This modality also provides anatomical detail of the other intra-abdominal structures. In patients with haematuria, urine cytology, renal tract ultrasound and cystoscopy provide an adequate work up. If the above fails to demonstrate a cause, a reasonable approach is to observe the patient over time. Radiological studies of the small bowel frequently add little to diagnosis.

haemoglobin. A normal diet provides about 15mg of iron daily, of which 5 - 10% is absorbed, principally in the duodenum and upper jejunum, where the acidic conditions aid absorption of iron in the ferrous form. Absorption is helped by the presence of other reducing substances, especially ascorbic acid. The body has the capacity to increase its iron absorption in the face of increased demand, for example in pregnancy, lactation, growth spurts and iron deficiency.

Once absorbed from the bowel, iron is transported across the mucosal cell to the blood, where it is carried by the protein transferrin to developing red cells in the bone marrow. Iron stores comprise ferritin, a labile and readily accessible source of iron and haemosiderin, an insoluble form found predominantly in macrophages. This process is unchanged in older people. Tea and coffee consumption reduce iron absorption and vitamin C enhances it. Dietary iron deficiency can occur in older patients with atrophic gastritis and hypochlorhydria since an acidic milieu enhances absorption. About 1 mg of iron a day is shed from the body in urine, faeces, sweat, and cells shed from the skin and gastrointestinal tract.

Causes of iron deficiency anaemia
The main cause of iron deficiency anaemia is blood

TABLE 7
DIFFERENTIAL DIAGNOSIS OF HYPOCHROMIC ANAEMIA

Haematological indices	Iron deficiency anaemia	Anaemia of chronic disorders	Thalassaemia trait (α or β)	Sideroblastic anaemia
Degree of anaemia	Any	<9.0g/dl	Mild	Any
Mean cell volume	↓	N or ↓	↓↓	N ↓ or ↑
Serum ferritin	↓	N or ↑	N	↑
TIBC	↑	↓	N	N
Serum iron	↓	↓	N	↑
Marrow iron	Absent	Present	Present	Present

N = normal; TIBC = total iron binding capacity

Iron therapy in iron deficiency anaemia

Treatment of an underlying cause should prevent further iron loss but all patients should have iron supplementation both to correct anaemia and replenish iron stores. This is achieved most suitably and cheaply with ferrous sulphate 200mgs three times daily although ferrous gluconate and ferrous fumarate are equally effective. A liquid preparation may be tolerated when tablets are not. Ascorbic acid also enhances iron absorption and should be considered when response is poor. Parenteral iron treatment should only be used when there is intolerance to at least two oral preparations or non-compliance. Intramuscular iron is painful, expensive and may cause local and anaphylactic reactions. The rise in haemoglobin concentration is no quicker than with oral preparations. Failure of the haemoglobin concentration to rise by 2g/dl in 1 - 2 months is usually due to poor compliance, misdiagnosis, continued blood loss or malabsorption. Iron supplementation should be continued for three months after correction of anaemia to replenish the iron stores.

Anaemia of chronic disease (ACD)

The term anaemia of chronic disease is often used to explain anaemia associated with some other major disease process. Occasionally, the anaemia may be the initial manifestation of an occult disease. This anaemia is the most common in hospitalised older patients. Certainly, the specific diseases that are known to give rise to ACD, namely cancer, infection and chronic inflammatory diseases such as rheumatoid arthritis are more common in older people. Several mechanisms combine to produce ACD. There is mild ineffective erythropoiesis. There is also a decrease in red cell survival, the compensatory erythropoietic response to which is suboptimal due to the increase of inhibitory cytokines. The net effect is an impaired ability of the reticuloendothelial cells to recruit iron derived from phagocytosed red blood cells. Iron released from the phagocytosed red cell is diverted to iron stores in the form of ferritin and haemosiderin. The haemoglobin level is usually above 9g/dl and the serum iron is usually reduced. In contrast to iron deficiency anaemia the serum ferritin is normal or increased as shown already in Table 7. A bone marrow evaluation reveals abundant iron stores but reduced iron incorporation into maturing erythroblasts. The common disorders associated with anaemia of chronic disease are shown in Table 8.

The management of patients with ACD should focus on identifying and treating the underlying disorder. In patients with chronic renal disease, erythropoietin 50 to 100U/kg given parenterally 3 times per week, with doses increasing to 150U/kg if there is no response after three weeks has been shown to reduce the need for red cell transfusion.

Megaloblastic anaemia

Megaloblastic anaemias were initially characterised over one hundred years ago. The term identifies patients with anaemia and macrocytic red cells whose mean corpuscular volume is greater than 100. The bone marrow shows intense erythroid hyperplasia with an abnormal morphology. The megaloblast, the morphologic hallmark of the syndrome, is a product of impaired DNA formation which in turn is due to deficiencies of vitamin B_{12} or folic acid. Other causes of impaired DNA or RNA formation such as antimetabolite drugs and myelodysplastic syndrome can also lead to megaloblastic anaemia.

TABLE 8
DISORDERS ASSOCIATED WITH ANAEMIA OF CHRONIC DISEASE

Congestive cardiac failure (NYHA III/IV)
Chronic renal failure
Hepatic failure
Chronic infections
    Infective endocarditis
    Chronic pyelonephritis
    Tuberculosis
    Osteomyelitis
Neoplasm
    Renal cell carcinoma
    Colonic carcinoma
    Pancreatic carcinoma
    Lymphoma
    Leukaemia
    Multiple myeloma
Collagen vascular disease
    Rheumatoid arthritis
    Polymyalgia & Temporal arteritis
    Systemic lupus erythematosus
Endocrine disorders
    Hypothyroidism
    Addison's disease
    Hypopituitarism
Skin disease
    Chronic venous ulcers
    Pressure sores

The body's requirement for vitamin B_{12} is about 3µg daily. This is amply supplied by a normal Western diet which has a vitamin B_{12} content of 10 - 30µg daily. A strict vegan diet which excludes all animal produce including milk, eggs and cheese does not contain adequate vitamin B_{12}. Absorption of vitamin B_{12} is through the ileum, facilitated by intrinsic factor, which is secreted by the parietal cells of the stomach. Absorption is limited to 2 - 3µg daily. Total body stores of B_{12} are 2 to 5 milligrams, approximately one-half of which is in the liver. As a result, it takes years to develop vitamin B_{12} deficiency after absorption of dietary B_{12} ceases. In the stomach peptic digestion at low pH is a prerequisite for Vitamin B_{12} release from food protein. This is of clinical significance in the 70 – 80-year-old population, among whom hypochlorhydria or achlorhydria is frequently present (25 – 50% of patients) leading to inadequate release of protein-bound vitamin B_{12} via proteolysis with pepsin. Vitamin B_{12} deficiency is usually due to pernicious anaemia which now accounts for up to 80% of all cases of megaloblastic anaemia. The incidence of the disease is 1:10,000 in northern Europe and the disease occurs in all races. The underlying mechanism is an autoimmune gastritis that results in achlorhydria and the absence of intrinsic factor. The incidence of pernicious anaemia peaks at age 60, the condition has a female to male incidence of 1.6:1.0 and is more common in those with early greying, blue eyes and blood group A. It is also more common in those with a family history of the disease or of diseases that may be associated with it, for example vitiligo, myxoedema, Hashimoto's disease, Addison's disease and hypoparathyroidism.

Folates are widely distributed in nature in reduced and polyglutamated forms. They are synthesised by microorganisms and plants. Leafy vegetables such as spinach, lettuce, broccoli and beans, fruits such as bananas, melons and lemons, yeast, mushrooms and animal protein especially liver and kidney are rich sources of folate. Folates are extremely thermolabile; prolonged cooking for >15 minutes in large quantities of water, in the absence of reducing agents, destroys folate. Oxidation of food folate by nitrites reduces its bioavailability. The recommended daily intake for folate is 3µg/kg/day. A balanced Western diet contains adequate amounts of folate but the net dietary intake of folate in many developing countries is often insufficient to sustain folate balance. Dietary folates in some foods such as cabbage, lettuce and oranges are not well absorbed. Most other dietary folates are nutritionally available.

The causes of vitamin B_{12} and folate deficiencies are shown in Tables 9 & 10.

Deficiency of either vitamin B_{12} or folic acid can produce megaloblastic anaemia. Because Vitamin B_{12} stores are so large in relation to daily intake, years of inadequate intake or absorption are required before the onset of symptoms. On the other hand, symptoms of folate deficiency can occur within a few months after intake is diminished. Pernicious anaemia (PA) is more common in whites and usually affects older patients, possibly because of the superimposition of age-related chronic atrophic gastritis. The classic picture of vitamin B_{12} deficiency due to PA was that of a prematurely grey woman of Northern European descent who was lemon coloured reflecting anaemia and icterus, mentally sluggish, had a shiny tongue from atrophic glossitis and

TABLE 9	TABLE 10
CAUSES OF VITAMIN B$_{12}$ DEFICIENCY	**CAUSES OF FOLATE DEFICIENCY**

GASTRIC ABNORMALITIES	**NUTRITIONAL DEFICIENCY**
Pernicious anaemia	Alcoholism
Gastrectomy	Poor dietary intake
Gastritis	Overcooked foods
	Depression
SMALL BOWEL DISEASE	Nursing home residents
Malabsorption	
Coeliac disease	**MALABSORPTION**
Ileal resection	Coeliac disease
Crohn's disease	Crohn's disease
Bacterial overgrowth syndrome	Infiltrative bowel disease
	Short bowel syndrome
PANCREATIC DISEASE	
Pancreatic insufficiency	**DRUGS**
	Methotrexate
	Trimethoprim
DIETARY	Ethanol
Strict vegans	Phenytoin
AGENTS THAT BLOCK ABSORPTION	**INCREASED REQUIREMENTS**
Neomycin	Haematological disease with increased red cell production
Biguanides	eg. haemolysis
Proton pump inhibitors	Malignant disease
	Exfoliative dermatitis

a shuffling broad gait due to associated neurological deficits. The patient may have hard-to-characterize neuropsychiatric problems consisting of paraesthesiae, numbness, weakness, loss of dexterity, impaired memory and personality changes. The neurological problems may consist of the classic picture of subacute combined degeneration of the dorsal and lateral spinal columns. This lesion is due to a defect in myelin formation of unknown mechanism. The neuropathy is symmetrical and affects the legs more than the arms. It begins with paraesthesiae and ataxia associated with loss of vibration and position sense and can progress to severe weakness, spasticity, clonus, paraplegia and even faecal and urinary incontinence.

Both vitamin B$_{12}$ and folic acid are required for the metabolism of homocysteine to methionine. As a result deficiencies in these vitamins can lead to elevations in plasma homocysteine levels; a risk factor for the development of atherosclerosis and venous thromboembolism. Recent evidence suggests that an increased homocysteine level is a strong, independent risk factor for the development of dementia and Alzheimer's disease. Vitamin therapy with folic acid, alone or in combination with vitamin B$_{12}$ and dietary supplementation with folate enriched cereal-grain products and breakfast cereals can significantly reduce plasma homocysteine levels.

Treatment of vitamin B$_{12}$ and folate deficiency

Attempts should be made to identify an underlying cause such as coeliac disease or inflammatory bowel disease. Potential offending drugs should be stopped and a nutritional assessment sought to assess for dietary deficiency. Folate deficiency is treated with folic acid 1 to 5 mg/day orally for one to four months. Vitamin B$_{12}$ deficiency is typically treated with B$_{12}$ injections in a dose of 1000µg every day for one week, followed by 1mg every week for four weeks and then, if the underlying disorder persists, as in PA, 1mg every month for the remainder of the patient's life.

Conditions worth special mention in older patients

Multiple myeloma

Myeloma is due to unregulated, progressive proliferation of a monoclonal population of B lymphocytes and their evolution into abnormal or malignant plasma cells. These monoclonal plasma cells accumulate in the marrow, leading to anaemia and marrow failure. Myeloma is a disease which mainly affects older people. It is increasing in incidence and its age-adjusted mortality has increased almost fivefold in the last three to four decades. Its incidence is up to 21 per 100,000 in the over 75 year group. It is more than twice as prevalent in African Americans as in white Americans and Europeans. The median age at diagnosis is 69 years, with males being more affected than females. 60% of patients are anaemic at the time of presentation. Myeloma cells produce and secrete a monoclonal protein, usually intact immunoglobulin. IgG paraprotein is present in 60% of cases and IgA in 20 - 25%. In 15 - 20% of cases free immunoglobulin light chains alone are produced. Myelomas whose cells secrete IgD, IgM, two clonal proteins or no protein are rare. Free light chains are detectable in urine as Bence Jones protein.

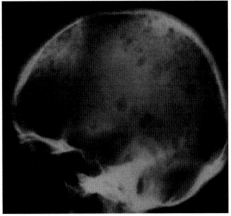

Figure 1: Pepper Pot skull in a patient with multiple myeloma

Clinical features

Occasionally myeloma is a chance finding, however most patients present in one of a number of classical patterns. They can be grouped as follows;
- Skeletal
- Neurological
- Renal
- Metabolic

Skeletal manifestations

Bone destruction is characteristic and the associated bone pain a major cause of morbidity in myeloma. Conventional radiographs revealed an abnormality in the majority of patients at the time of diagnosis. Myeloma is associated with abnormal bone remodelling due to increased osteoclastic bone resorption and inhibition of osteoblastic bone formation. Stimulation of osteoclastic activity by adjacent myeloma cells is thought to result from cytokine production. Various factors have been implicated including interleukin-1-beta, lymphotoxin, tumour necrosis factor, interleukin (IL)-6 and macrophage colony stimulating factor. This results in pronounced bone loss and the characteristic osteolytic lesions predispose to pathological fractures. Radiological manifestations may vary from a single vertebral collapse to multiple punched-out lesions in the skull, the so-called pepper-pot skull, (Figure 1).

Neurological manifestations

Peripheral neuropathy, mononeuritis multiplex and cord compression due to vertebral collapse are recognised neurological manifestations. Concomitant amyloidosis may contribute to neuropathy. Less common are symptoms of hyperviscosity with impaired central nervous system function, headache and visual disturbances.

Renal manifestations

25% of cases at presentation have evidence of renal impairment with tubular damage by light chain deposition, renal infections, hypercalcaemia and amyloidosis contributing. Impaired renal function at presentation indicates a poor prognosis.

Metabolic manifestations

Generalised bone involvement may lead to hypercalcaemia which is present in 20% of patients at presentation and is associated with a poor prognosis. The incidence of infection is increased in multiple myeloma with Streptococcus pneumoniae and gram-negative organisms being the most frequently implicated pathogens. The propensity to infection results from an impairment in the antibody response due to suppression of normal plasma cell function.

TABLE 11
DIAGNOSTIC CRITERIA FOR MULTIPLE MYELOMA
> 10% plasma cells in bone marrow or plasmacytoma on biopsy plus at least one of: Serum M band (IgG >30 g/l; IgA >20 g/l) Urine M band (Bence Jones proteinuria) Osteolytic lesions on skeletal survey

TABLE 12
FEATURES OF POOR PROGNOSIS AT DIAGNOSIS OF MULTIPLE MYELOMA

Low haemoglobin concentration (<8.5 g/dl)
Hypercalcaemia at presentation (>3.0mmol/l)
Advanced lytic bone lesions
High M protein production rates (IgG >70 g/l; IgA >50 g/l; Bence Jones protein >12 g/24h)
Abnormal renal function
High plasma cell proliferative index
Low serum albumin concentration (<30 g/l)
High β2-microglobulin concentration (>5.5 mg/ml)

Diagnosis of multiple myeloma

In older patients, the diagnosis may be delayed. The presenting features are often insidious and non-specific.

Treatment of multiple myeloma

Oral melphalan and prednisolone administered in four day pulses at intervals of four to six weeks produce >50% reduction in the M protein concentration in 50% of patients. The treatment is well tolerated but complete responses are rare. The median survival is about three years. During the plateau phase clinical and laboratory results should be reviewed at regular intervals to identify progression at the earliest opportunity. Further treatment with melphalan may then induce another plateau phase. Combination intravenous chemotherapeutic regimens may produce higher response rates of up to 70% and may improve survival. Combination regimens may be more effective in younger patients with high tumour loads, although they may be more toxic in older patients. Autologous stem cell transplantation and allogenic bone marrow transplantation are poorly tolerated in older patients. Certain factors are associated with a poor prognosis as shown in Table 12.

Other treatment modalities such as radiotherapy for painful bone lesions and bisphosphonate therapy are useful in older patients.

Myelodysplastic syndromes (MDS)

The term myelodysplastic syndrome was introduced in 1975 by a group of French, American and British haematologists, the FAB group, to describe a group of disorders with characteristic abnormalities of peripheral blood and bone marrow morphology and impaired bone marrow function, which tend to evolve into acute myeloid leukaemia. Although the myelodysplastic syndromes may occur at any age, they are predominantly diseases of older people. These disorders may occur de novo or arise years after exposure to potentially mutagenic chemotherapy. Patients with MDS are usually older than 60 years and there is a slight preponderance of men. Clinically, patients present with signs and symptoms related to a decrease in their peripheral blood counts. Symptoms related to anaemia may range from tiredness to frank congestive cardiac failure. Recurrent localised or systemic infections are associated with granulocytopaenia or poorly functioning granulocytes and monocytes. Bleeding manifestations such as petechiae or gross haemorrhage can occur with thrombocytopenia.

The French-American-British, FAB, Cooperative Group initially defined refractory anaemia with excess blasts (RAEB) and chronic myelomonocytic leukaemia (CMML) as preleukaemic states. Six years later, the FAB group added three more categories to this classification scheme and adopted the present term 'myelodysplastic syndromes'. The FAB group divided the myelodysplastic syndromes into five subgroups based on (a) the percentage of immature myeloid cells; blast cells and ring sideroblasts; immature red cells with iron granules arranged in a ring around the nucleus, in the bone marrow and (b) the presence or absence of a raised peripheral blood monocyte count:

• Refractory anaemia (RA)
• Refractory anaemia with ringed sideroblasts (RARS)
• Refractory anaemia with excess blasts (RAEB)
• Refractory anaemia with excess blasts in transformation (RAEB-t)
• Chronic myelomonocytic leukaemia (CMML)

The clinical course of the myelodysplastic syndromes is extremely variable even among patients of the same subgroup. About two thirds of patients die of marrow failure of whom half undergo leukaemia transformation and one third die of unrelated causes. The median survival of patients with myelodysplastic syndrome is 20 months. Although the FAB classification has prognostic significance, a more accurate prediction of survival can be achieved by using a scoring system that incorporates the presenting haemoglobin concentration, neutrophil and platelet counts, the percentage of blasts in the bone marrow and chromosome abnormalities. The treatment of the myelodysplastic syndromes is generally unsatisfactory, which partially accounts for the variety of therapeutic options. Before the most appropriate treatment can be determined, several factors must be taken into consideration. These include the patient's age and general fitness, the severity of the disease at presentation, prognostic factors and whether the disease is stable or progressive. Consequently, whenever possible there should be a period of observation before a decision about long-term treatment is made. The cornerstone of the treatment of the myelodysplastic syndromes remains the judicious use of red cell and platelet transfusions and antibiotics for older patients with symptomatic disease. Iron chelation therapy should be considered for patients who need red cell transfusion long term. Recombinant growth factors such as granulocyte-colony stimulating factor or granulocyte-macrophage colony stimulating factor can improve the neutrophil count in over 90% of patients. Erythropoietin with or without either of these colony stimulating factors can improve the haemoglobin concentration in 20-40% of patients. Intermittent administration of either colony-stimulating factors may be considered in patients with severe neutropenia and recurrent infections. Low dose and intensive chemotherapy is generally considered in only a minority of patients.

Haemolytic anaemia

Haemolytic anaemia is anaemia due to shortened survival of circulating red blood cells (RBCs). Although the time of RBC senescent death in adults is approximately 120 days, it is convenient to define haemolysis as a shortening of RBC survival to a value of less than 100 days. While haemolysis can be a lifelong asymptomatic condition, it most often presents as anaemia when erythrocytosis cannot match the pace of red cell destruction. Haemolysis also can manifest as jaundice, cholelithiasis or isolated reticulocytosis. There are two mechanisms of haemolysis. Intravascular haemolysis is the destruction of red blood cells in the circulation with the release of cell contents into the plasma. Mechanical trauma from a damaged endothelium, complement fixation and activation on cell surfaces and infectious agents may cause direct membrane degradation and cell destruction. The more common extravascular haemolysis is the removal and destruction of red blood cells with membrane alterations by the macrophages of the spleen and liver. A detailed list of causes is outlined in Table 13.

TABLE 13
CAUSES OF HAEMOLYTIC ANAEMIA

EXTRAVASCULAR DESTRUCTION OF RED BLOOD CELLS

Intrinsic red blood cell defects
Enzyme deficiencies
Haemoglobinopathies
Membrane defects

Extrinsic red blood cell defects
Liver disease
Hypersplenism
Infections (bartonella, babesia, malaria)
Oxidant agents (dapsone, nitrites, aniline dyes)
Other agents (lead, snake and spider bites)
Microangiopathic (DIC, TTP-HUS)
Autoimmune haemolytic anaemia (warm or cold reacting, drugs)

INTRAVASCULAR DESTRUCTION OF RED BLOOD CELLS
Microangiopathy (aortic stenosis or prosthetic valve)
Transfusion reactions (ABO incompatibility)
Infection (clostridial sepsis, severe malaria)
Paroxysmal nocturnal haemoglobinuria
Following intravenous infusion with hypotonic solutions
Snake bites

A systematic approach, starting with an accurate history and physical examination is the cornerstone of the patient's evaluation. While there are no symptoms specific for the diagnosis of haemolytic anaemia, recognising haemolysis is not difficult in the classical patient, who may have many or all of the following:
• New onset of pallor and anaemia
• Jaundice with increased indirect bilirubin concentration
• Gallstones
• Splenomegaly
• Presence of circulating spherocytic red cells
• Increased serum lactate dehydrogenase (LDH) concentration
• Reduced (or absent) level of serum haptoglobin
• A positive direct antiglobulin test (Coomb's test)
• Increased reticulocyte percentage or absolute reticulocyte number, indicating the bone marrow's response to the anaemia

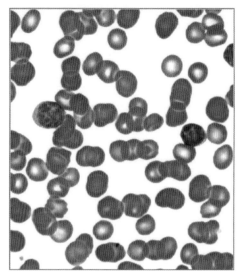

Figure 2: Blood film CLL

- Unintentional weight loss of over 10% of body weight within the previous six months
- Fevers of over 38°C for over 2 weeks without evidence of infection
- Night sweats without evidence of infection
- Extreme fatigue

Most patients with CLL consult a physician because they have noted painless swelling of lymph nodes, most often in the cervical area which spontaneously wax and wane but do not altogether disappear. There may be a mixture of features as outlined below:
- Lymphadenopathy - 87%
- Splenomegaly - 54%
- Hepatomegaly - 14%
- Total white blood cell count greater than 100,000/μl - 30%
- Haemoglobin concentration less than 11.0 g/dl - 31%
- Platelet count greater than 100,000/μl - 16%

The diagnosis is usually reasonably clear when combined with peripheral blood film analysis. In general bone marrow evaluation is not required. Phenyotyping of peripheral lymphocytes can give useful clinical information from a diagnostic and prognostic perspectives. Many older patients will not require treatment as many will have a smouldering form of their disease which remains stable for many years.

Indications for therapy
- Disease-related symptoms such as weakness, night sweats, weight loss, painful lymphadenopathy or fever
- Symptomatic anaemia or thrombocytopenia
- Progressive disease as demonstrated by increasing lymphocytosis with a lymphocyte doubling time less than six months
- Autoimmune haemolytic anaemia
- Repeated episodes of infection

Treatment options for elderly patients usual involve watchful waiting or the use of a combination of corticosteroids and chlorambucil. In selected patients more significant chemotherapy or use of newer agents such as rituximab can be undertaken under the supervision of a haematologist.

Summary
Weight loss is a common presenting symptom in older patients presenting to both primary and secondary

Haematology consultation should be obtained in virtually all patients with new onset of haemolysis since sudden and life-threatening worsening of anaemia may occur requiring urgent coordination between clinicians, clinical pathologists and blood bank personnel for appropriate management. Haemolysis may also be the first sign of an underlying systemic disorder, such as thrombotic thrombocytopenic purpura, lupus erythematosus, or chronic lymphocytic leukaemia, and may require urgent intervention to prevent death or disease-related complications.

Chronic lymphocytic leukaemia
Chronic lymphocytic leukaemia (CLL) is one of the chronic lymphoproliferative disorders or lymphoid neoplasms. It is the most common leukaemia in Western countries. The male to female ratio is 1.7:1 with a higher incidence among whites compared to blacks. CLL is considered to be mainly a disease of the elderly with a median age at diagnosis of 70 years. Approximately 25 percent of patients feel entirely well with no symptoms when a routine blood count reveals an absolute lymphocytosis, leading to a diagnosis of CLL. On the other end of the spectrum, approximately 5 to 10 percent of patients present with typical 'B' symptoms of lymphoma formally defined for protocol purposes as one or more of the following:

care. It is associated with at least a two-fold increase in mortality compared with age-matched controls. There is often an underlying physical cause associated with these 'failure to thrive' syndromes. The cause should become apparent after structured assessment. This assessment is based on a focused history, physical examination and targeted investigations. Anaemia is also common in older people and it becomes more so with advancing decades. Because the older population is increasing, the prevalence of anaemia and consequently its impact on health and healthcare expenditure is expected to rise. Although the causes and consequences of anaemia have not been fully elucidated and its aetiology is occasionally elusive, clinical evidence has indicated that anaemia itself is a cause of morbidity and it can complicate other health conditions. The clinical approach to anaemia is evolving. In the past anaemia was mainly seen as a sign of underlying disease; today anaemia is considered to be a cause of severe deterioration of quality of life, morbidity and decline in physical function and a risk factor for death. A better understanding of anaemia in the elderly will lead to improved treatment strategies including the more judicious use of transfusion.

Suggested further reading

- Ania BJ, Suman VJ, Fairbanks VF, et al. Incidence of anaemia in older people: an epidemiological study in a well defined population. J Am Geriatr Soc 1997; 45: 825–831.
- Antony AC. Megaloblastic anaemias. In Hoffman R, Benz EJ Jr., Shattil SJ et al (eds): Hematology: Basic Principles and Practice, 2nd ed. Churchill Livingstone, New York, 1995, pp. 552–586.
- Bennett, JM, Catovsky, D, Daniel, MT, et al. Proposals for the classification of the acute leukaemias. French-American-British (FAB) co-operative group. Br J Haematol 1976; 33: 451.
- Bennett, JM, Catovsky, D, Daniel, MT, et al. Proposals for the classification of the myelodysplastic syndromes. Br J Haematol 1982; 51: 189.
- Dinant HJ, de Matt CEM. Erythropoiesis and mean red-cell lifespan in normal subjects and in patients with the anaemia of active rheumatoid arthritis. Br J Haematol 1978; 39: 437-444.
- Eschbach JW, Kell MR, Hayley NR, et al. Treatment of the anaemia of progressive renal failure with recombinant human erythropoietin. N Engl J Med 1989; 321: 158-163.
- Freedman ML, Marcus DL. Anaemia in the elderly: Is it physiology or pathology? AM J Med Sci 1980; 280: 81-85.
- Garry PJ, Goodwin JS, Hunt WC. Iron status and anaemia in the elderly: new findings and a review of previous studies. J Am Geriatr Soc 1993; 31: 389-399.
- Green, R, Kinsella, LJ. Editorial: Current concepts in the diagnosis of cobalamin deficiency. Neurology 1995; 45: 1435.
- Guyatt GH, Patterson C, Ali M, et al. Diagnosis of iron deficiency in the elderly. Am J Med 1990; 88: 205-209.
- Hallerg L, Brune M, Rossander-Hulthen R. Is there a physiological role of vitamin C in iron absorption. Ann NY Acad Sci 1987; 498: 324-323.
- Izaks GJ, Westendorp RGJ, Knook DL. The definition of anaemia in older persons. JAMA 1999; 281: 1714-1717.
- Joosten E, Hiele M, Ghoos Y, et al. Diagnosis of iron deficiency anaemia in a hospitalised geriatric population. Am J Med 1991; 90: 653-654.
- Kirkeby OJ, Fossum S, Risoe C. Anaemia in elderly patients. Incidence and causes of low haemoglobin concentration in a city general practice. Scand J Prim Health Care 1991; 9: 167-171.
- Kyle RA. Multiple myeloma: Review of 869 cases. Mayo Clin Proc 1975; 50: 29.
- Liu L, Bopp MM, Roberson PK, et al. Undernutrition and risk of mortality in elderly patients within 1 year of hospital discharge. J Gerontol A Biol Sci Med Sci 2002; 57(11): M741-6.
- Moses PL, Smith RE. Endoscopic evaluation of iron deficiency anaemia; a guide to diagnostic strategy in older patients. Postgrad Med 1995; 98: 213-224.
- Salmon SE, Durie BGM. Myeloma and related disorders. Clin Haematol 1985; 2.
- Salvie ME, Cornoni-Huntley J, Guralnik JM et al. Anaemia and haemoglobin levels in older persons: relationship with age, gender, and health status. J Am Geriatr Soc 1992; 40: 489-496.
- Sears DA. Anaemia of chronic disease. Med Clin North Am 1992; 76: 567-579.
- Selhub, J, Jacques, PF, Wilson, PW, et al. Vitamin status and intake as primary determinants of homocysteinemia in an elderly population. JAMA 1993; 270: 2693.
- Seshadri S, Beiser A, Selhub J, et al. Plasma Homocysteine as a Risk Factor for Dementia and Alzheimer's Disease. N Engl J Med 2002 346: 476-483.
- Smith AG. Prescribing Iron. Prescribers' J 1997;37:82-87.
- Sumner, AE, Chin, MM, Abrahm, JL, et al. Elevated methylmalonic acid and total homocysteine levels show high prevalence of vitamin B12 deficiency after gastric surgery. Ann Intern Med 1996; 124: 469.
- Thompson MP, Morris LK. Unexplained weight loss

in the ambulatory elderly. J Am Geriatr Soc 1991; 39: 497-500.

- *Wallace JI, Schwartz RS, La Croix AZ, et al. Involuntary weight loss in older outpatients: incidence and clinical significance. J Am Geriatr Soc. 1995; 44: 465-466.*
- *Zauber NP, Zauber AG. Haematological data of healthy very old people. JAMA 1997; 257: 2181–2184.*

🗀 Case Study I

An 86 year old female attends her General Practitioner with symptoms of reduced vitality and recent involuntary weight loss. She has noticed 8 kilogram weight loss over six months with her current weight 46 kgs. She denies upper or lower gastrointestinal symptoms nor does she complain of any other constitutional symptoms. She has a background history of hypertension and stable coronary artery disease. Physical examination reveals evidence of mild tenderness in her epigastrium. Bloods are performed and yield mild normochromic anaemia of 10.3g/dl associated with elevation of serum creatinine at 177 umol/l with an ESR of 68mm/hr. An upper GI endoscopy was performed which showed moderate gastritis. She was commenced on triple therapy and returned to outpatients 2 months later. She related that she felt no better. On review of her renal function there had been a progressive decline over 18 months with her current creatinine measured at 186umol/l. Estimation of her glomerular filtration rate (eGFR) using the MDRD equation demonstrate a GFR 20mls/min consistent with Stage 4 Chronic Kidney Disease.

Weight loss is frequently a symptom of progressive renal disease. One should be wary of interpretation of "mild" abnormalities in serum creatinine in elderly patients. Calculation of estimated GFR is more useful in estimating the burden of disease. This can be done simply by using an on line calculator from the Renal Association, UK at http://www.renal.org/eGFRcalc/GFR.pl

🗀 Case Study 2

An 82 year old male attends his General Practitioner with symptoms of fatigue, dyspnoea and dizziness on standing. He has a history of long standing rheumatoid arthritis and hypertension. His medications include Aspirin 75 mgs daily, Celecoxib 200mgs daily and Bendrofluazide 2.5mgs daily. On examination he is pale, has evidence of recent weight loss and epigastric tenderness. An FBC reveals haemoglobin of 7.6g/dl typical of iron deficiency. He is referred to local hospital for investigation. An upper GI endoscopy reveals patchy gastritis and colonoscopy reveals diverticular disease only. He is transfused with five units of packed cells and discharged on a proton pump inhibitor and oral iron. Six months later his haemoglobin is 10.7g/dl and his weight has fallen further. He is referred back to hospital and a repeat gastroscopy shows normal oesophagus, stomach and duodenum. His iron supplements are increased. After discharge his General Practitioner performs a urinalysis that shows a large amount of blood. Urine cytology confirms malignant cells and a subsequent CT scan of abdomen shows a right-sided bladder mass, (Figure 3). Subsequent cystoscopy reveals a large bladder cancer, which was resected.

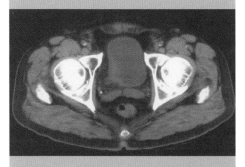

Figure 3

This case clearly confirms the usefulness of urinalysis as part of a routine anaemia workup and demonstrates that minor changes found at gastroscopy should not necessarily be accepted as definite proof of a bleeding site.

Case Study 3

An 81 year old female with a six month history of altered bowel habit associated with significant iron deficiency anaemia is referred by her general practitioner to a gastroenterologist for evaluation. She has a history of a previous hip fracture and chronic lower back pain. Physical examination reveals evidence of weight loss only. She does not have hepatomegaly or splenomegaly. A colonoscopy is performed which shows mild inflammation in the sigmoid colon. Histology is non-specific. The entire colon was otherwise visualised and no further abnormality was seen. She is prescribed Imodium for her symptoms as well as oral iron. She returns to the clinic six months later with continuing symptoms and persisting anaemia. On closer review of her history she has had intermittent diarrhoea for 5 – 7 years. She is also noted to be of short stature. Subsequently she is admitted for further evaluation. An OGD shows loss of duodenal folds with granular appearance, (Figure 4), and histology confirms subtotal villous atrophy, (Figure 5)

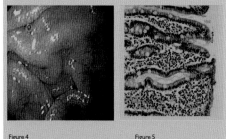

Figure 4   Figure 5

Subsequent coeliac related antibodies were strongly positive. With the introduction of a gluten free diet her weight, diarrhoea and haematological parameters improved.

Coeliac disease is a common disorder possibly affecting 1 in 200 of the general population, the majority of patients being diagnosed in adulthood. Up to a quarter of new cases are diagnosed in those over the age of 65 years and many are asymptomatic. Diagnosis is aided by availability of coeliac related antibodies including anti-endomysial and tissue transglutaminases.

Case Study 4

An 88 year old female attends the day hospital for monitoring of heart failure and recurrent anaemia. She has a background of critical aortic stenosis and peptic ulcer disease. Over a period of five years she has had numerous admissions with upper gastro-intestinal bleeding. She had endoscopically proven gastric and duodenal ulcers and is maintained on a proton pump inhibitor. Over a four month period she has three admissions with melaena. On her most recent admission a bleeding arterio-venous malformation is visualised. This is injected with adrenaline and bleeding stops. However three weeks later the problem recurs and repeat endoscopy shows another bleeding vessel that is injected.

This lady has upper gastro-intestinal angiodysplasia with recurrent upper GI haemorrhage. There are three therapeutic options available;

• Laparotomy with gastrectomy: due to her coexisting severe aortic stenosis this would be associated with unacceptable peri-operative mortality
• Periodic transfusion: due to the increasing frequency of bleeding episodes the patient's quality of life is

affected and an alternative option is pursued
- Coeliac axis angiography: during the patient's subsequent bleeding episode she undergoes angiography, which identifies three bleeding points. The distal portion of her left gastro-duodenal artery is embolised. As a consequence her bleeding settles and remains inactive over the subsequent 12 month follow-up period.

🗁 Case Study 5

An 82 year old female is seen by her General Practitioner with bilateral shoulder girdle pain of 3 months duration. She has a background of hypertension and hypothyroidism. She takes Atenolol 50mgs daily and Pravastatin 20mgs daily. Physical examination revealed limited shoulder abduction bilaterally, more marked on the right. Investiga-

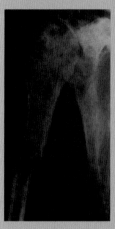

tions reveal a markedly elevated ESR at 108mm/hr. Other laboratory tests show a normochromic anaemia of 10.2g/dl and a creatinine of 208µmol/l. A diagnosis of Polymyalgia Rheumatica is made and the patient is commenced on Prednisolone 15mgs daily. There is no significant response and indeed her shoulder pain deteriorates particularly on the right side. A shoulder x-ray is performed, (Figure 6).

Figure 6

The x-ray shows multiple lytic lesions and a pathological fracture of proximal third of right humerus. Subsequent investigation demonstrates a large IgG paraprotein band in serum with suppression of other immunoglobulins. Bone marrow aspiration demonstrates an excessive population of plasma cells confirming a diagnosis of IgG multiple myeloma, (Table 11).

Data Interpretation

Question 1

A 78 year old man with a background history of hypertension and chronic stable angina presents with involuntary weight loss of 12 kilograms over 8 months. He denies upper or lower gastrointestinal symptoms. He is an ex-smoker for 5 years with a 40 pack year history. He has a tanned complexion and obvious signs at his left lung base. His blood results are illustrated below.

Na	118mmol/l
K+	6.7mmol/l
Urea	18.5mmol/l
Creat	216µmol/l
Albumin	27g/l
Calcium	2.78mmol/l

a. What is likely explanation for electrolyte for the disturbance?
b. What simple test will most likely confirm answer to A?

Question 2

A 76 year old female presents with increasing fatigue over a six month period. She denies any constitutional symptoms. She has a background history of seizure disorder treated with phenytoin and hypertension controlled with amlodipine. Her blood tests are shown below.

Hb 7.8g/dl
MCV 110fl
PLTs 340 x10⁹/l

a. Describe the haematological abnormality
b. What is the likely aetiology?
c. What would be a reasonable approach to management?

Question 3

A 78 year old female presents with increasing fatigue and is found to have normochromic anaemia of 8.2g/L with an ESR of 112. Serum biochemistry shows normal renal function with a slightly raised alkaline phosphatase. She complains of reduced mobility and difficulty getting out of bed in the morning.

a What is the most likely diagnosis?
b. What is a likely beneficial intervention?
c. What special precautions should accompany this intervention?

Best of five questions

Question 1

An 83 year old man who is a heavy drinker presents with a short history of weight loss and diarrhea. He has extensive lower GI investigations which are normal and negative coeliac antibodies. His random glucose is found to be 13mmol/l.

What is the most likely diagnosis?

a   Cirrhosis
b.   Gastric ulceration
c.   Pancreatic insufficiency with diabetes secondary to alcohol
d.   Diverticular disease
e.   Latent coeliac disease

Question 2

Involuntary weight loss with a reduced appetite is found in

a.   Coeliac disease
b.   Thyrotoxicosis
c.   Diabetes mellitus
d.   Depression
e.   Angina pectoris

Question 3

The following are not typical of a diagnosis of multiple myeloma

a.   Paraprotein band in serum
b.   Recurrent infections
c.   Thrombocytopaenia
d.   Sclerotic lesions on x-ray
e.   Hypercalcaemia

Answers are on page 311

Dyspnoea and chest pain

C O'Brien, C Henry, C Twomey, R Liston

Introduction

Cardiorespiratory diseases account for significant morbidity in older patients and are a leading cause of death in this group. Statistics from the American health care system show that 80% of patients hospitalised with heart failure are more than 65 years old while COPD is the fourth leading cause of chronic morbidity and mortality in the United States. The incidence of both these illnesses increases with age. Diminishing reserve in cardiorespiratory function makes older patients more vulnerable to the effects of these diseases and indeed the medication used to treat them. Ischaemic heart disease, chronic obstructive pulmonary disease (COPD) and congestive cardiac failure (CCF) may all present with dyspnoea and chest pain alone or in combination. As with other disease processes however these symptoms are often absent in older patients making assessment difficult. For instance older patients may not readily report exertional symptoms because over time they have curtailed their exercise to avoid symptoms or because their mobility has already been affected by comorbid conditions. Equally chest pain may be absent in myocardial infarction due to altered sensory perception associated with ageing. In the acute phase of these illnesses cognitive impairment may prevent older patients from volunteering these symptoms again making assessment difficult and in the absence of classical presentations a high index of clinical suspicion is required. In this chapter, we will highlight the approach to older patients who presents with dyspnoea or chest pain, focusing on the commoner conditions.

Changes in respiratory and cardiac function with age

Although there are clearly observed changes in both structure and function of the ageing respiratory and cardiovascular systems, these do not apply uniformly to all older people. The reserve capacity of the lungs is vast so that a significant reduction in function can occur with only a minimal effect on normal breathing. Ageing causes a decline in elastic recoil of the small airways with a resulting decline of 0.2% per year in the FEV_1/FVC ratio from 70% at the age of 45 years. Symptoms will occur when FEV_1 falls below 50%. This loss of elastic recoil can lead to an increase of ventilation-perfusion mismatch because there is an increasing tendency of the smaller airways to collapse in dependent areas of the lung in expiration.

Factors other than age may also be influential. Smokers, for instance, tend to demonstrate a much more rapid decline in Forced Expiratory Volume (FEV_1) than would be seen in non-smokers. Likewise, those people who had significant respiratory disease in childhood may never have achieved their maximum respiratory potential and the naturally occurring fall in FEV_1 may result in the manifestation of symptoms at an earlier than expected age. With 'normal' ageing, the normal lungs become stiffer and less compliant resulting in a larger residual volume. These changes are more exaggerated in smokers. In parallel, there is a reduction in respiratory muscle strength and endurance, blunting both the maximum inspiratory and expiratory pressures achieved. Alterations in forced expiratory volumes are well described and again are exaggerated in smokers. Figure 1, which comes from the Fletcher and Peto paper on the natural history of airflow obstruction, demonstrates that 'impairment' is reached at an earlier age in smokers and that even late changes in smoking habits may result in halt of decline in respiratory formation. The changes accelerate with age. These physiological and smoking-related changes become relevant in the presence of intercurrent illness such as pneumonia or left ventricular failure when this loss of reserve results in earlier respiratory distress, longer times to recovery and altered physiological responses to medication.

In tandem with these changes, the ageing process leads to a reduction in the numbers of glandular epithelial cells with a resultant decrease in protective mucus which impairs the defences against infection. As well as this, the respiratory centre, located in the pons and medulla, shows altered responses to both hypoxia and hypercapnia. These responses result in a more blunted ventilatory response to the metabolic

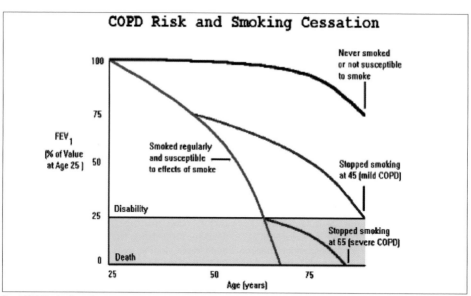

COPD Risk and Smoking Cessation

Never smoked or not susceptible to smoke

FEV₁ (% of Value at Age 25)

Smoked regularly and susceptible to effects of smoke

Stopped smoking at 45 (mild COPD)

Disability

Stopped smoking at 65 (severe COPD)

Death

Age (years)

Figure I COPD risk and smoking cessation

changes seen in severe respiratory illness. The clinical result is a higher risk of respiratory failure.

As with the respiratory system, age-related changes in the cardiovascular system show a lot of inter-individual variation in older people. Again diminished reserve may be exposed by intercurrent illnesses. These physiological changes may be further compounded by the increased prevalence of cardiovascular disease in the older population most noticeably coronary artery disease. Ageing is associated with a reduction in the compliance of large elastic arteries causing an increase in mean blood pressure and in pulse pressure. Ageing also prolongs the duration of left ventricular contraction and relaxation. There is a resultant increase in afterload leading to an increase in left ventricular wall thickness and systolic hypertension. A less compliant left ventricle results in diminished rapid early ventricular filling and increased dependency on late atrial filling. Although this may not impact on cardiac function in healthy states, this dependency on atrial preload leaves the older person vulnerable to reduced output states in atrial fibrillation, a condition which is much more common with age. Beta-adrenergic responsiveness of the cardiovascular system also alters with age. This is reflected at times of cardiovascular stress, for example during exercise, when there are blunted responses

in terms of maximum heart rates and peak ejection fractions. Because of reduced cardiac and vascular responsiveness to beta stimulation, the vasodepressor effects of many drugs have a more penetrative effect, commonly presenting as orthostatic hypotension. Unfortunately, both respiratory and cardiac diseases are more common with age and will continue to be a leading cause of disability, morbidity and mortality in older age for the forseeable future.

Assessment of dyspnoea and chest pain
It is important to bear in mind that clinical features, which may be somewhat imprecise in younger patients, lack even more sensitivity and specificity in terms of identifying a particular diagnosis when dealing with older patients. In this section, we will examine the usefulness and discriminatory qualities of the different facets of dyspnoea and chest pain and illustrate the particular challenges of clinical assessment in older age with real case histories.

Asthma
Older people with asthma may present with typical features of shortness of breath, cough and intermittent wheeze but not as commonly as in younger patients where a more obvious bronchospasm may be evident. Older patients tend not to be as aware of the symptoms of bronchoconstriction as younger

patients and frequently underestimate their presence and severity. Intermittent wheeze at night is often thought to be paroxysmal nocturnal dyspnoea. The clinical signs of basal crepitations and oedema are common and non-specific in older individuals with a low positive predictive value for CCF. Asthma however is a common condition in older age and may occur de novo where there is a tendency to confuse all airflow obstruction with COPD. A high level of clinical suspicion is required in order not to miss it. The key features of asthma are variability in symptoms, intermittent deterioration especially at night, provocation by triggers such as exercises or specific medications such as NSAIDs, aspirin or beta-blockers. The most useful sign, if found, is wheeze, which may be variable and associated with a reduced Peak Expiratory Flow Rate (PEFR) and an obstructive pattern on spirometry with the FEV_1/FVC ratio < 70%. In addition, a personal or family history of asthma may be a pointer. British Thoracic Society and SIGN guidelines recognise the importance of objective measurements when diagnosing asthma as shown in Table 1.

Arriving at a diagnosis is all the more difficult because of the high prevalence of COPD. There is a great deal of overlap between both conditions, not least because smoking can act as a provoking agent in asthma. In addition, patients with COPD can also suffer exacerbations. The diagnosis of asthma requires not just careful history taking but also objective measurements in the form of spirometry. It is important to remember that acute asthma carries a higher mortality rate in old age partly because older patients underreport the severity of their symptoms and also because they tend to develop less tachycardia and tachypnoea for the same degree of bronchconstriction. Reversibility testing should be considered in all supposed cases of COPD as chronic asthma in older age may present with persistent and not intermittent airflow obstruction.

Treatment of asthma in older adults follows the same principles as in younger patients. Their condition needs to be monitored, factors that precipitate attacks need to be avoided and pharmacological therapies are similar. Symptom relief is provided by short acting beta agonists, with inhaled glucocorticoids offering the same benefits as in younger patients. Step up therapy generally follows the same guidelines as in younger patients. However in those patients with coexistent CHF increasing inhaled corticosteroids

| TABLE 1 |
DIAGNOSIS OF ASTHMA
>20% diurnal variation on > 3 days in a week for two weeks on PEFR diary
OR
FEV_1 ≥ 15% and 200ml increase after short acting beta 2 agonist (salbutamol 400ug by metered dose inhaler + spacer or 2.5mg by nebuliser)
OR
FEV_1 ≥ 15% and 200mls increase after trial of steroid tablets (prednisolone 30mg/day for 14 days)
OR
FEV_1 ≥ 15% decrease after six minutes of exercise

may be better than introducing long acting beta agonists. Oral steroids should only be used in short bursts and chronic oral steroid therapy only as a last resort. Steroid sparing therapy with a leukotriene antagonist is successful in older adults. Theophyllines are not recommended for treatment of asthma in this group of patients. Inhaler technique may be difficult for some older adults where a metered dose inhaler or breath-activated inhaler or indeed a nebuliser will provide better drug delivery.

Bronchial carcinoma

Ageing is a major risk factor for the development of lung cancer. Individuals with bronchial carcinoma may present with infective exacerbations of COPD with associated resistant respiratory tract infections. Because of a shared aetiology, patients with lung cancer frequently have co-existing COPD as well as ischaemic heart disease. Patients who are current or ex-smokers should have a chest x-ray if they present with new or deteriorating respiratory symptoms. In addition, sputum cytological analysis may yield a diagnosis in over 40% of cases with suspicious chest x-rays or suspicious clinical features. One of the peculiarities of lung cancer in older people is that it is less likely to have spread by time of diagnosis. Rather than reflecting any particular resistance to spread in older people, this may occur simply because older people are more likely to have a chest x-ray for concomitant disease, thus picking up pathology at an earlier stage of its natural history. The presence of other respiratory symptoms, particularly haemoptysis or pleuritic pain as well as systemic symptoms such as weight loss or anorexia should

TABLE 2
THE GOLD GUIDELINES

STAGE	CHARACTERISTICS	RECOMMENDED TREATMENT
At risk	Chronic symptoms Exposure to risk factors Normal spirometry	Avoid risk factors (tobacco smoke etc) Influenza vaccination
Mild COPD	$FEV_1/FVC < 70\%$ $FEV_1 \geq 80\%$ of predicted With or without symptoms	Avoid risk factors Influenza vaccination Short acting bronchodilator when needed
Moderate COPD (a)	$FEV_1/FVC < 70\%$ FEV_1 - 50% to 80% of predicted With or without symptoms	Avoid risk factors Influenza vaccination Regular treatment with bronchodilators Rehabilitation Inhaled steroids if significant symptoms and lung function response
Moderate COPD (b)	$FEV_1/FVC < 70\%$ FEV_1 - 30% to 50% of predicted With or without symptoms	Avoid risk factors Influenza vaccination Regular treatment with bronchodilators Rehabilitation Inhaled steroids if significant symptoms and lung function response or if repeated exacerbations
Severe COPD	$FEV_1/FVC < 70\%$ $FEV_1 < 30\%$ of predicted or presence of respiratory failure or right heart failure	As above plus: Long-term oxygen if indicated Treatment of complications Surgical treatment if necessary

heighten the suspicion of an underlying malignancy. The presence of pleural effusion, lymphadenopathy or persistent consolidation may also point towards this diagnosis. Patients occasionally present with specific localising syndromes such as Horner's syndrome in association with a Pancoast's tumour, hoarseness due to recurrent laryngeal involvement or superior vena caval syndrome due to obstruction. Older patients are less likely to be referred for bronchoscopy than younger patients although the procedure is safe and generally tolerated very well. However caution is advocated for those with significant comorbidities and those not fit for any follow-on interventions. In the case of squamous cell carcinoma, the 5 year survival rates for those who undergo surgery are similar to younger patients.

Chronic obstructive pulmonary disease

As stated above, there is a progressive decline in lung function with age. This is more marked in smokers or in those who never achieved maximum lung function. There is considerable overlap between what is termed COPD, emphysema which is essentially a pathological term and asthma. It is now accepted that COPD should be considered in any patient who complains of dyspnoea that is persistent, progressive, usually worse with exercise, accompanied by a chronic cough which may be intermittent and may or may not be productive. Chronic sputum production or a history of exposure to risk factors such as tobacco smoke or industrial dust or chemicals should also raise suspicions. The diagnosis should be checked with spirometry where a FEV_1/FVC ratio below 0.7 (70%) after bronchodilator therapy confirms the diagnosis.

Many patients with COPD may demonstrate some reversibility in spirometry. However it is only when changes in FEV_1 of greater than 12% or 200ml occur after bronchodilator therapy that the diagnosis of asthma becomes a greater likelihood. In some older patients it is likely that both asthma and COPD coexist. Therefore all patients with suspected COPD should have reversibility studies.

The aims of management are to relieve symptoms, improve exercise tolerance and overall health status. The aim should be to prevent and treat exacerbations and complications and reduce mortality. Unfortunately COPD is a progressive disease with a reduction in lung function expected over time. The patient's symptoms and measurements of airflow limitation should be monitored to determine when to modify treatment and identify complications. Co-morbidities are common in older patients and should be actively identified as they will complicate management and influence the course of the disease. According to the Global Initiative for Chronic Obstructive Lung Disease (GOLD) guidelines, patients should be stratified according to symptoms and spirometry results. The level of severity dictates the level of treatment (Table 2). Clearly, stopping smoking is a priority and there is increasing evidence that rehabilitation programmes can benefit many individuals.

Interstitial lung disease

While COPD and asthma or a combination of both account for the majority of respiratory cases seen in the older population, other respiratory illnesses including interstitial lung diseases increase in prevalence with age. This group includes pneumoconioses such as silicosis, asbestosis and extrinsic allergic alveolitis eg. farmers lung. Asbestosis tends to present in the older population because of the long latency period between exposure and disease. Lung fibrosis may occur in association with other autoimmune disorders such as rheumatoid arthritis and Wegener's granulomatosis. A drug-induced variant can develop as a response to cytotoxic agents and other more commonly used drugs such as amiodarone. By virtue of the fact that some drug usage increases with age, the frequency of such reactions may also increase.

Another large group of interstitial lung diseases of uncertain aetiology are the idiopathic interstitial pneumonias. They are characterised by inflammation and a tendency to fibrosis of the lung parenchyma. The most common of these is interstitial pulmonary fibrosis

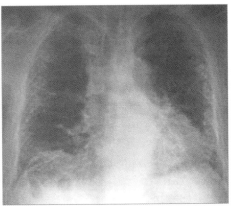

Figure 2: Chest x-ray of 69 year old man with UIP. There are coarse reticular infiltrates with associated honeycombing in the periphery of the lungs and lung bases

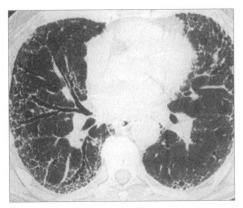

Figure 3: High resolution CT in a similar 75 year old patient with UIP. The image is taken at the level of the right middle lobe bronchus. There is extensive subpleural honeycombing with subpleural reticular opacities. There is also traction bronchiectasis in post-segmental branches of right middle lobe and superior segmental branches of right lower lobe

which is a disease of the elderly, rarely seen in patients less than 50 years. Radiologically and pathologically the findings are of a usual interstitial pneumonia (UIP). It is characterised clinically by progressive respiratory impairment culminating in respiratory failure. In older patients with interstitial lung disease the combination of pulmonary fibrosis with reduced chest wall compliance and respiratory muscle weakness and deconditioning exacerbate dyspnoea significantly. The typical presentation is with dyspnoea of exertion, often indistinguishable, in the early stages at least, from COPD. Clinical examination often reveals finger clubbing and late inspiratory crackles said to sound like velcro being unzipped. As the disease progresses there is central cyanosis and evidence of right heart

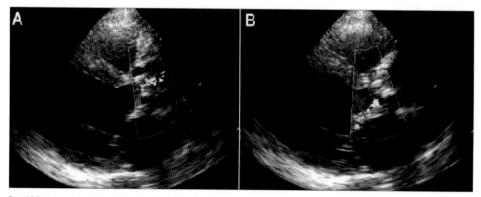

Figure 4: 2-D echo long axis view of calcific aortic stenosis in a 76 year old man who complains of increasing dyspnoea. There is turbulent flow at the aortic valve in systole (A). In B there is also a regurgitant jet seen in the outflow tract in diastole. As well as having thickened valve leaflets causing a degree of obstruction in systole, the leaflets are also failing to appose properly and so allowing a degree of regurgitation in diastole

failure. Pulmonary function tests may reveal a restrictive defect with reduced total lung capacity, reduced residual volume and diminished transfer factor. There is often poor correlation between clinical features and radiological changes. Chest radiographs may typically show widespread reticular shadowing in middle and lower zones differing from the upper zone involvement of tuberculosis and sarcoidosis. Nodular or 'ground-glass' patterns may indicate intra-alveolar oedema and focal areas of inflammation respectively. End-stage disease is associated with cystic change. High-resolution CT scanning is sensitive and can give estimations of the degree of activity of the disease process as well as predicting response to treatment. High dose steroids are the mainstay of treatment along with immunosuppressive therapy.

Aortic stenosis

In case 5 the expected symptoms of exertional dyspnoea, chest pain or exertional syncope were not present because the patient avoided exercise but these classical symptoms of aortic stenosis are common in older patients. Aortic stenosis particularly if associated with dyspnoea, fatigue, peripheral oedema or raised JVP is often progressive and death usually occurs within 2 to 3 years unless there is intervention. Milder degrees of aortic stenosis are common in older people mainly due to calcific degeneration of the valve. It is worthwhile repeating echocardiography on a yearly basis to identify these patients before the stenosis becomes too severe.

Heart failure

Heart failure is a common and disabling disease

which impacts greatly on quality of life and health care costs. The incidence of heart failure increases from 2% to 3% at age 65 years to more than 80% in persons over 80 years of age. Heart failure is associated with left ventricular systolic dysfunction (LVSD) and left ventricular diastolic dysfunction (LVDD). In LVSD the impaired left ventricle does not contract well enough to pump an adequate supply of oxygenated blood to the peripheral circulation. In LVDD the left ventricle is stiff and fails to relax properly which means that the left ventricle does not fill properly and so cannot pump a sufficient volume of blood to the peripheral circulation. LVDD is more common in the elderly. Diagnosis may be difficult because there are other causes of dyspnoea or fatigue in older people such as COPD or asthma and these conditions may co-exist.

Clinically heart failure is characterised by dyspnoea, peripheral oedema and fatigue; the latter being more common in older patients. Insomnia is also common, perhaps because of orthopnoea. By the time older patients present with overt symptoms, the disease process is often advanced. The usual scales used to assess severity may therefore not be particularly helpful in older people. In many patients, diagnosis may be simple if there are obvious clinical signs. In others, especially in milder cases, the diagnosis may not be so straightforward. The diagnosis is arrived at by assessing the combination of symptoms and signs and the presence of a likely cause of chronic heart failure (CHF).

The clinical features, which may be sensitive, are not

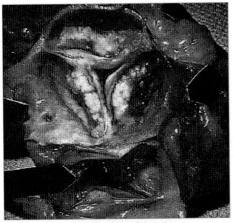

Figure 5: A pathological specimen showing a stenotic calcified aortic valve

TABLE 3
NEW YORK HEART ASSOCIATION FUNCTIONAL STATUS (NYHA)

Class I	No limitation: ordinary physical exercise does not cause undue fatigue, dyspnoea or palpitations
Class II	Slight limitation of activity: comfortable at rest but ordinary activity results in fatigue, palpitations or dyspnoea
Class III	Marked limitation of physical activity: comfortable at rest but less than ordinary activity results in symptoms
Class IV	Unable to carry out any physical activity without discomfort: symptoms of heart failure are present even at rest with increased discomfort with any physical activity

specific i.e. peripheral oedema and bibasal crepitations. However, those signs that are specific may not be so sensitive eg. raised JVP and the presence of a third heart sound. ECGs may reveal old myocardial infarction, left ventricular hypertrophy seen in hypertension or aortic stenosis or poorly controlled atrial fibrillation. In recent onset heart failure, it is essential to outrule a new myocardial infarct.

The common changes on the chest x-ray seen in heart failure are cardiothoracic ratio > 0.55, upper lobe venous diversion and Kerley B lines with or without bilateral pleural effusions. Echocardiography is a far more useful investigation, supporting the diagnosis where there is doubt, by giving an estimate of ventricular systolic function or by identifying diastolic dysfunction. Echocardiography will yield a cause of heart failure in many instances, for example by identifying regional wall motion abnormalities post myocardial infarction, left ventricular hypertrophy seen in hypertension or valvular problems, most notably aortic stenosis. In diastolic dysfunction there is normal systolic function on echocardiography but clinically patients present with signs and symptoms of heart failure. 51% of the Framingham cohort of patients with heart failure had an ejection fraction greater than 50%.

There is increasing interest in the use of brain natriuretic peptides in the diagnosis of left ventricular dysfunction. Brain natriuretic peptide and N terminal-pro-BNP (NT-proBNP) are peptide hormones produced in the heart by breakdown of a precursor protein (pro-BNP). These peptides have been shown to correlate well with left ventricular function. They are raised in patients with heart failure and the concentrations rise with NYHA class. This test has a strong negative predictive value but a lesser positive predictive value for systolic heart failure. It may be useful in a primary care setting or in a day hospital to discriminate dyspnoea caused by heart failure from other causes. There is also evidence that it may be used to guide dosage of ACE inhibitor therapy.

Heart failure has a mortality rate worse than many cancers and despite the introduction of new pharmacological agents and other interventions, it still carries a 1-year mortality rate of 45%. It is therefore important to identify and treat any reversible causes or aggravating factors including cardiac arrhythmias, thyrotoxicosis, anaemia or aortic stenosis. Treatment strategies for patients with heart failure aim to reduce cardiac work, reduce excessive plasma volume and cardiac dilatation and improve cardiac contractility. Table 4 outlines the current best guidelines for managing heart failure in older patients in both the acute and chronic setting. The priorities of management are:
• Stabilise the patient, relieve distress and begin definitive treatment
• Look for the underlying causes
• Optimise long-term therapy

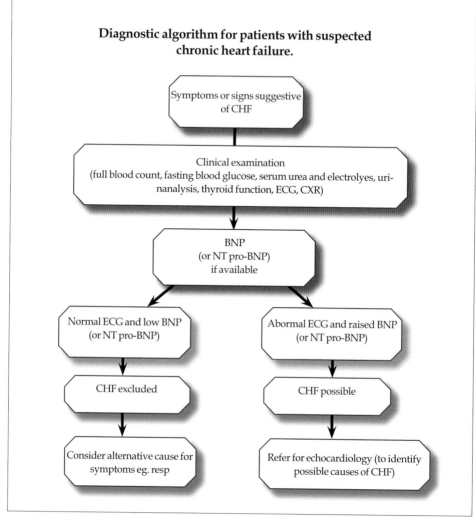

Diagnostic algorithm for patients with suspected chronic heart failure.

Symptoms or signs suggestive of CHF

Clinical examination
(full blood count, fasting blood glucose, serum urea and electrolyes, urinanalysis, thyroid function, ECG, CXR)

BNP
(or NT pro-BNP)
if available

Normal ECG and low BNP
(or NT pro-BNP)

Abormal ECG and raised BNP
(or NT pro-BNP)

CHF excluded

CHF possible

Consider alternative cause for symptoms eg. resp

Refer for echocardiology (to identify possible causes of CHF)

Figure 6: CHF diagnostic algorithm

Loop diuretics are recommended as first line diuretic therapy in older patients because of their effectiveness particularly at lower glomerular filtration rates and because they are less likely to cause hypokalaemia than thiazides. However in the management of chronic cardiac failure it is important to bear in mind the social difficulties older patients may experience because of the increasing frequency and volume of voiding. Treatment regimes should be discussed with patients so that they are allowed the flexibility to alter the timing of their diuretic medications to enable them to plan for leaving home for shopping trips etc, or if they are going on longer journeys to omit the diuretic for one day during the journey. For some patients a brisk diuresis over a shorter duration from a higher dose loop diuretic may allow them more freedom during the day while for others a slower, easier diuresis may be suitable. For older men with prostatic hypertrophy a brisk diuresis might lead to acute urinary retention. In general, patients with

1. Sit patient up
2. Give oxygen 40-60% and maintain oxygen saturation
3. Record an ECG, attach to ECG monitor, treat any arrhythmia
4. Give morphine 2.5mg IV and frusemide 40mg IV
5. Repeat at 5 min if no response
6. Further drug therapy depends on blood pressure and symptom response
    Systolic BP > 100mmHg and still symptomatic
    *   Give another dose of Frusemide 40mg
    *   Repeat in 5 min if no response
    *   If patient remains breathless and BP > 100mmHg start a GTN infusion (50mg GTN in 400mls 5% dextrose), start at $10\mu g$/min and increase by $10\mu g$ every 10 min to a maximum of $300\mu g$/min
    Systolic BP < 100mmHg
    *   Start dobutamine infusion (500mg in 500ml 5% dextrose) at $5\mu g$/kg/min and increase every 15 min to a maximum of $20\mu g$/kg/min
    *   A nitrate infusion can be added if patient still breathless & systolic BP can be maintained at greater than 100mmHg
7. Urgent investigations for all patients
    *   ECG - cardiac arrhythmia or myocardial infarction
    *   ABG - pulse oximetry can be inaccurate if peripherally shut down
    *   U&E – pre-existing renal failure and potassium level
    *   FBC - anaemia or leucocytosis indicating the precipitant
8. If patient has renal failure conventional doses of frusemide can be ineffective and higher dose required

urinary retention or incontinence manage better with low-dose loop diuretics or thiazide agents. ACE inhibitors and beta-blockers are essential particularly after myocardial infarction because they are associated with improvement in survival and quality of life. They also reduce hospitalisation rates and the incidence of sudden death. NSAIDs are commonly prescribed for older patients but should be avoided if possible because this class of drugs are associated with an increased incidence of heart failure and increased hospitalisation for heart failure.

Management of chronic heart failure (CHF)

In all patients with a clinical diagnosis of CHF the aim is to address non-pharmacological and lifestyle measures, review medication and if possible discontinue aggravating drugs.

Diuretics

These agents remain the mainstay of symptomatic control. The aim should be for optimal diuretic therapy, usually with either frusemide or bumetanide (1mg bumetanide = 40mg frusemide), to control dyspnoea and fluid retention without causing dehydration or renal dysfunction.

ACE inhibitors

These are the cornerstone of treatment in patients with all grades of symptomatic heart failure and in patients with asymptomatic left ventricular dysfunction. The contraindications to ACE inhibitor use include hypersensitivity, angioedema, known or suspected renovascular disease and aortic stenosis with a gradient >20mmHg.

Angiotensin II receptor blockers (ARBs)

ARBS are an acceptable alternative in patients who develop intolerable side effects from ACE inhibitors. Patients with left ventricular systolic dysfunction who remain symptomatic after treatment with ACE inhibition and a beta-blocker may benefit from the addition of an ARB.

Oral nitrates and hydralazine

Hydralazine plus isosorbide mononitrate is an alternative to ACE inhibitors and angiotensin II receptor blockers where these are contraindicated.

All patients

1. Patient & family education. Cognitive impairment is associated with CHF particularly in older patients so advice and education may have to be tailored to suit this
2. Advise to stop smoking and offer smoking cessation advice and support
3. Advise to avoid excessive alcohol consumption. Alcohol is a myocardial depressant. If the cause of heart failure is suspected alcohol cardiomyopathy then the advice is to stop alcohol completely
4. Dietary advice to include weight reduction if obese and appropriate diet if nutritional deficiencies found and salt restriction
5. Patients should be advised to undertake regular low intensity physical activity once heart failure is stable
6. Screen patients for depression. Common in patients with CHF and is associated with an increase in mortality
7. Review medication and stop any meds which may aggravate heart failure such as NSAIDs or calcium antagonists. If tricyclics are being used to treat depression substitute an alternative

Inpatients

8. Daily weights
9. Restrict fluid to 1-1.5l/24 hours
10. Tinazaparin 3,500U s/c daily

| TABLE 6 |
| USE OF DIURETICS IN CHF |

Mild HF (NYHA class I-II)
- Start loop diuretic eg. frusemide 40mg od PO

Moderate HF (NYHA class II-III)
- Increase loop diuretic eg. frusemide 80mg od PO/IV
- Consider changing to bumetanide if suboptimal response on frusemide

Severe HF (NYHA class IV) - diuretic therapy must be intravenous initially
- Frusemide 40mg iv bd x 24 hours - if no response
- Frusemide 80mg iv bd x 24 hours - if no response
- Add metolazone 2.5mg PO for 24 hours - if no response
- Metolazone 5mg PO daily
- Other therapies
  - Spironolactone
  - Digoxin
  - Hydrochlorothiazide
  - Bendrofluazide

The dose is hydralazine 75mg bd (37.5mg bd for the first 2 weeks) and isosorbide mononitrate is 60mg od (30mg od for the first 2 weeks).

Beta blockers

Patients with mild to moderate stable heart failure should be considered for beta blocker therapy (NYHA class II-III). Initiation should be under close supervision either in hospital or more likely at the Geriatric Day Hospital. They should be commenced on a low dose and gradually titrated upwards. Beta blockers are contraindicated in patients with asthma, symptomatic hypotension and in patients with second or third degree heart block. Cardioselective beta blockers may be used in patients with COPD. Carvedilol, bisoprolol or nebivolol are the drugs of choice. In the SENIORS trial nebivolol significantly reduced death and cardiovascular hospitalisations in elderly heart failure patients. In the short term there may be a mild deterioration in symptoms, which may require alteration of other therapies particularly diuretics.

The use of spironolactone should be considered in patients with severe chronic cardiac failure (NYHA class III-IV).

As well as the above pharmacological and non-pharmacological measures other goals of therapy in treatment of heart failure will include measures that treat concomitant disease processes such as hypertension or diabetes which influence myocardial function. The possibility of tachyarrhythmias should also be considered and treated if found. Many cases of heart failure in the elderly are due to underlying myocardial ischaemia which when treated will improve heart failure. A large proportion of these patients may even have preserved left ventricular function. The evidence for which pharmacological agents are best for these patients is lacking at present. While diuretics and increasingly ACE inhibitors are the mainstay of treatment as in systolic dysfunction, there is a danger that overdiuresis may lead to a

TABLE 8
DIGOXIN SHOULD BE CONSIDERED IN THE FOLLOWING CASES

- Patients in sinus rhythm and continued symptoms of heart failure despite optimal doses of diuretic and ACE inhibitor
- Patients in sinus rhythm with recurrent hospital admissions for heart failure
- Patients in atrial fibrillation will probably already be on digoxin

reduction in left ventricular filling pressures which should be kept high in diastolic dysfunction, to maintain a normal cardiac output. Results from the CHARM Preserve trial showed favourable trends for the treatment of these patients with ARBs. Careful control of blood pressure and good control of diabetes is also highly beneficial in this group.

Annual influenza vaccination is recommended for all elderly patients with CHF. These patients should also receive the pneumococcal vaccine. Studies have shown that episodes of acute heart failure have been provoked by influenza and pulmonary infections, which are significantly reduced in the vaccinated population. Cardiac resynchronisaton can be considered in patients in sinus rhythm with left ventricular ejection fraction ≤35%, and symptomatic heart failure despite optimal medical treatment with a prolonged QRS (>120 msec). Correcting ventricular dyssynchrony with bi-ventricular pacing has improved quality of life and reduced hospital admissions for heart failure and improved mortality. Similarly implantable cardiac defibrillators (ICD) will have a role to play in patients with heart failure and life threatening arrhythmias.

While full use of pharmacological regimes in the treatment of heart failure brings benefits to older patients some adjustments may have to be made for frail elderly patients. The existence of co-morbid conditions such as renal dysfunction, postural hypotension or COPD may influence drug choice. Multiple drug regimens and target dose titration may not be tolerated by these patients. These factors together with the presence of other life limiting disease will dictate that symptom control and improvement

in quality of life are the aims of treatment rather than the improvement of prognosis. As regards using devices such as ICD and cardiac resynchronisation, co-morbidities, life expectancy and quality of life issues must be addressed by the clinicians, patients and families. A guideline that may be used is that where there is a reasonable expectation of survival with a good functional status for more than one year it should be considered.

Indications for permanent cardiac pacing and ICDs

The primary reason for considering permanent cardiac pacing in older adults as in younger patients is identifying bradycardia as a cause of syncope. Sinus node disease (SND) is primarily a disease of the elderly. The ageing process causes degenerative changes in the sinus node and in the specialised conducting tissue of the atrium. This degeneration causes sinus bradycardia and sinus arrest. It also causes paroxysmal supraventricular tachycardia and paroxysmal atrial fibrillation ('tachy-brady syndrome'). Clinically patients can present with syncope, seizures, dizziness, palpitations, heart failure and confusion. A permanent pacemaker is needed for documented, symptomatic bradycardia

TABLE 9
SPIRONOLACTONE

- Prior to spironolactone consideration, patients should have loop diuretic therapy and optimal use of an ACE inhibitor if tolerated. Potassium-sparing diuretics and potassium supplements should be stopped
- Creatinine concentration >200mmol/l is a relative contraindication
- Use is contraindicated if potassium is > 5mmol/l
- Starting dose is spironolactone 25mg od

TABLE 10 PHARMACOLOGICAL MEASURES BY NYHA CLASS IN PATIENTS WITH LVSD	
CLASS	DRUGS
NYHA I	ACE inhibitor
	Beta blocker
	Diuretic for fluid retention
NYHA II-III	ACE inhibitor
	Beta blocker
	Diuretic for fluid retention
	ARB
NYHA III-IV	ACE inhibitor
	Beta blocker
	Diuretic for fluid retention
	ARB
In selected patients consider	
	Digoxin
	Hydralazine/Nitrates
	Spironolactone
Additional measures:	
	Biventricular pacing
	ICD

including frequent sinus pauses. For those patients with heart rates of less than 40bpm, with symptoms suggestive of bradycardia, but in whom the correlation between bradycardia and symptoms has not been documented, permanent pacemaker insertion is warranted. This is particularly relevant in elderly patients who have had syncope and are at risk of significant injury if they fall. If syncope occurs in SND in the elderly it is highly likely to recur.

The second commonest indication for pacemaker insertion is acquired AV block. In the elderly the most common reasons for acquiring it are ischaemic heart disease and calcification affecting the aortic or mitral rings. Certain drugs can cause AV block such as digoxin and calcium channel blockers. All drugs that potentially cause conduction abnormalities should be stopped if possible. However if these drugs are necessary then you can consider continuing them and inserting a pacemaker. This can occur in cases where treatment of tachyarrhythmias is necessary with medications which as a side effect may impair conduction significantly.

Older patients can be considered for implantable cardioverter defibrillators (ICD). Accepted indications for the devices included patients who are survivors of cardiac arrest due to ventricular fibrillation, or haemodynamically unstable sustained ventricular tachycardia. Patients who have been found to have life threatening arrhythmias post myocardial infarction with heart failure or patients with cardiomyopathy and life threatening arrhythmias should also be considered. As already stated if a patient's general condition is such that they have a reasonable expectation of a one year survival with good quality then these options should be discussed with the patient and their families.

The insertion of either a permanent pacemaker or ICD is well tolerated by elderly patients. In the future more consideration will have to be given to decisions about if and when these devices are extracted. This is especially relevant in the case of ICD where issues regarding switching off the defibrillator function of the device as patients approach end of life may need to be discussed. No current guidelines are in place at present regarding this issue.

Atrial fibrillation in older patients

Atrial fibrillation is the commonest sustained arrhythmia and its incidence increases with age. Atrial fibrillation is found in 2-3% of 70 year olds and approaches 10% in those aged over 80 years. Common causes for atrial fibrillation in older patients are coronary artery disease, valvular heart disease especially mitral valve disease and hypertension. It is also caused by hyperthyroidism and excessive alcohol intake which are important to remember as they are potentially reversible causes. Atrial fibrillation can be paroxysmal or persistent. Patients will complain of palpitations, weakness, dyspnoea and reduced exercise capacity. As atrial fibrillation can aggravate underlying angina and heart failure patients may present with chest pain, worsening heart failure or hypotension. Relevant investigations for patients in atrial fibrillation include ECG to confirm the diagnosis or holter monitoring for those with intermittent atrial fibrillation. An echocardiogram is useful to detect heart failure and structural heart abnormalities. Thyroid function tests will rule out hyperthyroidism. The most important issue in managing atrial fibrillation in older patients is choosing between rate and rhythm control and prevention of systemic embolisation.

The vast majority of these patients will be managed with rate control and anticoagulation with warfarin.

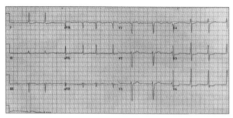

Figure 7: Atrial fibrillation

However in some patients with first presentation atrial fibrillation without any underlying cardiac structural abnormality rhythm control may be considered. Sinus rhythm can be restored by either DC cardioversion or antiarrhythmic medication. DC cardioversion can be used in patients with atrial fibrillation who are haemodynamically unstable and in whom it is of short duration. If time since onset is less than 48 hours cardioversion can be carried out without anticoagulation, otherwise the patient must be anticoagulated beforehand. Antiarrhythmic agents such as flecanide, or propafenone or amiodarone may restore sinus rhythm. DC cardioversion is less successful in older patients and is followed by high rates of recurrent arrythmia. Medications are also less successful and are not always well tolerated. Similarly catheter ablation for atrial fibrillation has been shown to offer less therapeutic benefit to elderly patients. Rate control is a more realistic target. Rate control is important to prevent haemodynamic instability improving symptoms of light headedness, palpitations, dyspnoea and reduced exercise capacity. In the long term this will help to prevent tachycardia mediated cardiomyopathy.

Recent studies have shown that rhythm control is no better than rate control in older patients either with or without heart failure. Rate control can be achieved by using beta blockers or calcium antagonists. Digoxin is useful in older patients with heart failure, however it is not as effective in achieving rate control during exercise as beta blockers or calcium antagonists. Adequate rate control is achieved where resting heart rates are < 80 bpm and heart rates are <110bpm following exercise.

Atrial fibrillation is found in 15% of all stroke patients and in 2 – 8% of those with TIAs. Anticoagulation reduces this risk significantly. The CHAD2 score is a validated score used to stratify patient risk of embolisation in atrial fibrillation and so guide therapy. The CHAD2 score is as follows:

TABLE 11 COMMON INDICATIONS FOR PERMANENT PACE-MAKER INSERTION IN OLDER PATIENTS

Sinus node disease
- Sick sinus syndrome

Acquired AV block
- Complete (third degree) heart block (CHB)
- Advanced second degree heart block (block of 2 or more p waves)
- Symptomatic Mobitz I or Mobitz II second degree AV block
- Mobitz II second degree block with widened QRS or chronic bifasicular block regardless of symptoms
- Bifasicular or trifasicular block with syncope that can be attributable to transient CHB
- Third degree and advanced second degree block in patients with a. fib and bradycardia and 1 or more pauses of >5 seconds

Neurocardiogenic syncope
- Recurrent syncope caused by spontaneously occurring carotid sinus stimulation and carotid pressure that induces ventricular asystole of > 3 seconds
- Syncope without clear, provocative events and with a hypersensitive cardioinhibitory response of 3 seconds or longer on tilt testing
- Symptomatic neurocardiogenic syncope associated with bradycardia documented spontaneously or at the time of tilt testing.

Heart failure
- Cardiac resynchronisation therapy

Bradycardia induced ventricular arrhythmia

Symptom	Score
C Congestive cardiac failure	1
H Hypertension systolic BP >160	1
A Age > 75 years	1
D Diabetes	1
P Prior cerebral ischaemia	2

Patients with CHAD2 score of 0 are low risk and their anticoagulation can be achieved with aspirin. Patients with score = or > 3 are high risk and require warfarin. Patients with score of 1 -2 are low risk and have the option of using either aspirin or warfarin. However patients who have had a prior cerebral

| TABLE 12 |
| MANAGEMENT OF STABLE ANGINA |

Control of symptoms
* Sublingual nitrates
* Aspirin +/- clopidogrel
* Oral nitrates
* Beta-blockers
* Calcium antagonists

Treatment of aggravating factors
* Anaemia
* Thyrotoxicosis
* Rhythm disturbance
* Heart failure
* Hypertension
* Hypoxaemia
* Valvular heart disease

Risk factor management
* Smoking cessation
* Low cholesterol diet and lipid lowering therapy - statins
* Adequate blood pressure control
* Good diabetic control
* Weight control
* Regular exercise up to but not beyond chest discomfort

ischaemic event should be anticoagulated with warfarin. Target INR should be kept below 3 in patients over 75 years to avoid the risk of intracranial haemorrhage in this group.

Ischaemic heart disease

Coronary heart disease (CHD) has a high prevalence in older people. In American studies 70 to 80% of elderly men and 50% of elderly women were found to have evidence of obstructive coronary artery disease at post-mortem. The condition may be underdiagnosed because of atypical presentation such as in case 6 where pain was absent. Ischaemia as well as age alters diastolic function in older patients making them more likely to experience symptoms of dyspnoea rather than pain. With decreased activity and co-morbidity, ischaemia may frequently be 'masked'. There is also an increase in the incidence of silent ischaemia in older patients. The presentation in older patients of myocardial ischaemia as dyspnoea or worsening heart failure is now regarded as an 'angina equivalent' and carries a worse prognosis. The principle risk factors at a younger age, namely

hypertension, dyslipidaemias and smoking remain powerful predictors in older age. There is increasing evidence that an increased pulse pressure, a reflection of decreased aortic compliance mentioned above, may be a particularly important predictor of disease. In terms of investigation, exercise stress testing is generally well tolerated in older people and yields similar information. However, because of co-morbidity and perhaps also because of symptom severity, pharmacological stress testing can be of value. Thallium perfusion scans are particularly useful prognostically in addition to their capability of identifying ischaemic areas on exercise. Finally, angiography is well tolerated and coronary artery disease is often more extensive than that seen in younger people.

Acute myocardial infarction may present with chest pain in older patients but may be atypical and localised to non-praecordial sites. It is important to remember to outrule myocardial infarction as a cause of new onset heart failure or sudden episodes of heart failure in previously well-controlled patients. Acute myocardial infarction, presenting with a history of chest pain or chest pain equivalent in the elderly, ST elevation or evolving Q waves on ECG or new bundle branch block and a rise in cardiac enzymes, CK-MB and Troponin T, is classified as an ST elevated myocardial infarction (STEMI) and represents one end of the spectrum of acute coronary syndrome. Non ST elevated MI (NSTEMI) refers to those with symptoms of myocardial ischaemia with a rise in cardiac enzymes and ischaemic changes on ECG other than ST elevation. At the other end is what used to be referred to as unstable angina; a patient with chest pain, ischaemic changes on ECG tracings but no rise in cardiac enzymes. All of the entities of acute coronary syndrome (ACS) share similar pathophysiological mechanisms and may result in little or no myocardial damage or a full thickness (Q wave) infarct. In ACS there is a dynamic process whereby either thrombus formation or coronary artery spasm in an area of plaque formation leads to obstruction which may remain or regress.

The significance of differentiating STEMI from NSTEMI lies in the choice of therapy for each group. Thrombolysis or percutaneous coronary intervention (PCI) are the main treatment options in STEMI. Thrombolysis has many beneficial effects in older patients but has a number of limitations. Older patients are not always suitable candidates for thrombolysis due to contraindications such as severe hypertension or recent cerebrovascular events or because of atypical symptoms resulting in delayed presentations. There is a higher incidence of complications with thrombolysis in older patients but it must be remembered that these patients can also benefit hugely from this treatment. The benefit of thrombolysis has been proven up to the age of 75 years. Primary PTCA seems to offer some advantage over thrombolysis in the very elderly. Either treatment option gives significantly better outcomes than conservative care.

Myocardial infarction carries an increased mortality in older patients. Contributors to this increased mortality other than late or atypical presentation include an increased incidence of comorbid conditions and a lesser use of beneficial therapies including thrombolysis and PCI even in patients who are clearly eligible. In patients over 75 years more than 50% will develop heart failure from either systolic or diastolic dysfunction. All patients should be commenced on an ACE inhibitor and beta blockers unless contraindicated. These medications have been shown to improve survival post MI. Nitrates are also valuable in elderly patients because of their advantageous effects on preload, afterload and recurrent ischaemia.

Low molecular weight heparin and nitrates are the treatments of choice in ACS including NSTEMI. Aspirin and clopidogrel are always given if there are no contraindications. Elderly patients have been shown to gain from early PCI in ACS. In recent years the rapid development of newer techniques and increasing experience in dealing with multi-vessel disease by angioplasty and stenting means more older patients are gaining symptomatic improvement. There is not enough information available for the age group greater than 80 years to decide on what is best practice at present. Glycoprotein 11b/111a inhibitors prevent recurrent myocardial infarction in high risk patients when given prior to revascularisation procedures and have been used successfully in older patients (< 75 years). The tendency to greater bleeding with this treatment may limit its use but more data needs to be collected before it can be widely recommended. As in the case of heart failure, any aggravating factors such as anaemia, hyperthyroidism or arrhythmias should be identified and treated. Good control of blood pressure and CHF will also improve symptoms and once corrected may return patients to their previous symptom-free position.

Risk stratification post ACS and myocardial infarction should follow similar steps to younger patients. Consideration is given to symptoms, left ventricular function and results of stress testing. However due regard has to be given to patients' general wellbeing and the existence of other cardiovascular disease or other medical conditions. It is important to carefully weigh up risks and benefits before embarking on further invasive cardiac tests. Table 12 deals with the management of angina in stable patients whose symptoms are not accompanied by acute ischaemic changes.

In stable angina coronary perfusion is impaired by fixed or stable atheroma. The approach to management should not differ substantially from that recommended for younger patients. The aims of therapy are to:
• Relieve symptoms
• Prevent or slow down coronary vascular disease
• Prevent future cardiovascular events (ACS, MI, CHF)
• Improve survival

Medical management relies on the use of nitrates to control symptoms and aspirin or clopidogrel to reduce the number of ischaemic events. Nitrates may cause hypotension in the elderly and lower doses may have to be used. If there is concern about the possibility of GI bleeding because of aspirin a proton pump inhibitor may be used. The use of additional medication will be dictated by concomitant conditions. Beta-blockers and calcium channel antagonists are useful if hypertension is a concern or in the post-myocardial infarction setting but their negative inotropic effects may limit their use in heart failure. It is recommended that the influenza vaccine should be given to all patients > 65 years who have cardiovascular disease.

The importance of risk factor management in the prevention of coronary artery disease in the younger population is well established. It is now becoming evident that primary and secondary prevention of cardiovascular disease in older population also has a valuable role to play. However epidemiological studies continue to show that cardiovascular risk in the older patients is under-managed. In the Systolic Hypertension in the Elderly Program Trial, treatment

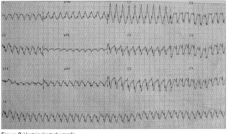

Figure 8: Ventricular tachycardia

of systolic hypertension in people older than 60 years lead to a 32% reduction in all major cardiovascular events. However other investigators have shown that some caution is necessary in lowering diastolic pressure below 85mmHg, as diastolic readings lower than this were associated with some increase in adverse outcomes in patients known to have CHD. In a meta-analysis of the older subgroups of 5 landmark statin trials which included 4S study, LIPID study and WOSCOPS, the relative risk reductions for older patients on statin therapy were similar to younger patients although absolute risk was greater for those >65 years. There was reluctance to extrapolate these findings to all elderly patients. However the PROSPER study has shown that treatment with pravastatin reduced the relative risk for coronary death, non-fatal MI and fatal or non-fatal stroke significantly by 15% and CHD death by 24% in those aged 72 to 80 years. The presence of diabetes is a powerful predictor for the occurrence of secondary events in older patients. Good glycaemic control is beneficial. Weight management and exercise programmes form part of the management principles of good diabetes control and will have the added benefit of reducing cardiovascular risk in CHD patients. Even outside the setting of diabetes and CHD, exercise programmes have been shown to improve functional capacity in

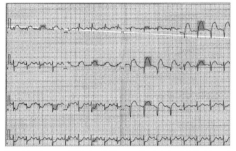

Figure 9: Anterior myocardial infarction with ST segment elevation in the anterior leads (orange) and reciprocal ST segment depression in the inferior leads (blue)

older patients. Clearly these programmes have to be designed to take into account the general status and comorbid conditions of the individual older patient. Smoking is a modifiable risk factor and if tackled will lead to a reduction of cardiovascular events for the older population.

Risk stratification of older patients with stable angina is the same as in younger patients. High risk patients include those with post-infarct angina, poor effort tolerance, CHF and ischaemia at low workload demonstrated on exercise stress testing. These patients warrant coronary angiography to assess the extent and severity of disease. This information will direct what further interventions may be necessary. As in the setting of ACS, PCI is successful in older patients with stable angina although it does carry a higher complication rate. Cornary artery bypass grafting (CABG) is tolerated very well by older patients although they do have a higher mortality in the early post-operative phase. However for those who survive this they can expect the same life expectancy as those of a similar age group who have not had the procedure. The decision to carry out intervention rather than using optimal medical therapy is one which requires careful discussion with patients.

Infective endocarditis

In the older patient, infective endocarditis generally has an insidious onset and will present most often with non-specific symptoms such as general malaise, anorexia and vomiting. Pyrexia will not always be present but older patients may develop confusion either due to the infective process or through embolic complications which may be mistaken for cerebrovascular disease. Organisms are not always cultured in cases of infective endocarditis in the older patient but the sources of infection are commonly urinary tract, bowel, teeth and gums. A high index of suspicion is needed and the diagnosis should be considered when tests suggest an infection but no obvious source is found. Patients may have an elevated WCC, normochromic normocytic anaemia, raised ESR and C-reactive protein. Many older patients have minor abnormalities of their valves which makes infection more likely but impaired immunity of advancing age and the presence of other diseases such as diabetes also contribute. Unfortunately echocardiography will not always make the diagnosis. Minor irregularities of valves that occur with age make the definitive finding of

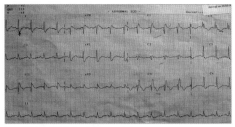
Figure 10: Classical ECG findings of pulmonary embolism

vegetations difficult. Large vegetations are seldom found in cases of infective endocarditis in older patients. Intravenous antibiotics followed by a prolonged course of oral antibiotics is the treatment. Where organisms are cultured the choice of antibiotic should be guided by the advice of a microbiologist. Surgical intervention is only considered in cases of uncontrolled sepsis, where there is abscess formation, acute valve regurgitation or where vegetations are so large that they present a risk of significant embolisation.

Pulmonary embolism

Pulmonary emboli are notoriously difficult to diagnose. Older people are particularly at risk for pulmonary emboli because of the higher prevalence of risk factors in this population. In case 8, the symptoms and signs of pulmonary embolism were attributed to other conditions, namely COPD and CCF. The patient already suffered from dyspnoea of mild exertion and did not complain initially of chest pain. It was only when he suffered circulatory collapse that the diagnosis was considered. D-dimers are raised in many conditions other than pulmonary emboli. Often, the diagnosis of pulmonary embolus is only made at post-mortem and thus a high degree of vigilance is required. In those patients who have emboli large enough to cause circulatory collapse the mortality rate is as high as 80%. The clinical features and investigations are often imprecise and a high degree of suspicion is required. Ventilation/ perfusion scanning may give high false positives and high false negative rates. The existence of previous respiratory disease, which many older patients will have, reduces the accuracy of the test. Spiral CT scanning of the pulmonary vessels is becoming more commonly used to make the diagnosis, particularly for those emboli occurring in the larger vessels.

Pulmonary emboli usually originate in ileo-femoral veins, although most patients have no symptoms of lower limb involvement. The common clinical features in older people are the same as in younger patients and include dyspnoea, chest pain, tachycardia and tachypnoea whether alone or in combination. The ECG and CXR changes are usually non-specific. The most frequent ECG findings are sinus tachycardia, ST and T wave abnormalities, right bundle-branch block or atrial fibrillation, all relatively common and non-specific findings in older patients. The classical ECG findings of an S wave in lead 1 and a Q wave with T wave inversion in lead 3 are not seen very often. Chest radiographs are normal in most cases thus helping to outrule other causes of symptoms but may show linear atelectasis, pleural effusions or wedge-shaped defects. Arterial blood gas measurements may show hypoxia with hypocapnia. Attempts to stratify risk were made in the PIOPED study. Against a gold standard of pulmonary angiography, patients were stratified according to clinical features and ventilation/perfusion scan. The particular risk factors identified were:

- Immobilisation
- Surgery within the past three months
- Lower extremity paralysis
- Venous embolism
- Malignancy especially pelvic
- Recent lower limb fracture

Patients in this study were deemed clinically to have low, intermediate or high probability for pulmonary embolism. However, the majority of patients were deemed to be intermediate, highlighting the difficulty in achieving a degree of certainty. In addition, in the subgroup of patients with chronic cardiac or respiratory disease, the positive predictive value of the perfusion scan was much lower. D-dimers are often measured but are very non-specific when raised. If negative, the diagnosis of pulmonary embolus is much less likely. The presentation of massive pulmonary embolus is similar to that of younger people with right heart failure and cardiovascular collapse. Treatment with supportive measures including oxygen and fluids may be necessary in cases of hypotension, as patients require high filling pressure in right heart failure. Caution is necessary as patients may also have pre-existing left heart failure. Anticoagulation will take the form of intravenous or subcutaneous heparin for 5 to 7 days when maintenance oral anticoagulants such as warfarin will commence. The international normalised ratio (INR) should be kept between 2 and 3. Anticoagulation for pulmonary emboli should continue for a minimum

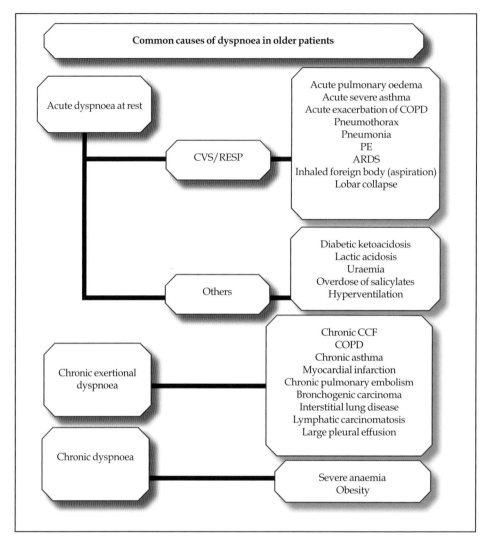

Figure 11: Common causes of dyspnoea in older patients

of 6 months. To date there has not been enough data to show if thrombolytic therapy in massive PE is beneficial to older patients.

Sleep apnoea in older patients

Changes in sleep patterns are part of the ageing process with total time spent sleeping decreasing with age. Patients will not experience difficulty in getting to sleep but tend to wake early. Older patients sleep less in the early morning hours and experience increased sleepiness in the evening. Reduction in nocturnal sleep may be compensated by an increase in daytime napping. These changes in sleep pattern make it difficult to separate disease processes from the normal ageing process. Snoring is more common in old age and its significance in sleep apnoea is not clear. Although identifying sleep apnoea is difficult many consider sleep apnoea to be present in a significant number of patients although there have not been many conclusive studies to prove

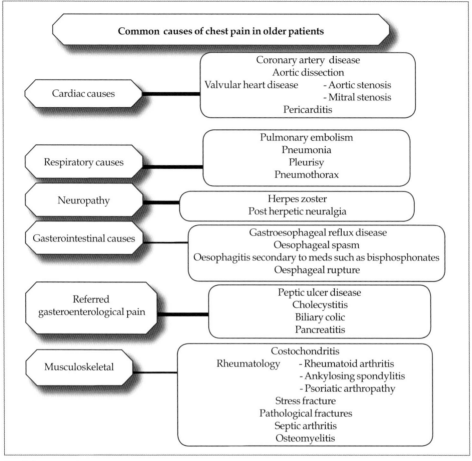

Common causes of chest pain in older patients

Cardiac causes
Coronary artery disease
Aortic dissection
Valvular heart disease   - Aortic stenosis
                           - Mitral stenosis
Pericarditis

Respiratory causes
Pulmonary embolism
Pneumonia
Pleurisy
Pneumothorax

Neuropathy
Herpes zoster
Post herpetic neuralgia

Gasterointestinal causes
Gastroesophageal reflux disease
Oesophageal spasm
Oesophagitis secondary to meds such as bisphosphonates
Oesphageal rupture

Referred gasteroenterological pain
Peptic ulcer disease
Cholecystitis
Biliary colic
Pancreatitis

Musculoskeletal
Costochondritis
Rheumatology   - Rheumatoid arthritis
                 - Ankylosing spondylitis
                 - Psoriatic arthropathy
Stress fracture
Pathological fractures
Septic arthritis
Osteomyelitis

Figure 12: Common causes of chest pain in older patients

this. A new finding of snoring or disturbed sleep in an older patient who previously did not complain of sleep difficulty should be considered significant. Treatment options are similar to those for younger patients. Nasal CPAP, weight reduction, avoidance of sedatives and a tricyclic antidepressant such as protriptyline may improve symptoms.

Iatrogenic dyspnoea

Iatrogenic dyspnoea can be caused by a variety of mechanisms affecting pulmonary function. Pulmonary oedema of ARDS can be caused by hydochlorothiazides or thrombolytics such as streptokinase. Overdose of aspirin and opiates can also have the same effect. Aspirin, beta blockers and NSAIDs are all commonly prescribed for elderly patients and may cause dyspnoea by increasing bronchoconstriction in asthma. Amiodarone, methotrexate and cytotoxic agents can lead to alveolitis with consequent dyspnoea. As well as alveolitis, amiodarone and methotrexate can give rise to pleural disease. Patients may rarely develop pulmonary eosinophilia after exposure to cytotoxic agents such as bleomycin and methotrexate. This has also been seen with carbamazepine and phenytoin. It is believed to be an immunological response to these drugs and patients will present with dyspnoea, cough and fever with patchy shadowing on CXR. Finally drugs such as phenytoin, hydralazine and isoniazid, by inducing SLE, may cause dyspnoea when this disease process affects the lungs.

Other conditions

There are a host of potential causes when considering the older person with dyspnoea or chest pain as shown in Figures 11 and 12. Much depends on the particular context and patient profile. However, as many of the main culprits are particularly prevalent in older people, one must always consider myocardial ischaemia or thromboembolic disease particularly in acute presentations. Other conditions such as community-acquired pneumonia will often be quickly identified with routine investigations even if there are no symptoms of chest pain or dyspnoea. Other less common conditions such as pneumothorax present with similar clinical features, though surprisingly with less pleuritic pain. Malnutrition is frequently seen in the older person presenting with pneumonia and may be associated with tuberculosis. Older people are particularly at risk for this condition as they may have been exposed to tuberculosis at an earlier age without overt clinical manifestation. Subsequent illness or immunosuppression may uncover a tuberculous pneumonia, which may present in protean ways with loss of weight, anorexia and confusion often in the absence of respiratory symptoms. Bacteriological identification of causative organisms is difficult not just in tuberculosis but also in community-acquired pneumonias and treatment is more often based on clinical suspicion than definitive bacteriological culture. Older patients may present with chest pain or vague chest discomfort due to upper gastrointestinal pathology. This is particularly important in patients with known CHD, taking aspirin, when their symptoms should not always be attributed to cardiac disease. Gastro-oesophageal reflux disease is particularly common in older patients often exacerbated by medications such as NSAIDs. Musculoskeletal disorders may also present with chest discomfort and should not be attributed to cardiac causes. Osteoarthritis, osteoporosis and metastatic bone lesions are all seen with increasing frequency in this age group and should not be forgotten in the differential of chest pain.

In summary, the presence of dyspnoea or chest pain is often associated with potentially serious illness in older people and should always be taken seriously. However, these symptoms are often under-reported or atypical. As with most disease states in older people, the presentation may be vague and poorly specific. A patient simply 'gone-off' or confused can have a wide differential of potential conditions, including most respiratory or cardiac illnesses. The absence of 'expected' symptoms and signs does not safely outrule pathology.

Suggested further reading

- *Ahmed H. Abdelhafiz. Heart Failure in older people: causes, diagnosis and treatment. Age and Ageing 2002; 31: 29-36.*
- *Berman AR. Pulmonary embolism in the elderly. Clin Geriatr Med 2001;17(1): 107-30.*
- *British Thoracic Society/ SIGN Guidelines British Guideline on the Management of Asthma May 2008 SIGN 101 http:www.sign.ac.uk.*
- *Management of Chronic Heart Failure. February 2007 SIGN 95 http://www.sign.ac.uk.*
- *Flather MD, Shibata MC, Coats AJS, et al Eur Heart J 2005; 26: 215-225 Randomized trial to determine the effect of nebivolol on mortality and cardiovascular hospital admission in elderly patients with heart failure (SENIORS).*
- *Cruickshank JM, Thorp JM, Zacharias FJ. Benefits and potential harm of lowering high blood pressure. Lancet 1987;(1) 8533: 581-584.*
- *Fletcher C, Peto R. The natural history of chronic airway obstruction. Br Med J 1977; 1(6077): 1645-1648.*
- *Global Initiative for Chronic Obstructive Lung Disease (GOLD). National Institutes of Health, National Heart, Lung and Blood Institute, Bethesda, Maryland, USA. http://www.goldcopd.com*
- *Kelly J and Hunt BJ. Role of D-dimers in diagnosis of venous thromboembolism. Lancet 2002; 359: 456-458.*
- *Liston R, McLoughlin R and Clinch D. Acute pneumothorax: a comparison of elderly with younger patients. Age and Ageing 1994; 23: 393-5.*
- *Masotti L, Ceccarelli E, Cappelli R, Guerrini M and Forcono S. Pulmonary embolism in the elderly: clinical, instrumental and laboratory aspects. Gerontology 2000; 46: 205-11.*
- *Selton-Suty C, Hoen B, Grentzinger A, et al. Clinical and bacteriological characteristics of infective endocarditis in the elderly. Heart 1997; 77(3): 260-3.*
- *Sheifer SE, Girsh BJ, Yanez ND et al. Prevalence, predisposing factors and prognosis of clinically unrecognised myocardial infarction in the elderly. J Am Coll Cardiology 2000; 35: 119.*
- *SHEP Cooperative research Group: Prevention of stroke by antihypertensive drug treatment in older persons with isolated systolic hypertension. JAMA 1991; 265: 3255-3264.*
- *LaRosa , HeJ, Vupputuri S. Effects of statins on risk of coronary disease: a meta-analysis of randomized controlled trials. JAMA 1999; 282: 2340-2346.*
- *Shepherd J, Blauw GJ, Murphy MB, Bollen EL, Buckley*

BM, Cobbe SM, Ford I, Gaw A, et al for the PROSPER Study Group: Prospective Study of Pravastatin in the Elderly at risk of vascular disease (PROSPER): a randomised control trial. Lancet 2003; 360: 1623-1630.

- Stuart D, Hutcheon ND, Gillespie AD et al. B-type natriuretic peptide in the diagnosis of cardiac disease in elderly day hospital patients. Age and Ageing 2002; 31: 295-301.

- The PIOPED investigators. Value of the ventilation/perfusion scan in acute pulmonary embolism. Results of the prospective investigation of pulmonary embolism diagnosis (PIOPED). JAMA 1990; 263: 2753.

- Sadeghi HM, Grines CL, Chandra HR et al PCI in octogenarians glycoprotein 11b/111a receptor inhibitors profile. J Am Coll Cardiol 2003; 42: 428-432.

- Conaway DG, House J, Bandt K et al. The elderly: health benefits and recovery of function one year after coronary artery bypass surgery. J Am Coll Cardiol 2003; 42: 1421-1426.

- Secondary prevention of Coronary Heart Disease in the Elderly (WITH Emphasis on Patients > 75 years of Age) An American Heart Association Scientific Statement from the Council on Clinical Cardiology Subcommittee on Exercise, Cardiac Rehabilitation and Prevention. Circulation 2002; 105: 1735-17434.

- ACC / AHA/ HRS Task force on Practice Guidelines. JACC. 2008; 51 e1-62 Guidelines for Device-based Therapy of Cardiac Rhythm Abnormalities.

- Gage BF, Waterman AD, Shannon W et al. Validation of clinical classification schemes for predicting stroke: results from the national Registry of Atrial Fibrillation. JAMA 2001; 285: 2864-2870.

Case Study 1

An 82 year old man presented to his General Practitioner complaining of worsening breathlessness, especially at night. He was a retired teacher and ex-smoker of 10 pack years. He had no history of respiratory or cardiac disease. On further questioning, he admitted to episodes of chest tightness and what sounded like paroxysmal nocturnal dyspnoea. During the day, he had reasonable exercise tolerance. On examination, he was obese, and was not in any respiratory distress. His colour was normal and he had no clubbing. Chest examination revealed slightly reduced expansion. There were mild diffuse rhonchi and bibasal crepitations, JVP was not raised and heart sounds were normal. He had mild bilateral ankle oedema. He was commenced on Frusemide 40mgs daily but represented two weeks later with unchanged symptoms. Chest x-ray was reported as normal with no signs of cardiac failure and ECG showed sinus rhythm and no changes of ischaemia. He proceeded to spirometry which revealed the following results:

FEV_1:	0.9 l (40% predicted)
FVC:	1.74 l (60% predicted)
FEV_1/FVC ratio:	52%

He was placed on beta-agonist inhalers initially with good symptomatic relief but subsequently gained better relief from steroid inhalers after testing demonstrated reversibility. This case demonstrates the difficulty of arriving at a diagnosis of asthma in older people based on clinical assessment alone.

Case Study 2

A 75 year old man presented with history of worsening cough and recurrent respiratory tract infections, particularly in winter. He was a retired bar-worker who stopped smoking in his early 40s. He was not taking any medications. On examination, he was not cyanosed or distressed but was cachectic. There was no clubbing or lymphadenopathy. Respiratory examination revealed a barrel-shaped chest with poor inspiratory expansion. He had diffuse rhonchi but no localising signs. Spirometry revealed a marked obstructive picture with an FEV_1 < 1.5l. Following two weeks of steroids, there was a small but significant improvement. Sputum cultures grew Haemophilus influenzae and were negative for acid-fast bacillus. He was placed on regular beta-agonist and steroid inhalers and responded reasonably well from a symptomatic perspective. He represented two months later with a chest infection that failed to clear despite two courses of antibiotics. A chest x-ray revealed a large cavitating mass near the hilum. Routine bloods showed hyponatraemia of 122mmol/l with normal potassium, glucose and urea. He was referred for further assessment.

In this case history clinical course together with chest x-ray findings makes the probable diagnosis either lung tumour or lung abscess. The past history of smoking and cachexia are in keeping with a diagnosis of lung carcinoma. The hyponatraemia with normal potassium, normal glucose in the absence of medication points strongly to a diagnosis of Syndrome of inappropriate ADH (SIADH) secretion. Addison's disease from adrenal metastases would be another possibility but glucose would be expected to be low and potassium high. Further management included repeat sputum for culture and sensitivity and cytology, serum calcium, serum and urine for osmolarity and ECG. Bronchoscopy and biopsy was arranged and CT scan of chest and upper abdomen to identify tumour extent and any evidence of metastases in lymph nodes or liver or adrenals was also performed. Biopsy revealed a bronchogenic carcinoma which was deemed to be inoperable due to its position. If the tumour had been operable the patient would have required a full respiratory and cardiac assessment to quantify operative risk.

Case Study 3

A 75 year old lady presented with a recurrent cough productive of sputum each winter. During these episodes, she tended to become more breathless and wheezy. Over the preceding two years, she had become breathless climbing one flight of stairs between exacerbations. She was an ex-smoker with a total of 40 pack-years. She felt cigarettes had caused 'noisy breathing' even when younger and that every cold 'went to my chest'. On examination she was thin with a hyperinflated chest. She was clearly using accessory muscles of inspiration. There was poor chest expansion and breath sounds were distant. There were no audible rhonchi. She grew a coliform on sputum culture and chest x-ray was reported as showing hyperinflated lung fields and a narrowed mediastinum. Spirometry showed the following results with no significant changes after two weeks of oral steroids:

FEV$_1$:	0.6l (60% predicted)
FVC:	1.1l (80% predicted)
FEV$_1$/FVC ratio:	55%

The diagnosis is COPD. She was placed on regular combined beta-agonist and anticholinergic inhalers. Steroid inhalers were not given initially because of the failure of reversibility studies. However, these were later added as she developed frequent exacerbations. Thereafter her exercise tolerance declined. When she was found to have developed baseline hypoxia with a pO$_2$<7.3kPa in the setting of right heart failure, she was provided with domiciliary oxygen.

Case Study 4

A 69 year old man, who has been treated for many years with COPD, complained of worsening shortness of breath over the previous 1 year. He was on no medications apart from his inhalers and antihypertensives. In an effort to relieve his symptoms, his GP had tried a variety of bronchodilators. Although he had a partial response initially, his deterioration had been relentless. Addition of steroid inhalers made no difference and there was no clinical evidence of infective exacerbations. He was referred to outpatients where a chest x-ray was performed. This showed reticular shadowing throughout both mid and lower zones. Investigations revealed the following findings:

PO$_2$:	7.5 kPa
PCO$_2$	4.5 kPa
FEV$_1$	1.96 l (70% predicted)
FVC	2.56 l (69% predicted)
FEV$_1$/FVC	76%

As shown pulmonary function tests showed reduced total lung capacity and residual volume and a lowered DLCO (transfer factor) was later identified. A high-resolution CT scan confirmed the clinical suspicion of interstitial lung disease.

Case Study 5

An 84 year old man presented to his GP complaining of worsening fatigue. His only past medical problem had been hypertension. He was a retired council worker. He lived alone in a terraced house on a hill and had been active until 3 months prior to presentation when he stopped going out and relied on relatives to do his shopping. He admitted to sleeping poorly, despite feeling 'washed out' all of the time. He had smoked 20 cigarettes a day until 5 years previously. On examination, he appeared thin and pale. Blood pressure was 160/100mmHg and pulse rate 90 and irregular. He had a raised JVP and a displaced apex beat. There was a soft systolic murmur heard best over the aortic area radiating to both carotid arteries. There were bibasal crepitations and also pitting ankle oedema. Initial investigations were as follows:

FBC and biochemistry	Normal
Chest x-ray	Upper lobe venous diversion Enlarged heart Interstitial oedema
ECG	Atrial fibrillation Left ventricular hypertrophy
Echocardiogram	Poor left ventricular function Ejection fraction 30% Aortic stenosis with gradient of 100mmHg

The diagnosis was left ventricular failure secondary to severe aortic stenosis and atrial fibrillation. The patient was admitted for treatment of heart failure and cardiac assessment with a view to aortic valve replacement. His heart failure responded to diuretic therapy and his atrial fibrillation was treated with digoxin. Subcutaneous anticoagulation was commenced in view of heart failure and atrial fibrillation. In this instance vasodilators or ACE inhibitors could not be added to heart failure treatment, as it would further increase the gradient across the aortic valve with catastrophic results. His heart rate was monitored with telemetry to rule out any significant bradyarrhythmias associated with aortic stenosis and serial cardiac enzymes and ECGs ruled out any recent myocardial infarction. The patient was observed carefully for pyrexial illness in view of the risk of endocarditis. When his heart failure was controlled, the subcutaneous heparin was stopped and the patient had cardiac catheterisation carried out to further assess the gradient across the valve along with coronary angiography to identify concomitant coronary artery disease, which could be grafted at the time of surgery. Exercise stress testing was clearly contraindicated in the setting of aortic stenosis. In order to quantify the risk of aortic valve replacement, an assessment of respiratory function was performed and the extent of other vascular disease especially carotid disease was made with Doppler studies. The patient subsequently survived aortic valve replacement and triple vessel bypass surgery.

Case Study 6

A 76 year old man was admitted to hospital for further assessment. His GP was concerned because of recent onset breathlessness and chest discomfort. He had no history of respiratory or cardiovascular disease and had been generally fit and well for most of his life. He had stopped smoking many years before and had never taken alcohol. His only medication was an NSAID which he took for osteoarthritis. His wife had died a few months previously following a long illness and he had become depressed and withdrawn. On examination he was not distressed but pale. Blood pressure was 150/95mmHg and pulse regular. There were no signs of heart failure or respiratory disease. Following admission, the nursing staff confirmed that he appeared exhausted and breathless after walking the length of the ward. His investigations were as follows:

FBC	Hb 7.4g/dl MCV and MCH both low
Haematinics	Ferritin low, B_{12} and folate normal
ECG	Non-specific ST and T wave changes
CXR	Heart size upper level of normal, lung fields clear
Echo-cardiogram	No valvular abnormality Some impairment of anterior and septal wall motion. Ejection fraction 55%

It was felt that he had developed dyspnoea secondary to his anaemia. He underwent a gastroscopy, which showed a large prepyloric ulcer. He tested negative for Helicobacter pylori. He was commenced on proton pump inhibitor and his NSAIDs were stopped and alternative pain relief was given. He was transfused to a haemoglobin level of 11g/dl. Despite this his breathlessness persisted. Arterial blood gases showed a pO_2 of 15kPa and pCO_2 of 3.4 kPa on room air. These were much better than might be expected for his age. Despite these readings, a CT pulmonary angiogram was arranged and this showed small but definite emboli throughout both lung fields. There was some doubt as to whether this finding could have accounted for his presentation. After 1 minute of an exercise stress test, he collapsed with hypotension and marked ST depression throughout all leads. Coronary angiography demonstrated widespread coronary vessel disease which was amenable to bypass surgery. The result of surgery was beneficial in terms of his dyspnoea.

Case Study 7

An 86 year old woman returned to her GP with complaints of general malaise and anorexia. She was accompanied by her daughter, with whom she lived, who confirmed that the patient had not returned to her baseline state of health since a urinary tract infection 9 weeks earlier. Her GP had treated this with antibiotics and had given her a further course of antibiotics a month later when her symptoms persisted and she complained of temperature and 'shivering'. Her daughter was also concerned that her mother had become mildly confused in recent days which was a new finding for her and her glucometer readings were elevated in the past 2 days. In her background history she had Type 2 diabetes for 5 years, which was well controlled on oral hypoglycaemics and diet. She had not developed any complications from her diabetes. She had been fit and fully independent in the activities of daily living until 9 weeks previously. Her only hospital admission had been for pneumonia 5 years previously during which her diabetes and mild hypertension were also diagnosed. Her medications were oral hypoglycaemics, ACE inhibitor and a statin. On examination she was alert and oriented and well hydrated. She had a mild pyrexia of 37.5^{0}C. Pulse and BP were satisfactory. There was a soft systolic murmur noted in the aortic area, which had been noted before. Her chest was clear to auscultation and there were no signs of heart failure. Nil of note was found on abdominal examination and there were no focal neurological signs. Urinalysis showed proteinuria, trace haematuria and a large amount of ketones and glucose. In view of the pyrexia, poorly controlled diabetes and ongoing symptoms she was referred to hospital. Additional investigations in hospital were as follows:

FBC	Hb 10.1g/dl
	WCC 18.2 x10^9/l
	PLTS 155 x10^9/l
	MCV and MCH normal
	Sodium 137 mmol/l
	Potassium 4.1 mmol/l
	Urea 11.3 mmol/l
	Creatinine 124 μmol/l
	Glucose 20 mmol/l
ABGs	Normal
ESR	100
CXR	Cardiothoracic ratio upper limit of normal
	Clear lung fields
ECG	Sinus rhythm, no acute ischaemia

In hospital no new clinical findings were found, although the patient was noted to be mildly confused and refused to eat and drink adequate amounts. She had urine sent for culture and sensitivity and 3 sets of blood cultures taken. Other investigations such as liver function tests, thyroid function and calcium were normal. C-reactive protein was significantly elevated. She was commenced on broad-spectrum antibiotics, IV fluids and subcutaneous insulin.

Subsequently her confusion settled but she continued to have low-grade pyrexia. Blood cultures grew Streptococcus but urine was negative for infection. Her antibiotics were changed to give more specific cover for the streptococcal infection. In view of the blood culture findings a diagnosis of infective endocarditis was made and echocardiography was carried out. This showed a calcified aortic valve with the suspicion of vegetations. There was good opening of the aortic valve with no evidence of aortic regurgitation. Left ventricular function was good. Her IV antibiotics were continued for 2 weeks, at which stage the patient was well on full diet and her usual medication. Her antibiotics were continued for a further 4 weeks. She made a full recovery.

Case Study 8

A 78 year old man with a long history of COPD and CCF presented to the Accident and Emergency department complaining of worsening shortness of breath. He admitted that he was usually short of breath with minimal exertion but stated that he had noticed a definite deterioration in the previous four days. He was a long-term heavy smoker who had stopped the previous winter. He had been admitted on several occasions with exacerbations of COPD and CCF. Recently he had been supplied with home O_2 as his steady-state PO_2 had fallen below 7.3 kPa. On systems review, he admitted to urinary frequency and dizziness when standing. On examination, he was in respiratory distress with a respiratory rate of 28. Blood pressure was 130/60 and pulse rate 110 beats per minute. He had a raised JVP but no third heart sound. There were diffuse rhonchi and bibasal crepitations. He also had pitting ankle oedema. Previous admissions had documented similar signs. Investigations were as follows:

Chest x-ray	Upper lobe venous diversion with interstitial oedema
ECG	Sinus tachycardia. No signs of acute ischaemia

Arterial blood gas	PO$_2$ - 6.8kPa
	PCO$_2$ - 5.8kPa
	pH - 7.4
Full blood count	WCC - 12.7 × 10^9/l
	Hb - 14.7 g/dl
D-dimer	>500

A diagnosis of exacerbation of COPD and CCF was made and he was commenced on intravenous antibiotics and diuretics after blood cultures were taken. He was transferred to the general medical ward once his condition was seen to be stable. Later that night, he became more breathless and had central chest pain. On this assessment, he was found to be hypotensive and cyanosed with no new findings on cardiorespiratory examination. ECG showed rapid atrial fibrillation but no evidence of acute ischaemia or myocardial infarction. He was given additional diuretics, but remained unwell. ABG showed a marked deterioration with PO$_2$ = 5.7kPa, PCO$_2$ = 6.4kPa and pH = 7.2. He was transferred to CCU but sustained a cardio-respiratory arrest. The attempted resuscitation was unsuccessful. A post-mortem examination revealed a saddle pulmonary embolus with right heart failure. In addition to findings in keeping with COPD and CCF, he was found to have prostatic adenocarcinoma with widespread metastases.

Data Interpretation

Question 1
A 78 year old woman returned to her GP complaining of weakness and nausea. She had a background history of atrial fibrillation, CHF NYHA II and hypertension. She had been well controlled on digoxin, a loop diuretic, an ACE inhibitor and warfarin. Her loop diuretic had been increased 2 weeks previously to control increasing dyspnoea and ankle oedema. She was apyrexial, BP138/72 mmHg and pulse irregular 45/min. No evidence of heart failure and no ankle oedema.

Na$^+$	138mmol/l
K$^+$	4.9mmol/l
Urea	14.5mmol/l
Creatinine	210μmol/l
ECG	atrial fibrillation rate 46/min no acute ischaemic changes seen

a. What are the most likely causes of the abnormalities?
b. What other blood tests would you consider?
c. What corrective measures would you take?

Question 2
A 71 year old man attends his GP for review following a recent hospital admission for an uncomplicated inferior myocardial infarction. He was compliant with his new medication of aspirin, nebivolol and pravastatin. He was asymptomatic apart from muscle soreness which had started just after hospital discharge. Routine bloods showed;

FBC	normal
U&E	normal
ALT	120 U/l
AST	90 U/l
Bilirubin	10 μmol/l
Total cholesterol	6.3 mmol/l

a. Describe the abnormalities
b. What blood test should be done and why?
c. How would you manage myalgia?

Question 3
This 74 year old male smoker presented with a history of productive cough, dyspnoea, fever, weight loss and excessive sweating. His CXR is shown below

a. Describe the abnormalities
b. What are the causes for these abnormalities?

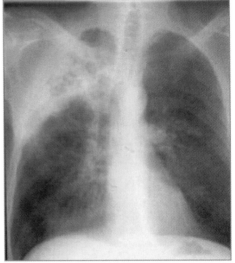

Figure 12

Best of five questions

Question 1

A 74 year old woman attends surgery with complaints of exertional chest tightness which began 8 weeks previously while she was out for her regular walk. In the past week she has not been able to walk more than 200 yards without getting the pain which went after a few minutes rest. She never had this before and has not had any episodes at rest. Which of the following is the optimum course of management in her case?

a. If ECG does not show acute ischaemia prescribe aspirin and GTN and review in a few days

b. Refer to rapid access chest pain clinic where stress testing and angiography can be arranged.

c. Refer to cardiology OPD

d. Refer to A&E for urgent hospital admission

e. Check ECG, cardiac enzymes, lipids, glucose, prescribe aspirin, GTN and review with results

Question 2

A 70 year old man with long-term atrial fibrillation makes a full neurological recovery after a presentation with right arm weakness with lasted less than 24 hours. This patient had been unsuccessfully treated with DC cardioversion in the past and he was intolerant of flecanide, propafenone and amiodarone. Echocardiogram demonstrated a mildly dilated left atrium and carotid dopplers all normal. Fasting glucose 4.9mmol/l cholesterol 6.2mmol/l. His a. fib and hypertension were well controlled on a beta blocker and calcium antagonist and he had previously been on aspirin. Optimum pharmacological therapy in this case would be?

a. Add clopidogrel to his aspirin, continue beta blocker and calcium antagonist and add statin

b. Stop aspirin, anticoagulate with warfarin, add ACE inhibitor and statin to his beta blocker and calcium antagonist regime

c. Stop calcium antagonist, add warfarin, statin and ACE inhibitor to his usual beta blocker and aspirin

d. Stop aspirin, commence warfarin and statin, continue beta blocker and calcium antagonist

e. Stop aspirin, commence warfarin, continue beta blocker and arrange for DC cardioversion

Question 3

A 72 year old man with a long-term diagnosis of asthma attends asthma clinic for review. Three months ago he had been admitted with acute coronary insufficiency which required PCI and stenting. He had no further angina symptoms but he was told that he had mild heart failure. An ACE inhibitor, aspirin, diuretic and statin had been added to his usual salbutamol inhaler and steroid inhaler. His asthma symptoms had become more troublesome in the past month and he was using his salbutamol inhaler twice as much as usual despite being on 1000μg per day of his inhaled steroid. Which is the next most appropriate step in the management of his asthma?

a. CXR to check if there is any evidence of pulmonary oedema and increase diuretic dose

b. Add long acting beta 2 agonist

c. Increase inhaled steroids incrementally up to a dose of 2000μg daily

d. Give short dose of oral steroids and commence theophylline

e. Increase dose of inhaled steroid and add in an ipratropium bromide inhaler

Answers are available on page 311

Abdominal problems

B Moynihan, L O'Donnell, R Liston

Assessment of gastrointestinal symptoms in older patients

Symptoms attributable to the gastrointestinal tract (GIT) are common to patients of all ages. The stereotypical image of an older adult focused on bowel habit belies the serious impact that symptoms of constipation, abdominal discomfort and faecal incontinence have on quality of life. The high prevalence of co-morbidities and serious pathology in older adults increases the challenge for the physician. Getting the right balance between excessive investigations and missing serious diagnoses is the key to this challenge. The importance of specifically asking about gastrointestinal symptoms cannot be overestimated as many patients will not readily volunteer this information. Open discussion regarding the probable diagnoses and appropriate investigations will allow an informed choice to be made by the patient. In general, older adults tolerate endoscopy as well as younger adults and a positive approach to diagnosis and treatment is advisable. In this chapter we address three main themes; a) age-related changes in the gastrointestinal tract, b) symptom based assessment of older adults, c) disease-specific information regarding older adults.

Age-related changes in the gastrointestinal tract

The most externally obvious change in older adults is change in dentition and associated gum atrophy. This has important consequences for nutritional intake. In otherwise healthy adults, changes in the GIT due to ageing are quite subtle. Reduced taste and olfaction may lead to reduced oral intake. Diseases such as Alzheimer's disease and Parkinson's disease lead to more pronounced loss of olfaction and are associated with anorexia. Angiotensin converting enzyme inhibitors and other medications can cause dysgeusia; a distortion or reduction in the sense of taste. Swallowing also changes as we grow older; the oropharyngeal phase of swallowing and time to opening of the upper oesophageal sphincter are prolonged in older adults. In healthy older adults however, these changes do not affect oesophageal function. Gastric emptying is slower, especially with large meals, in older adults and is even more slowed by drugs such as opioids and calcium channel blockers. Gastric acid production is maintained in healthy older adults but the high prevalence of Helicobacter pylori associated atrophic gastritis and over-prescription of proton pump inhibitors leads to hypochlorhydria in many older adults. The small intestine is largely unchanged in healthy older adults. The number of Peyer's patches is somewhat reduced. Motility and absorption of nutrients are well maintained in old age. Large intestinal transit time is frequently increased in older adults, but changes due to medications, fluid intake and mobility are more significant than the effects of ageing and may lead to constipation. The microflora of the large intestine is more diverse in older people with an increase in fungi being notable. Bifidobacteriae from healthy older adults bind less well to intestinal mucosa

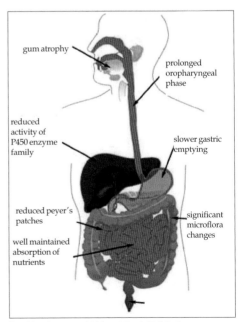

gum atrophy

prolonged oropharyngeal phase

reduced activity of P450 enzyme family

slower gastric emptying

reduced peyer's patches

significant microflora changes

well maintained absorption of nutrients

Figure 1: Some important age-related changes to the gastrointestinal tract

TABLE I	
COMMON CAUSES OF ABDOMINAL PAIN IN OLDER PATIENTS	
ACUTE	**CHRONIC**
Biliary pain	Oesophagitis
Diverticulitis	Duodenal ulcer
Pancreatitis	Gastric ulcer
Appendicitis	Gallstones
Perforated peptic ulcer	Irritable bowel syndrome
Intestinal obstruction	Functional abdominal pain
Mesenteric infarction	Gastritis
Ruptured abdominal aortic aneurysm	Gastroenteritis

than those from younger adults and may explain the reduced number of bifidobacteriae in the older large intestine. The lumina of the pancreatic and biliary ducts are increased in older people and biliary stasis is more common. Liver function is normally unchanged in healthy older adults but the metabolism of drugs is affected by reduced activity of the cytochrome P450 enzyme family. In summary, the effects of diseases and medications are of far more importance than age-related changes in structure and function when assessing older people with gastrointestinal complaints.

Acute abdominal pain

Common causes of abdominal pain in the older patient are tabulated in Table 1. Gallstone related pain accounts for approximately 25% of cases of acute abdominal pain in older individuals. Although appendicitis is uncommon in older patients, it is often associated with a high morbidity and mortality. Silent presentations of appendicitis and peptic ulcer disease are well described in older adults. Pain may be localised, generalised or referred depending on the degree of peritoneal involvement. The history taker needs to be aware of these three possibilities and careful examination of the abdomen is paramount.

Very sudden onset of severe pain occurs with perforation, abdominal aneurysm leak or rupture or acute mesenteric ischaemia or infarction. Pain due to inflammation such as appendicitis or diverticulitis is usually more gradual in onset and may take 24 to 48 hours to reach peak intensity. Patients with peritonitis prefer to lie still whereas those with renal colic or biliary pain move around to try and get comfortable. Associated symptoms such as vomiting, diarrhoea, constipation, jaundice, dysuria or constitutional symptoms such as fevers and rigors are important

symptoms to elicit. Of course, older patients may have pre-existing cognitive impairment or may develop delirium as part of their acute illness making history taking difficult and a collateral history will be required from a relative or carer in this situation.

Chronic abdominal pain

Population based epidemiological surveys indicate that irritable bowel syndrome (IBS) symptoms are only marginally less common in the over seventies than in the 20 to 40 year old age group. Health seeking behaviour for irritable bowel syndrome, however, is less in older patients. The diagnosis of irritable bowel syndrome and functional gastrointestinal disease in older patients is not necessarily a diagnosis of exclusion but is reliant on positive features in the history; the Rome III Criteria (Table 2) and absence of alarm symptoms such as rectal bleeding or weight loss. Consideration of serious alternative pathologies causing IBS-like symptoms is vital in older adults; negative investigations can help reassure the patient and physician.

Meticulous history taking is the bedrock of a precise diagnosis of chronic abdominal pain (Table 3). The retrosternal position of the pain, a burning nature and aggravation by posture and large meals are discriminating for oesophagitis. Gastric ulcer pain commonly occurs half an hour after eating and is associated with anorexia. Duodenal ulcer pain is often nocturnal, classically awakening patients at 2.00am and is aggravated by long fasts and relieved by eating.

An important part of the history in abdominal pain is the social history. Stress is a major aetiological factor in many patients with irritable bowel syndrome and functional abdominal pain. Family tragedies, concerns regarding accommodation or death of a spouse are common causes of emotional distress which can give rise to abdominal pain.

Dysphagia

Dysphagia may be best considered as either oro-pharyngeal or oesophageal. Oro-pharyngeal dysphagia occurs either due to neuromuscular dysfunction or a local pathological process in the pharynx or upper oesophageal sphincter. Early diagnosis of oro-pharyngeal dysphagia is imperative as this is the type of dysphagia which may easily give rise to aspiration pneumonia. Coughing after fluids or food is highly suggestive but formal assessment is important. Common causes include stroke, motor neurone disease and parkinsonian disorders. If the dysphagia occurs in the body of the oesophagus the patient will complain of difficulty in getting food to pass down the oesophagus and they often complain that food is stuck behind the lower end of the sternum. Benign oesophageal stricture is the commonest cause of dysphagia in older patients. There is usually an accompanying history of heartburn and the dysphagia develops gradually. More rapid onset of dysphagia in the absence of heartburn suggests the

TABLE 2
ROME III CRITERIA FOR DIAGNOSIS OF IRRITABLE BOWEL SYNDROME

Recurrent abdominal pain or discomfort at least 3 days per month in the last 3 months associated with 2 or more of the following:
1. Improvement with defecation
2. Onset associated with a change in frequency of stool
3. Onset associated with a change in form (appearance) of stool

possibility of oesophageal carcinoma. Hiccoughing, dysphagia for solids, smoking and alcohol history or previous Barrett's oesophagus are all suggestive for oesophageal cancer. With achalasia, dysphagia of both liquids and solids occurs from an early stage and the patient often has learned trick manoeuvres such as standing up during eating, bending backwards or using a valsalva manoeuvre to relieve the dysphagia. Painful swallowing, odynophagia, is usually due to inflammation of the oesophagus with candida, herpes or cytomegalovirus. Diverticulae, scleroderma and

TABLE 3				
SYMPTOM PATTERNS IN CHRONIC ABDOMINAL PAIN				
	Oesophagitis	**Gastric ulcer**	**Duodenal ulcer**	**Irritable bowel syndrome**
Site	Retrosternal or epigastric	Epigastric	Epigastric	Upper or lower abdomen
Radiation	Retrosternal	Back	Back	Variable or throat
Frequency	Variable	Variable	Variable	Variable
Onset	Variable	Gradual	Gradual or nocturnal	Variable
Duration	1/2 - 1 hour	1-2 hours	1-2 hours	Variable
Periodicity	Constant	Constant	Constant	Variable
Intensity	Variable	Variable	Variable	Variable
Character	Burning	Gnawing	Gnawing	Crampy or spasmodic
Aggravating or relieving factors	Worse lying flat	Worse after food	Worsened by fasting	Relieved by defaecation
Relationship to meals	Aggravated by	Pain after meals, large meals	Relieved by eating	Variable
Associated symptoms	Dysphagia, haematemesis,	Weight loss, anorexia, anaemia		Constipation, diarrhoea, mucus rectally, abdominal bloating, feeling of incomplete rectal evacuation

TABLE 4
CAUSES AND ASSESSMENT OF CONSTIPATION IN
OLDER PATIENTS

CAUSE	ASSESSMENT
Low dietary fibre intake	Dietary history
Immobility	Timed get up and go
Faecal impaction	Digital rectal exam
GI pathology	Abdominal exam
	Colonoscopy
	Abdominal x-ray
Autonomic neuropathy	Lying and standing BP
Spinal lesions	Neurological
	examination
Depression	Geriatric Depression
	Score
Confusional states	Abbreviated Mental Test
	Score
Hypothyroidism	TSH
Hypercalcaemia	Serum Ca^{++} & Mg^{++}
Drug history	opiates
	anti-cholinergics
	anti-depressants
	anti-convulsants
	calcium antagonists
	iron
	anti-parkinsonian drugs

fibreoptic endoscopic evaluation of swallowing (FEES) are helpful for the precise definition of oro-pharyngeal dysphagia in these patients and may be particularly beneficial in assessing whether silent aspiration is occurring.

Constipation

Constipation has been defined as the passing of two or less bowel motions per week. In practice, other criteria, such as straining at defaecation, hard stool and tenesmus are frequent associated complaints. The critical point however is that constipation affects both quality of life and the functional independence of older adults. The prevalence of constipation increases with age and frailty. Community surveys of older patients indicate that one third describe constipation occurring at least once a month but only 2 - 3% report that their mean stool frequency is less than three per week. Reduced mobility, food and fluid intake and medication use are common themes associated with constipation. Warning symptoms that should prompt urgent assessment include rapid onset, weight loss, bleeding per rectum and features of iron deficiency. Constipation may be due to slow colonic transport or ano-rectal dysfunction or a combination of both. Although both of these functions can be measured objectively by transit studies with radio-opaque markers, defaecation proctography and assessment of ano-rectal pressures and sensory thresholds, this is rarely necessary as symptomatic assessment is usually accurate enough for clinical purposes. When patients complain of constipation, they usually are referring to infrequent passage of stool, straining at defaecation or a feeling of bloatedness. Most cases of constipation in older patients are 'simple' constipation and in most patients it is appropriate to assume this and treat with lifestyle and dietary measures. Constipation not responding to these measures requires further assessment and more detailed appraisal of causation (Table 4).

Faecal impaction, which is nearly always rectal, occurs due to decreased rectal sensitivity, with consequent accumulation of faeces. There may be an overflow incontinence of faecal liquid. Diagnosis is made by digital examination which reveals a rectum full of faeces which is usually soft, not hard. Treatment initially is by use of laxatives, enemas and in the long-term by use of dietary measures, bulking agents and toilet training; sitting on the toilet twice a day after meals for 10 minutes. Occasionally, manual evacuation is required.

webs associated with iron deficiency anaemia are less common causes of dysphagia in older patients.

Radiological contrast studies and endoscopy are the investigations of first choice for oesophageal dysphagia. Subtle dysphagia for solids may be demonstrated by radiologically observing swallowing with either bread or marshmallow which has been dipped in contrast.

Oro-pharyngeal dysphagia in older patients is most commonly due to stroke. Left hemisphere strokes tend to cause oral phase dysphagia and the pharyngeal phase tends to be affected by right hemisphere lesions. Dysarthria is commonly associated with dysphagia but the two disorders do not necessarily occur together. Dysphagia also occurs frequently with brainstem strokes. Dysphagia associated with stroke often settles within the first three months. Patient may be supplemented with nasogastric tube feeding while formal assessment of swallow continues. Some patients will require PEG tube insertion. Video-fluoroscopy and

TABLE 5
COMMON CAUSES OF DIARRHOEA IN OLDER PATIENTS

ACUTE (< 4 weeks)	CHRONIC		
	Watery	Inflammatory	Fatty
Infective:			
Clostridium difficile	Diverticulitis	Diverticulitis	Coeliac disease
Salmonella	Faecal Impaction	Ulcerative colitis	Pancreatic dysfunction
Campylobacter			
Shigella	SBBO	Crohn's disease	Whipple's disease
Norovirus			
Giardiasis	Post-Surgery	Ischaemic colitis	
Cryptosporidium	Diabetes	Persistent C diff	
Antibiotic related	Microscopic colitis	Tuberculosis	
(non Clostridium difficile)			
Acute dietary intolerance	Laxative abuse	Yersinia	
	Hyperthyroidism		
	Addison's disease		
	VIPoma		
	Carcinoid syndrome		

General measures in the treatment of constipation include advice on a balanced diet, increased fibre and fluid intake and regular exercise. Patients should be advised to never neglect a call to stool. Bulk laxatives, such as wheat bran, isphaghula or methylcellulose may be particularly helpful where dietary factors are important in the causation. Senna or other stimulant laxatives can be useful as short-term treatments only. Many patients find lactulose in a dose of 30-90 mls per day useful. Unabsorbed polyethylene glycol electrolyte (PEG) solutions can be used in the acute setting or for long-term treatment. These solutions appear to be particularly effective for faecal impaction as long as the patient can drink the large volumes involved. In patients with impaction, it may also be necessary to use rectal preparations such as phosphate enemas or stimulant suppositories such as glycerine, bisacodyl or oxyphenisatin.

Diarrhoea

In the western hemisphere, diarrhoea is usually defined as passage of stools greater than 200gms in weight in a 24-hour period. Other definitions include excessive liquidity or frequency of stools. Real diarrhoea needs to be distinguished from pseudo-diarrhoea where there is frequent passage of small amounts of stool but daily weights do not exceed 200gms per day. Pseudo-diarrhoea is a feature of IBS and other functional gastrointestinal disorders.

The differential diagnosis of diarrhoea, with its multiple causes, is very broad. Table 5 shows a scheme of causation based on the duration of the diarrhoea and on stool form.

In the evaluation of older patients with diarrhoea, the most important features are environmental context, duration, stool format and relationship of the diarrhoea to fasting. Older patients are particularly prone to get diarrhoea due to drug side effects (Table 6). Acute rapid onset diarrhoea is usually due to an infectious agent. Norovirus outbreaks have become commonplace in recent years. Vomiting is a prominent feature of norovirus outbreaks and precipitates admission for intravenous fluid resuscitation until it settles. Good hygiene limits the spread of infection but outbreaks place great demands on patients, staff, nursing homes and hospitals. The vast majority of patients with diarrhoea have an acute episode due to an infectious agent which usually settles spontaneously. The diagnosis of this common cause of diarrhoea is easily confirmed by stool culture if necessary. As it is self-limited, maintenance of hydration is all that is usually needed. Unfortunately, immunity is short-lived. Diarrhoea lasting longer than

TABLE 6
DRUGS CAUSING DIARRHOEA IN OLDER PATIENTS

Antibiotics
Chemotherapeutic agents
NSAIDs
β–Blockers
Mg^{++} containing antacids
Colchicine
Theophylline
Metformin
Clopidogrel
Proton-pump inhibitors
Digoxin

a month is almost never infectious, apart from rare infections with amoebae, giardia and shistosoma.

As shown in Table 5, assessment of stool format, whether it is watery, inflammatory or fatty is helpful in narrowing down the differential diagnosis of chronic diarrhoea. The presence of blood or pus in the stool suggests inflammatory diarrhoea. Fatty stool is characterised by a pale, whitish colour, its foul odour, the associated presence of oil droplets and the fact that it floats. The clinician should not rely on the patient's description of their stool but should personally inspect the stool in a bedpan in cases of protracted diarrhoea. Fatty stool occurs when there is greater than 7g of fat in the stool of a patient ingesting at least 100g of fat a day; usually a 2 - 3 day collection is necessary for this estimation and patients should be on a high fat diet for 2 - 3 days before collection. If only a random sample of stool is available, a Sudan stain of a faecal smear may be helpful. Risk factors for pancreatic insufficiency include chronic pancreatitis due to alcohol or other causes. With diverticulitis, there is usually a history of alternating constipation and diarrhoea and pain is often prominent.

Each day, approximately 9 litres of ingested food and secretions (saliva, gastric, intestinal and pancreatic, and bile) pass through the intestine with approximately 99% being absorbed resulting in a stool output of approximately 150g. Increased secretion (eg. Vipoma induced, cholera toxin, cytokine or inflammatory induced) or decreased absorption (eg. small intestinal malabsorption or surgical resection) or a combination of the two may result in a secretory diarrhoea. Osmotic diarrhoea, which is characterised by disappearance of the diarrhoea on fasting, is usually due to increased ingestion of magnesium (eg. antacids or mineral supplements), lactose deficiency or ingestion of poorly absorbed carbohydrates (lactulose, sorbitol, mannitol, fructose – often used as artificial sweeteners or in chewing gum).

Because the differential diagnosis is so wide, it is best to adopt a stepwise approach to investigation (Table 7). With a good history and the simple tests involved in Phase I, it should be possible to diagnose the majority of instances of diarrhoea in older patients. If it is necessary to proceed to Phase II, an estimation of daily stool weights at the outset may indicate pseudo-diarrhoea and obviate further unnecessary tests. Stool pH is usually alkaline but the presence of stool with a pH less than 6 suggest carbohydrate malabsorption in the small intestine, with consequent fermentation by colonic bacteria and the production of fatty acids. Northern Europeans, unlike Asians and Africans, are exceptional in that they retain lactase activity in the brush border of the intestinal epithelium into adult life but this activity may fall off in older individuals. The malabsorption of lactase gives rise to an acid stool. Secondary lactose intolerance may persist for a long period after infectious gastroenteritis in older patients and be a cause of chronic diarrhoea. Low stool pH may also be due to the ingestion of poorly absorbed sugar alcohols used as artificial sweeteners (eg. sorbitol or mannitol) or ingestion of fructose which has a limited absorptive capacity.

Any suggestion that the diarrhoea is inflammatory should lead to Phase II investigations of colonoscopy and barium follow through. In patients with diarrhoea, it is essential always to take biopsies at colonoscopy; the mucosa may have a normal gross appearance but be abnormal microscopically with microscopic colitis, collagenous colitis, amyloidosis, Whipple's disease or shistosomiasis. When diarrhoea is due to acute diverticulitis, pain is usually a prominent feature. At ultrasound, there may be thickening of the bowel wall, an associated collection or thickening of the mesentery.

If at this stage the diagnosis is not clear, many experienced clinicians attempt serial therapeutic trials with a variety of agents; co-amoxiclav, metronidazole, pancreatic enzyme supplements and/or bile acid sequestrants such as cholestyramine. The evidence for this approach is lacking and these therapeutic trials often are difficult to assess clinically. However, the use of opiates and loperamide may produce a welcome relief for the patient.

Phase III investigations may then be introduced but it is usually wise to obtain specialist review at this stage. Despite all investigations, about 5% of cases of chronic diarrhoea remain undefined. Many of these have what is termed 'idiopathic secretory diarrhoea'. Epidemiologically, this condition behaves like infectious diarrhoea but as yet no infectious agent has been identified. Onset is abrupt and there may be substantial weight loss. This form of diarrhoea, although prolonged, is self limiting and usually settles over a 9 - 12 month period.

Diarrhoea in nursing homes

Diarrhoea in nursing homes is common and institutionalised elderly are a selected population. In general, this group have more problems with mobility, cognition and co-morbidities than community living older adults. Diaries with visual or descriptive scales can be useful to identify true diarrhoea. Faecal impaction is the commonest cause. Laxative or drug-induced diarrhoea is also common. Clusters of cases should prompt testing for norovirus or Clostridium difficile. It should be remembered that norovirus can cause isolated cases as well. Colonisation rates with Clostridium difficile among residents of nursing homes may be as high as 70%. People with IgG antibodies against Toxin A are protected from clinical disease and have asymptomatic carriage. Chronic diarrhoea should prompt referral for assessment as described above.

Faecal incontinence

The involuntary loss of stool, liquid or solid is an embarrassing event for adults. It needs to be specifically asked for as it is rarely volunteered. Concomitant urinary incontinence is also common. Faecal incontinence places great strains on carers and is strongly associated with eventual placement in long term care. Continence requires several factors; awareness of the need to go, the ability to get to the toilet on time and good sphincter control. Factors such as cognitive impairment, reduced mobility, pain and access to carers all play a role. Medications such as analgesics, hypnotics or anti-psychotic agents can contribute to faecal incontinence. Prior pelvic surgery such as hysterectomy or prostate surgery can alter pelvic floor function. Faecal incontinence affects quality of life, mental health, skin integrity and limits the social life of patients and their carers. Associated constipation can be managed with regular enemas or other measures as outlined above

TABLE 7	
STEPWISE INVESTIGATION OF DIARRHOEA	
PHASE I	FBC
	ESR
	U&E, TFTs, LFTs, Ca^{++} & Glucose
	Stool cultures
	Stool viral studies
	Clostridium difficile stool toxins A&B
	Stool microscopy for ova, parasites, shigella &
	white cells
	Abdominal x-ray
PHASE II	Stool weights
	Stool pH
	Duodenal biopsies
	Saline smear - Giardiasis
	H&E stain - Coeliac disease
	PAS stain - Whipple's disease
	Colonoscopy with colon and terminal ileum
	biopsies
	Ultrasound of abdomen for acute
	diverticulitis
	Small bowel barium follow through
	Trial of metronidazole or tetracycline or
	ciprofloxacin
PHASE III	GI hormones - VIP & gastrin
	5-HIAA 24hr urine collection
	Stool laxative screen
	Urine laxative screen
	CT abdomen for pancreatic enlargement
	or atrophy
	3 day faecal fat collection
	Stool electrolytes & osmolality
	HIV testing
	Amoebic serology
	Pancreo-lauryl test for pancreatic
	insufficiency
	SeHCAT test for bile acid malabsorption
	Trial of cholestyramine or pancreatic
	enzyme replacement

not just to improve the patient but also to reduce carer workload thus helping to maintain patients at home for longer. The Royal College of Physicians national audit on continence care for older people identified urinary incontinence, dementia, stroke and impaired mobility as the commonest risk factors for faecal incontinence, anorectal incontinence being uncommon.

Investigation starts with a stool diary. Offending medications should be withdrawn and faecal impaction and diarrhoea should be treated. Efforts to improve mobility and access to commodes and toilets should be made. Scheduled toileting after meals may be effective. Pelvic floor exercises including biofeedback should be offered to cognitively intact individuals. Where anatomical reasons exist, such as sphincter damage, surgical repair should be considered. With attention to these details, successful treatment can be provided to many for this debilitating condition.

Gastrointestinal disease in older patients

Mouth

Currently about 50% of people in Ireland and Britain are edentulous at 70 years of age. In the future, it is likely that this percentage will fall due to better standards of oral hygiene and fluoridation of water. Degenerating, rotting teeth may be hazardous giving rise to local abscess formation, anaerobic lung infections including lung abscess, bronchial foreign bodies and endocarditis. Dentures may have their own problems. Dentures may give rise to candidiasis, mouth ulceration and fibrous hyperplasia of the gums. Oral candida, which is characterised by white curd like flecks on the tongue and gums which when removed leave a reddened or bleeding mucosa, is common in debilitated hospitalised older patients or those who have had antibiotics, steroids or have diabetes. Angular stomatitis may be due to iron, B_{12} or folate deficiencies.

Oesophagus

Oesophagitis and gastro-oesophageal reflux disease (GORD) are increasing in prevalence throughout the population. Unlike duodenal ulcer, oesophagitis cannot be easily eradicated and thus there are many modalities of treatment. These range from lifestyle modification to simple antacid usage to powerful suppression of gastric acid secretion with proton pump inhibitors (PPIs). The principle of management is to use the medication which is least expensive, has the best side effect profile and gives relief of symptoms. This can often be achieved with simple antacids or coating agents or the 'as required' use of proton pump inhibitors. Oesophagitis should not be overlooked as a cause of unexplained iron deficiency anaemia in older patients. Dysphagia due to peptic stricture should, in the first instance, be treated with up to two months of high dose proton pump inhibitor as this may obviate the need for endoscopic oesophageal dilatation which carries a small but definite risk of oesophageal perforation.

Barrett's oesophagus, in which there is intestinal metaplasia and primitive sub-mucosal crypt formation, in the lower oesophagus, is a pre-malignant condition. Although surveillance endoscopy is advocated by many for this condition, no evidence has emerged that this approach affects outcome and prevents cancer development. Thus, in older patients who are prone to multiple pathologies, surveillance endoscopy for Barrett's oesophagus may not be worthwhile. Oesophageal carcinoma, especially adenocarcinoma of the lower oesophagus, is increasing in incidence, especially in older patients. Prognosis is dismal with a one and five year average survival of 27% and 9% respectively. Surgery with or without chemotherapy offers only slight improvements in the prognosis but perhaps with better selection of patients in combination with new imaging techniques such as PET scanning, survival may improve.

Upper gastrointestinal bleeding

Despite the introduction of selective COX-2 inhibitors, these drugs and the non-selective NSAIDs remain a common aetiological factor in upper GI haemorrhage in older patients causing gastric erosions, gastric ulcer and duodenal ulcer. Non-drug induced duodenal ulcer and gastric ulcer also remain common causes of upper GI haemorrhage in this age group with oesophagitis, Mallory-Weiss tear, variceal bleeding and carcinoma being less common.

At the time of initial presentation, a clear distinction between those with long standing chronic anaemia and those with acute blood loss needs to be made. The less experienced clinician often makes the mistake of diagnosing acute blood loss in patients with chronic anaemia who have developed relatively minor co-existing gastrointestinal upset such as diarrhoea or vomiting. Assessment of the blood film, especially the red cell mean corpuscular volume (high in B_{12} or folate deficiency, low in iron deficiency) and direct inspection of vomitus or stool are important. If at the time of presentation, there is doubt about this differential, assessment of iron, ferritin, B_{12} and folate should be performed.

Volume resuscitation in older patients may be hazardous due to the possibility of fluid overload, and fluid replacement therefore needs to be monitored carefully and occasionally central venous pressure monitoring will be required. Patients with upper GI haemorrhage are best treated in a joint fashion, with a defined protocol, by surgeons and physicians who have easy access to endoscopy. In those patients with significant haemorrhage, early endoscopy within 24 hours of presentation is advocated. The injection of 1 in 10,000 adrenaline into a bleeding duodenal or gastric ulcer has dramatically reduced the need for surgery. High dose intravenous proton pump inhibitors lower the complication, re-bleeding and surgical rates in patients who have had endoscopic injection therapy. Surgical mortality for patients over 80 years with upper gastrointestinal haemorrhage is about 25 to 30%.

Stomach and duodenum

Peptic ulcer disease (PUD) is a common diagnosis in older adults. Pain may not be a prominent feature in its presentation and a high index of suspicion will be required when assessing older patients, particularly those who present with anaemia. The revolutionary discovery of Helicobacter pylori (H. pylori) as the cause of PUD allowed successful treatment of PUD with 95 - 99% cure rates following triple therapy eradication regimes. Two such regimes are suggested in Table 8. H. pylori infection is encountered more frequently in older adults. Concomitant prescription of aspirin, warfarin or NSAIDs complicate the clinical presentation. Although COX-2 selective agents may have a lower risk of GI bleeding, this benefit is lost in patients taking aspirin. There have also been concerns regarding cardiac effects of this class of drugs which may reduce prescriptions significantly.

Gastroscopy should be performed in patients with suspected PUD. Antral biopsy can be tested for H. pylori with the CLO test (rapid urease test). This can allow immediate identification and treatment of infection. Gastric ulcers should be biopsied to exclude malignancy. Up to 10% of the general population are taking PPIs, many for non-ulcer dyspepsia which is the commonest cause of dyspepsia in all age groups. Patients with non-ulcer dyspepsia present with typical symptoms but no mucosal lesions are detected at endoscopy. PPIs have not been shown to produce a clear-cut benefit in non-ulcer dyspepsia or functional abdominal pain. It is debatable whether they should be prescribed prophylactically in patients taking aspirin, warfarin or NSAIDs; however in patients with prior documented PUD, it is reasonable to co-

| TABLE 8 |
| HELICOBACTER PYLORI ERADICATION REGIMES |

7 Days Treatment

1. Lansoprazole 30mg bd
   Metronidazole 400mg bd
   Clarithromycin 250mg bd

2. Esomeprazole 40mg bd
   Amoxicillin 1g bd
   Clarithromycin 500mg bd

prescribe a PPI. Where possible, infection with H. pylori should be sought and eradicated.

Prolonged infection with H. pylori results in a migration of the bacteria from the antrum of the stomach towards the body and fundus of the stomach. Due to the prolonged inflammation, atrophic gastritis is often seen in older patients who have H. pylori infection. This type of atrophic gastritis may be a prelude to gastric carcinogenesis and gastric cancer. The World Health Organisation regards H. pylori as a Class I carcinogen but the vast majority of people with H. pylori infection never develop gastric cancer and the incidence of this cancer is actually decreasing. Nevertheless an advantage of performing endoscopy for suspected PUD is early diagnosis of gastric cancer. H. pylori is also associated with mucosal associated lymphoid tumours (MALToma) and in the early stages of this cancer, cure may occur if eradication is successful.

Percutaneous endoscopic gastrostomy (PEG) in older adults

Percutaneous endoscopic gastrostomy (PEG) placement provides a route for long-term enteral feeding in patients that can no longer maintain effective or safe oral nutrition.

The benefit of PEG insertion is clear-cut in conditions where recovery is expected such as stroke. However, the results of the FOOD trial advocates against early (< 7 days) PEG placement, presumably as swallow often recovers in the first few weeks after stroke. Where PEG placement is performed, it is important to review the need for the PEG tube at intervals as the tube can often be removed when spontaneous swallow recovery occurs. PEG insertion may also be

TABLE 9

COMPLICATIONS FOLLOWING PEG TUBE INSERTION

Tube failure, slippage or blockage

Vomiting, abdominal distension, cramping and diarrhoea

Heavy bruising over the site

Local or abdominal infection

Gastro-intestinal bleeding

Bowel perforation

Aspiration pneumonia

Mortality rates in the first month is up to 30% in high risk groups

considered in conditions where there is a physical blockage to swallowing such as cancer of the larynx or oesophagus. The benefit of PEG insertion is controversial in conditions where no recovery is expected such as Alzheimer's disease and other dementias and swallow failure in this group of patients can to some extent be regarded as a terminal event. Anorexia is a common feature of cognitive impairment and PEG feeding has not been shown to improve outcomes. A 'feed when well' approach may be more appropriate in patients with end-stage disease. Similarly, severely disabled stroke patients, or those with terminal illness such as cancer will need individualised decisions on PEG feeding.

There are of course problems associated with PEG insertion and they are not suitable for all patients. Absolute contra-indications include the inability to access the stomach either endoscopically or trans-abdominally due to a large previous gastric resection for instance. Other relative contraindications include extensive previous abdominal surgery, poor general condition of the patient and intercurrent illness.

All medical and nursing staff should be aware of potential complications and these are listed in Table 9. Infection in the respiratory and urinary tract, as well as advanced age are the most potent predictors of mortality at 30 days. Of note, the mortality rates for PEG tube insertion at 30 days are approximately 17.9% and as high as 30% in high risk patients. The decision to insert one should therefore never be taken lightly.

PEG tubes can become blocked and the commonest reasons are failure to flush adequately, the use of crushed tablets instead of liquid solutions and viscous feed or medications.

If a PEG tube is blocked the clinican should ensure that all clamps are open and the tubing is not kinked and try to manually locate and break down the blockage. Then attach a 50ml syringe and try to aspirate feed or fluid. If the tube is still blocked the next step is to flush the tube with 50mls of warm water and leave for 30 minutes and add some bicarbonate of soda to the warm water while flushing the feeding tube using a 50ml syringe, leaving for 20 - 30 minutes. If necessary, flush the tube with diluted pineapple juice (contains proteolytic enzyme). Leave this in the tube for 20 - 30 minutes also. Finally for hospitalised patients, if the above measures fail to unblock the tube, empty the contents of one pancreatic enzyme capsule into a mortar and grind with a pestle and water. Syringe this mixture into the feeding tube and clamp the tube. Leave for 30 minutes and flush with water. Do not use cranberry juice or carbonated cola beverages to irrigate tubes as the acidity may exacerbate clogging. Never use sharp instruments or excessive force to unblock a tube.

Gallstones

The prevalence of gallstones in Western populations increases with age. Community based ultrasound studies indicate that up to 25% of women over 70 years of age currently have gallstones or previously have had a cholecystectomy. The vast majority of gallstones detected are asymptomatic (70 - 85%). Asymptomatic gallstones, especially in older patients, are unlikely to give rise to clinical problems and are best left alone. Abdominal ultrasound will often diagnose gallstones when performed for other reasons; the importance of this finding needs to be interpreted in the clinical context. Gallstones are a common cause of acute abdominal pain in older patients. Biliary colic occurs when a gallstone impacts in Hartman's pouch in the neck of the gallbladder and is the commonest presentation. Usually, the patient complains of severe right upper quadrant pain which is constant and not colicky and which typically lasts 2 to 4 hours after the evening meal. The patient is restless with the pain. Usually the stone falls back out of Hartman's pouch into the gallbladder and the episode of pain terminates. Acute cholecystitis can develop if a stone blocks the cystic duct for a prolonged time and inflammation develops in the gallbladder. In cholecystitis, pain persists for at least 24 hours accompanied by vomiting, fever and leucocytosis. In a small minority of patients an empyema of the gallbladder may develop. Acute cholecystitis is now treated with early laparoscopic

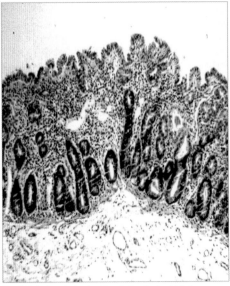
Figure 2: Coeliac disease showing subtotal villous atrophy and lymphocyte infiltration

cholangitis. Common bile duct exploratory surgery is associated with a high mortality in those over 75 years (5 - 15%), therefore ERCP with sphincterotomy and stone removal which has a lower mortality (1%) in this age group is recommended.

Coeliac disease

The traditional diagnostic criteria for coeliac disease are the demonstration of the typical small intestinal histology of subtotal villous atrophy and the demonstration that this has improved at re-biopsy after 3 to 6 months of gluten free diet. Serological tests, especially anti-endomysial and anti-tissue transglutaminase antibodies, have demonstrated that coeliac disease is more prevalent than that considered previously with a prevalence of approximately 1 in 150 in the population of Ireland and Great Britain. The spectrum of disease ranges from asymptomatic to the classical presentation of diarrhoea, anaemia and osteomalacia. Serological testing, however, has not replaced biopsy in the clinical arena and false negative tests do occur, particularly in the setting of IgA deficiency. Four endoscopic biopsies from the third part of the duodenum usually provide sufficient material on which to approach a diagnosis as mucosal changes can be patchy. Treatment is focused on excluding gluten from the diet. In patients who fail to respond, meticulous history taking usually reveals the source of ongoing gluten exposure. In older patients, asymptomatic disease or IBS like symptoms are common presentations. Anaemia, either iron deficient or associated with macrocytosis, or biochemical problems related to vitamin D and calcium malabsorption should prompt screening tests in older adults. Coeliac disease has been discovered in patients with ataxia, headaches, affective disorders and seizures. There is a higher incidence of intestinal lymphomas in coeliac disease and these may become manifest for the first time in older age.

Small bowel bacterial overgrowth

Recently it has been recognised that older subjects may have small bowel bacterial overgrowth (SBBO) without clinical problems, so called simple colonisation. However, SBBO may also cause significant clinical problems and may be the most common cause of malabsorption in older individuals. SBBO mainly manifests as diarrhoea, bloating and weight loss and has been associated with IBS type symptoms. Apart from age, SBBO occurs due to stagnation of small intestinal contents and compromise

cholecystectomy and intravenous antibiotics. If the patient presents late, surgery is often delayed for six weeks. If a gallstone escapes and become impacted in the hepatic or common bile ducts, right upper quadrant pain accompanied by jaundice is typical. A stone impacted in the lower end of the common bile duct may either pass through the sphincter of Oddi and ampulla into the intestine or may fall back into the dilated common bile duct. In both of these scenarios, the jaundice and pain will abate. However, the stone may remain impacted and infection of the stagnated bile may give rise to cholangitis presenting with Charcot's triad of fever, jaundice and right upper quadrant pain.

Ultrasound is more sensitive than either CT scan or MRI scan for detecting gallstones. It is also extremely good at detecting a dilated common bile duct but up to 20% of gallstones within a dilated common bile duct are not visualised by ultrasound. Magnetic resonance cholangiopancreatography (MRCP) can accurately assess the anatomy of the bile ducts and pancreatic ducts and has greater than 95% sensitivity for detecting gallstones within the bile ducts. Endoscopic ultrasound may also be helpful in difficult cases. Endoscopic retrograde cholangiopancreatography (ERCP) is occasionally complicated by pancreatitis and haemorrhage and is useful for retrieval of gallstones from the CBD and insertion of stents in obstructive of the gastric acid barrier to swallowed bacteria, often due to proton pump inhibitors. Thus patients who have blind loops due to previous gastric surgery, jejunal diverticulae, obstruction or dysmotility due to radiation, Crohn's disease, adhesions, scleroderma or diabetes are especially prone to SBBO. Blind loops are not however a prerequisite to the diagnosis in older patients and poor gut motility due to Parkinson's disease for instance may be equally important. The syndrome may be complicated by Vitamin B_{12} deficiency due to competitive utilisation of the B_{12} by small intestinal bacteria and carbohydrate, protein and fat malabsorption.

Definitive diagnosis requires specialised aerobic and anaerobic culture of aspirated proximal jejunal juices; this method is cumbersome and the specialised laboratory facilities required for culture may not be available. The ^{14}C-d-xylose breath test is the next best alternative but unfortunately requires the use of radioactive isotopes. The lactulose hydrogen breath test is an alternative but the sensitivity of this test is not high. Therapeutic trials with antibiotics may be necessary and a history of amelioration of symptoms with antibiotics for other infections may be a clue to diagnosis. The first aim of therapy should be to correct any anatomical underlying small bowel abnormality if possible. Nutritional support and review of medications that affect gut motility should be instituted. Depending on response, a weeklong course at monthly intervals or long-term antibiotics may be necessary. Co-amoxiclav is a common choice but there is no gold standard antibiotic. Metronidazole can also be useful. Probiotics may be useful but have not been tested in randomised trials thus far.

Large intestine

Colorectal cancer

Two-thirds of colorectal cancers (CRC) occur in adults over 65 years of age. The vast majority of colorectal cancers (CRC) in older patients are predated by adenomatous polyp formation, the so-called adenomacarcinoma sequence. It is highly unlikely that polyps less than 1cm in size in this age group will ever progress to a cancer, particularly a fatal cancer.

Associations with increased risk of CRC include IBD, diabetes, excess alcohol, smoking, obesity and possibly prior cholecystectomy. Aspirin or NSAID therapy (when required for other reasons) may be protective. Iron deficiency anaemia, weight loss, altered bowel habit or passing blood per rectum are well known red flag symptoms in older adults. The choice of investigation depends on local services, patient choice and general health. Tumour markers, CEA and CA 19.9, are not useful for diagnostic purposes but CEA levels may be useful in detecting recurrence. Colonoscopy has the advantage over barium enema and CT in providing histological diagnosis and potential for polyp removal. Frail, older adults may be best served by initial minimal preparation CT (MPCT). The Oxford experience suggests this is a safe practice and is associated with a lower technical failure rate than colonoscopy or barium enema. MPCT also provides some staging information and can also detect other pathologies.

Colon cancer in comparison to other cancers has a good prognosis. On average, five year survival for Duke's A carcinoma confined to the mucosa and sub-mucosa and Duke's B carcinoma confined to the bowel wall is greater than 90% and 75% respectively. Surgery is the primary treatment modality for colon cancer. Post surgery chemotherapy does not produce substantial benefit in patients with Duke's A or Duke's B colon cancer but may produce some limited survival benefit in patients with Duke's C carcinoma where there is extension of cancer cells to the lymph nodes. Rectal cancer behaves somewhat differently to colon cancer. It is more likely to be locally invasive and adjuvant chemotherapy and radiotherapy are considered prior to surgery. Patients are best served by a multidisciplinary assessment involving gastroenterologists, GI surgeons, GI radiologists and oncologists generating consensus plans for individual patients. Chemotherapy guidelines are based on the TNM method of staging and are subject to regular revision. There is no consensus on chemotherapy for adults over 80. Co-morbidities increase the probability of poor outcomes from neutropenic sepsis and other complications. Comprehensive geriatric assessment may facilitate the decision making process. Renally excreted chemotherapeutic agents should have the dose altered according to the estimated glomerular filtration rate (eGFR). Healthy older adults should be offered aggressive treatment with increased attention to possible side effects.

Intestinal ischaemia

The GIT is supplied by three main arteries, the coeliac, superior mesenteric and inferior mesenteric arteries. Despite a good collateral circulation, these vessels are frequently affected by vascular disease.

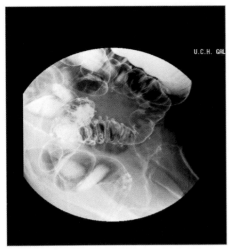
Figure 3: Diverticular disease on a barium enema

stool, known as haematochezia, although melaena may occur with right colon involvement. Physical signs include fever, hypotension and tenderness over the affected area. Typical radiographic features of 'thumb printing' in the region of the splenic flexure may be seen on plain abdominal x-ray but usually a barium enema or colonoscopy on the unprepared bowel is needed for diagnosis. These investigations should be performed within 48 hours of onset of symptoms as the findings become non-specific thereafter. Management is supportive and antibiotics can be used if pyrexia is prominent. Increasing abdominal tenderness, guarding, rising temperature and paralytic ileus indicate colonic infarction and demand immediate laparotomy and colon resection. In the majority of patients, the ischaemia resolves within 48 hours and the colon returns to normal over a number of weeks. Some patients, however, develop late strictures.

Acute mesenteric ischaemia causes acute abdominal pain, often secondary to cardioembolism associated with heart failure and atrial fibrillation. In-situ thrombosis of atherosclerotic vessels can also occur. The pain can be more severe than initial abdominal examination might suggest. Early diagnosis with CT or interventional angiography and early involvement of surgical colleagues is essential. Aggressive fluid resuscitation and antibiotics aim to optimise patients for early surgery. Despite increased awareness of the condition, mortality remains at around 70%. In survivors, the underlying cause must be treated. Chronic mesenteric ischaemia occurs in patients with atherosclerosis and causes post-prandial abdominal pain. Weight loss is common and an epigastric bruit may be heard. Occlusion of two of the three main vessels is present in the majority of, but not all, cases. Recently, CT angiography has shown sufficient sensitivity to largely replace conventional angiography. Treatment is via surgical revascularisation or percutaneous angioplasty.

Colonic ischaemia (ischaemic colitis) is a frequent disorder in older people and is more common in cardiac failure, hypertension, diabetes and nephropathy. Clinical manifestations range from transient alteration of bowel function to gangrene with bowel infarction. Approximately 50% of cases involve the 'watershed' area of the splenic flexure and left colon. Colonic ischaemia usually manifests as sudden onset crampy left lower quadrant abdominal pain and passage of bright red blood mixed with the

Diverticular disease

A diverticulum is a sac-like projection of the colon wall through the muscular layer of the colon; diverticulae develop where the vasa recta penetrate the bowel wall. The high incidence of diverticular disease in western societies is related to the low dietary fibre in western diets. Approximately 70% of Europeans have diverticular disease by the time they have reached 70 years of age. Diverticular disease predominantly affects the left colon, particularly the sigmoid colon. Mostly diverticular disease remains asymptomatic but in 10 to 25% of people with diverticular disease, it manifests as diverticulitis with usually left-sided abdominal pain and tenderness. A specific diagnosis of diverticulitis can be made with abdominal CT with contrast and these imaging techniques can also demonstrate associated complications. Thinning of the vasa recta can lead to significant haemorrhage in diverticular disease, mainly in right colon disease. Treatment is based on increasing the dietary fibre content and fluid intake. Acute diverticulitis is treated with fluids, antibiotics and surgery if there are signs of obstruction, peritonitis or perforation.

Inflammatory bowel disease

There are two populations of older people with inflammatory bowel disease (IBD). The first are the group diagnosed as younger adults who have reached their later years. The other group are those who develop IBD in later life that account for around 10% of cases. The full spectrum of IBD can be seen, although disease tends to be less severe in older individuals.

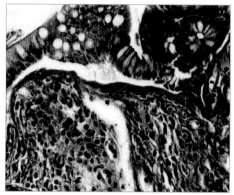

Figure 4: Collagenous colitis

Systemic and extraintestinal complications can also occur in older adults. In older patients, the diagnosis of IBD can be more difficult due to the higher incidence of other conditions presenting in a similar manner such as ischaemic colitis, pseudo-membranous colitis and diverticular disease. Treatment in older patients is the same as in younger patients with the exception that older individuals are more prone to the problem of osteoporosis and thus the use of steroids presents additional hazards. Azathioprine can be used in patients who have been tested for thiopurine methyltransferase activity. 5-aminosalicylates such as sulfasalazine and mesalazine are useful in ulcerative colitis but of unproven benefit in Crohn's disease. Tumour necrosis alpha antagonists such as infliximab are associated with serious adverse events in older adults and should only be instituted by specialists in IBD. Early surgical intervention can improve outcomes and surgical colleagues should be involved early in serious cases. In addition, older patients who have a long history of colitis, have an increased risk of colonic cancer. Surveillance programmes for the early detection of cancer in IBD are recommended, particularly for people with long-term disease.

Microscopic colitis

This condition is characterised by chronic watery diarrhoea. Colonoscopy is normal but biopsy shows colitis without ulceration. Two histological subtypes are recognised; lymphocytic and collagenous. The lymphocytic type has increased intraepithelial lymphocytes; both have evidence of a thickened layer of subepithelial collagen. The severity of the histological changes is greater in the proximal colon; biopsies should be taken from the right or transverse colon. The cause is unknown but NSAIDs

may precipitate the illness. They should be stopped but if the diarrhoea continues, a trial of steroids is warranted. Sulfasalazine and bismuth subsalicylate have been reported to be successful treatments.

Antibiotic-related diarrhoea and Clostridium difficile colitis

Antibiotics frequently cause alteration of bowel habit. Changes in the colonic flora which occur with antibiotic usage may also result in selective growth of Clostridium difficile. This Gram positive, spore forming organism can be a normal resident in the bowel and is not killed by hand washing with alcohol hand gels. Clostridium difficile associated diarrhoea (CDAD) is now a major concern in hospitalised older adults. Historically associated with clindamycin treatment, CDAD is now more often associated with cephalosporin and quinolone use but can be caused by any broad spectrum antibiotic. The diarrhoea is caused by toxins A and B and presents with a spectrum of illness from asymptomatic carriage to pseudo-membranous colitis and associated toxic megacolon. The incidence is increasing and the UK Office for National Statistics reported a 400% increase in the number of deaths attributed to CDAD in 2006 as compared to 2003. Part of this increase is presumably due to increased reporting of CDAD. However, increased prevalence of virulent strains such as the 027 ribotype is associated with increased severity of disease. There is an association with proton pump inhibitor usage with reduced gastric acid protection increasing the chance of faecal-oral transmission. CDAD should be suspected in hospitalised frail older adults with loose stools. Clinical features may be preceded by a leucocytosis. Generalised abdominal tenderness and features of a systemic inflammatory response with pyrexia, tachycardia and tachypnoea are strongly suggestive of CDAD. Abdominal x-ray may show dilated bowel loops and CT abdomen generally confirms colitis. Lower endoscopy can identify pseudo-membranous colitis but there is a risk of perforation so it should be performed only in certain circumstances. Diagnosis is routinely based on the detection of toxin A and B cytotoxicity in cell culture. Treatment is multilevel. The patient should be isolated with barrier nursing. Fluid resuscitation should be vigorous. Early commencement of metronidazole 400mg three times a day or vancomycin, 125mg to 250mg four times a day orally for 7 days should be instituted. The offending antibiotic should be stopped if possible. Oral therapy is preferred to parenteral therapy. Confirmed first recurrences can be treated with a 14 day course of antibiotics as above. A variety of regimes have been suggested for further recurrences with tapered courses of oral vancomycin over several weeks being one option. A recent meta-analysis of probiotics in CDAD found some evidence for treatment with Saccharomyces boulardii but this needs to be confirmed in larger studies. Toxin binding with cholestyramine, pooled human immunoglobulin and faecal therapy have all been reported to help in case reports but are not currently recognised as standard therapy. Surgical intervention with total colectomy is effective in selected patients with good pre-morbid status.

Abdominal aortic aneurysm

The aorta is considered aneurysmal if the diameter is greater than 3cm. The risk of rupture increases as diameter increases. AAA is more common in older men, patients with atherosclerotic disease elsewhere, hypertension, positive family history and smokers; 5% of men over 80 have an AAA. Screening for AAA in men aged 65 - 74 who have smoked is effective and endovascular repair is increasingly being advocated as an equally good therapy option to open repair for aneurysms larger than 5.5cm. Rupture of AAA has a mortality of roughly 80%. However, repair of AAA is only warranted for aneurysms larger than 5.5cm. The standard surgical technique for AAA repair is open repair. Recent trials have shown lower 30 day mortality with endovascular repair versus open repair (2% versus 5%) although longer-term follow up has shown no appreciable difference in mortality. Endovascular repair has an increased risk of recurrence as compared to open repair and up to 20% of individuals will require a further procedure. The choice of procedure should be based on fitness for surgery, patient choice and availability of appropriately skilled surgeons. Ongoing local audit of outcomes of both procedures will allow for more informed decision making for both patient and physician.

Suggested further reading

- Anonymous. Coeliac disease in the elderly (editorial). Lancet 1984; i: 775-776.
- Clinch D, Banerjee AK, Ostick G. Absence of abdominal pain in elderly patients with peptic ulcer. Age Ageing 1984; 13: 120-123.
- Collins JR. Celiac disease in elderly patients: Report of 13 cases with a note concerning drug absorption. Am J Dig Dis 1966; 11: 564-571.
- Eurogast Study Group: An international association between Helicobacter pylori infection and gastric cancer. Lancet 1993; 341: 1359-1362.
- Finucane PM, Arunachalam T, O'Dowd J, Pathy MS. Acute mesenteric infarction in elderly adults. J Am Geriatr Soc 1989; 37: 355-358.
- Fleischer DE, Grimm IS, Friedman LS. Inflammatory bowel disease in older patients. Medical Clin North Am 1994; 6: 1303-1319.
- Ganeshan A, Upponi S, Uberoi R, D'Costa H, Picking C, Bungay H. Minimal-preparation CT colon in detection of colonic cancer, the Oxford experience. Age and Ageing 2007; 36: 48–52.
- Korotinski S, Katz A, Malnick SD. Chronic ischaemic bowel diseases in the aged - go with the flow. Age and Ageing 2005; 34: 10-16.
- Kyne L, Kelly CP. Recurrent Clostridium difficile diarrhoea. Gut 2001; 49: 152-153.
- Lederle FA, Kane RL, MacDonald R, Wilt TJ. Systematic Review: Repair of Unruptured Abdominal Aortic Aneurysm. Ann Intern Med. 2007; 146: 735-741.
- Liston R, Pitt MA, Banerjee AK. Reflux oesophagitis and Helicobacter pylori in elderly patients. The Postgraduate Medical Journal 1996; 72: 221-223.
- Liston R, Pitt MA, Banerjee AK. IgG ELISA antibodies and detection of Helicobacter pylori in elderly patients. The Lancet 1996; 347: 269.
- Logan RPH, Dill S, Bauer FE et al. The European 13C-urea breath test for the detection of Helicobacter pylori. Eur J Gastroenterol Hepatol 1991; 3: 915-921.
- McEvoy AW, Fenwick JD, Boddy K, James OFW. Vitamin B12 deficiency from the gut does not decline with age in normal elderly humans. Age Ageing 1982; 11: 180-183.
- McEvoy A, Dutton J, James OFW. Bacterial contamination of the small intestine is an important cause of occult malabsorption in the elderly. Br Med J 1983; 287: 789-793.
- O'Keefe E, Talley NJ. The irritable bowel syndrome in the elderly. Gastroenterology Clinics of North America 1991; 20: 369-390.
- O'Riordan TG, Tobin A, O'Morain C. Helicobacter pylori infection in elderly dyspeptic patients. Age Ageing 1991; 20: 189-192.
- Reinus JF, Brandt LJ, Boley SJ. Ischemic diseases of the bowel. Gastroenterology Clinics of North America 1990; 19: 319-343.
- Roberts SH, James O, Jarvis EH. Bacterial overgrowth syndrome without "blind loop": A cause for malnutrition in the elderly. Lancet 1977; ii: 1193-1195.
- Thomas PD, Forbes A, Green J, Howdle P, Long R, Playford R, Sheridan M, Stevens R, Valori R, Walters J, Addison GM, Hill P, Brydon G. Guidelines for the investigation of chronic diarrhoea, 2nd edition. Gut

2003; 52 Suppl 5: v1-15.
• Wyatt JI, Shallcross TM, Crabtree JE, Heatley RV.
  Helicobacter pylori, gastritis and peptic ulceration in the
  elderly. J Clin Pathol 1992; 45: 1070-1074.

📁 Case Study 1

A 73 year old man with Parkinson's disease was admitted with rapid functional decline. While in hospital he had bouts of watery diarrhoea. This had been an intermittent problem over the preceding two years and was particularly troublesome if it coincided with one of his frequent 'off' periods or freezing episodes. The patient had had an anterior resection for Dukes A adenocarcinoma of the sigmoid colon 3 years earlier. He required a further laparotomy 6 months later after he developed intestinal obstruction secondary to adhesions. His current weight was steady and his appetite was good. He denied rectal bleeding. His routine blood tests were all normal including blood count, electrolytes and liver function tests. Total protein and albumin were also normal indicating that his nutritional status was also probably normal. Faecal occult blood was negative, stool cultures were negative and plain abdominal x-rays and ultrasound were normal. His serum B_{12} was low and his serum folate elevated. He was commenced on a course of co-amoxiclav and metronidazole and within one week his diarrhoea had stopped. His freezing episodes responded to increasing his doses of L-dopa and his quality of life was significantly improved.

Although no formal tests were performed in this case the diagnosis is almost certainly small bowel bacterial overgrowth syndrome. Prior surgery may have left 'stagnant' loops but it is important to remember that the syndrome can also occur in older patients with structurally normal guts. His Parkinson's disease and the poor intestinal transit associated with this also contributed in this case. The abnormal organisms cause diarrhoea by deconjugating bile acid which acts as an irritant in the colon. They also consume vitamin B_{12} and as a by-product of their metabolism they produce folate. The syndrome is common in older individuals and therapeutic trials of antibiotics are often successful.

📁 Case Study 2

A 78 year old man was admitted from a nursing home for investigation of anaemia. He had a background history of left hemiparesis, ischaemic heart disease and gout. Recently his gout had been troublesome and he required courses of NSAIDs. Although the gout had largely settled his prescription for indomethacin had been continued. On admission he was pale but denied any other symptoms and specifically there was no abdominal pain or dyspepsia. His initial blood tests confirmed iron deficiency anaemia with a Hb of 6.6g/dl, and MCV of 69 and low serum ferritin and iron with a high total iron binding capacity. His NSAID was stopped and an urgent gastroscopy was performed which confirmed the presence of a large gastric ulcer which was Helicobacter pylori positive. Histology was benign. The patient was transfused with 5 units of packed cells and was commenced on anti-helicobacter triple therapy, the proton pump inhibitor component of which was continued for 6 weeks. At follow-up his Hb had remained stable and he was discharged and advice was given that if the gout should become troublesome again NSAIDs should be avoided in favour of colchicine.

This case clearly illustrated the problems associated with assessment of peptic ulcer disease in older patients. Absence of pain is well recognised and makes assessment difficult. For many patients, a high index of clinical suspicion is required and many patients with active ulceration are asymptomatic and the first indication of a problem can be active bleeding or perforation. Most geriatricians are thus very cautious in their use of NSAIDs. Short courses (4 - 7 days) can be considered for acute gout. The interaction between NSAIDs and Helicobacter pylori is controversial. Some evidence suggests that because Helicobacter pylori produce prostaglandins as by-products of their metabolism a degree of protection from NSAID induced damage is given by the presence of the organism. Other evidence suggests that the ulcer should therefore be healed first before anti-helicobacter triple therapy is given. The investigation of choice for detecting Helicobacter pylori in older patients is the [13]Carbon urea breath test and serology is far less reliable in older individuals than in younger ones.

📁 Case Study 3

An 80 year old woman presented to hospital with a 6 week history of painless jaundice. This was associated with weight loss of almost one stone and the onset of mild ankle oedema. Her appetite was however normal. There were no associated features of vomiting, alteration in bowel habit or alteration in the colour of urine or stools. In her background she was on lisinopril for hypertension but was otherwise well. She was a non-drinker and a non-smoker. She lived in a warden controlled environment and had 2 supportive daughters. She was fully mobile and independent in the activities of daily living. Clinically she was icteric but there was no evidence of clubbing, lymphadenoapthy, scratch marks or xanthelasmata. There was however four finger hepatomagaly. Initial investigation revealed a bilirubin of 251, AST 770, alkaline phosphatase of 412, albumin of 24. Other bloods were normal. Abdominal ultrasound revealed two gallstones in the gallbladder with dilatation of the common bile duct and a stone present at the lower end of the common bile duct. The liver was noted to be diffusely enlarged with an irregular echo pattern. Free fluid was noted in the abdomen. Co-existing intrinsic liver disease was queried by the radiologist. ERCP was reported as showing the bile duct system to be moderately dilated with a simple calculus present in the common bile duct which was removed. The ducts appeared clear in the final film. The patient was discharged after a period of rehabilitation. The LFTs were repeated after one month with no significant improvement. The patient was readmitted for liver biopsy in view of increasing hepatomagaly but this was technically impossible due to ascites. Other investigations showed positive anti-smooth muscle antibodies and elevation of immunoglobulin IgG. Hepatitis serology and the rest of the liver screen was negative. The patient was tentatively labelled as autoimmune Chronic Active Hepatitis and responded well to corticosteroid therapy, spironolactone and frusemide with resolution of the ascites.

This case illustrates the importance of thorough assessment of older patients with jaundice. Gallstones are very common and although they were undoubtedly responsible for part of this lady's clinical presentation it was only when the underlying and coexisting intrinsic liver pathology was recognised that she improved with appropriate treatment. Autoimmune CAH usually presents in young women but is increasingly being recognised in older patients. Primary biliary cirrhosis is common in older patients however. It presents with malaise, itching, jaundice and evidence of liver failure. LFTs will demonstrate an obstructive picture with elevation of alkaline phosphatase and anti-mitochondrial antibodies are classically elevated

along with elevation of IgM. Prognosis is poor and treatment is with symptomatic measures and ursodeoxycholic acid.

Case Study 4

An 82 year old lady was admitted for investigation of iron deficiency anaemia. Her only complaint was tiredness but on closer questioning she admitted to occasional loose bowel motions which she had most of her adult life and which she thought were normal. She was on oral iron replacement. She had no other significant background history and had been well during childhood. She had been extensively investigated in another hospital with normal upper GI endoscopy, colonoscopy, barium enema, small bowel enema, ultrasound of abdomen, bone marrow biopsy and aspiration and routine bloods were normal apart from iron deficiency. She was admitted for repeat gastroscopy and duodenal biopsies along with coeliac antibodies. The biopsies showed clear evidence of villous atrophy and anti-endomysial antibodies were positive confirming the diagnosis of coeliac disease. She was commenced on a gluten free diet. Her energy levels significantly improved after a month and she subsequently commented that she had never known what it was like to be free of tiredness. Her anaemia completely resolved.

The above case illustrates the simple point that if clinicians do not specifically think of Coeliac disease as part of the differential diagnosis of iron deficiency anaemia in older patients, it will be missed.

Case Study 5

A frail 80 year old lady was admitted to hospital with a fractured left neck of femur. Four days after surgery, she was commenced on an oral cephalosporin for a presumed urinary tract infection. After a few days she developed a fever and profuse foul smelling diarrhoea and stool analysis confirmed the presence of toxin. The urine specimen showed no growth and her cephalosporin was stopped. She was commenced on oral metronidazole but her diarrhoea persisted. Vancomycin was tried with no significant improvement. Despite active supportive management and antibiotics as above she failed to respond to therapy and died. Following a review of antibiotic prescribing policy, prescription of cephalosporins was prohibited for urinary tract infections.

This case illustrates the dangers of using broad spectrum antibiotics in frail older patients. The antibiotics most likely to induce this condition are the cephalosporins, quinolones and fluoroquinolones and to a lesser extent penicillins. Strict enforcement of antibiotic prescription guidelines with support from clinical microbiology can reduce infection rates. Strict attention to infection control measures such as isolation of affected patients and attention to hand washing are essential to reduce CDAD in the hospital setting.

Data Interpretation

Question 1

An 82 year old woman presented with ataxia, low mood and lack of energy. This has developed over the preceding six months and was associated with abdominal discomfort and weight loss of 5kg. She had previously been diagnosed as having irritable bowel syndrome. Investigations show the following;

Hb	9.8g/dl
MCV	102fl
Na+	132mmol/l
K+	3.3mmol/l
Ca++	2.04mmol/l
Albumin	32g/l
Total protein	64g/l
TSH	normal

a.   Describe the abnormalities
b.   What is the differential diagnosis?
c.   What test would you order?

Question 2

A 78 year old man is admitted with an ischaemic left middle cerebral artery stroke with associated right hemiparesis and dysphasia. He is in sinus rhythm and carotid dopplers show 60% stenosis of the left internal carotid artery. He is commenced on aspirin and dipyridamole. He is unable to swallow safely and is fed through a nasogastric tube. One month later his full blood count shows anaemia;

Hb	8.6g/dl
MCV	68fl
Vitamin B₁₂	340ng/l
Folate	9ng/ml
Serum iron	10μmol/l

Serum ferritin	23ng/ml
ESR	42mm/hr

a.   Describe the abnormalities
b.   What test would you order?
c.   What treatment would you give?

Question 3

A 70 year old woman presents to the A&E with abdominal pain and diarrhoea for the last 2 days. She is dehydrated, her pulse is 120/minute, BP is 90/60mmHg, temperature is 39°C and abdominal exam reveals a soft distended abdomen with absent bowel sounds. She had a recent prolonged hospitalisat ion for severe community acquired pneumonia. Investigations showed the following;

WCC	30x10⁹/l (90% neutrophils)
Hb	12.7g/dl
Na+	147mmol/l
K+	3.5mmol/l
Urea	25mmol/l
Creatinine	204μmol/l
AXR	dilated loops of bowel
CXR	minimal left basal infiltrate, no free air under diaphragm

a.   What is the most likely diagnosis?
b.   What is your initial treatment?
c.   What action should also be considered?

Best of five questions

Question 1

A 72 year old woman was referred for investigation of raised LFTs. The investigations showed hypergammaglobulinaemia, ANA titre 1/160 and anti-SMA titre 1/320.
What is the most likely diagnosis?
a.   Alcoholic liver disease
b.   Coeliac disease
c.   Autoimmune hepatitis
d.   Primary biliary cirrhosis
e.   Fatty liver disease

Question 2

A 70 year old woman with a history of diabetes and heart failure presents with acute onset central abdominal pain and vomiting. The abdomen is tender without guarding and her BP is 76/40mmHg. ECG shows newly diagnosed fast atrial fibrillation. ABG shows a metabolic acidosis with a raised anion gap. Serum lactate is 2.4.
What is the most likely diagnosis?

a.   Ruptured abdominal aortic aneurysm
b.   Biliary colic
c.   Acute pancreatitis
d.   Acute mesenteric ischaemia
e.   Duodenal ulcer

Question 3

An 80 year old man presents to the A&E with a 6 hour history of abdominal pain radiating to the back. He is an obese ex-smoker and had a carotid endarterectomy 4 years previously. His abdomen is diffusely tender and there is a suggestion of a pulsatile mass in the epigastrium.

What is the most likely diagnosis?
a.   Perforated duodenal ulcer
b.   Leaking abdominal aortic aneurysm
c.   Gastric cancer
d.   Acute mesenteric ischaemia
e.   Acute pancreatitis

Answers are available on page 311

Continence

E C Mulkerrin, M Corcoran

Urinary incontinence

The prevalence of urinary incontinence (UI) in older patients varies according to the cohort of patients being studied. Between 18 - 30% of older people in the community suffer from UI, with prevalence rates rising to 35% in hospitalised older patients and 40 - 60% of patients in continuing care. It is associated with substantial morbidity and healthcare costs. Risk factors include:

- Central nervous system disease
- Impaired mobility
- Gender (more prevalent in females)

Ageing itself is not a risk factor as UI is never normal at any age. There are, however, age-related physiological changes in both sexes that may predispose to the condition. With advancing age, there is an increase in the percentage of daily fluid excreted at night, in residual urine and in uninhibited bladder contraction. Age-related changes pertinent to women alone include decreases in bladder capacity, contractility, inhibitory ability and urethral closure pressure. In the face of these physiological changes, any concomitant disease or medication may be enough to precipitate UI in predisposed individuals. It is important, therefore, for clinicians to ascertain the cause of new-onset UI which may be attributable to problems occurring outside the urinary tract and, as such, be responsive to medical intervention (table 1). Treatment, however, can reverse UI without necessarily addressing underlying lower urinary tract (LUT) abnormalities. If continence is not restored, pathology of the LUT must be suspected and the UI must be regarded as established.

Assessment of patients with UI

In patients with UI, clinicians must first consider the possibility of serious underlying conditions such as brain or spinal cord lesions, bladder or prostate cancer and hydronephrosis. Comprehensive details, such as the frequency and pattern of incontinence, sensation of bladder emptying, stranguary and the degree of urgency and straining, must be elicited from the history. The issue of polypharmacy is frequently

a consideration, particularly with regard to over-the-counter medications. A functional assessment of mobility and manual dexterity should include an appraisal of the impact on the patient's life-style. A targeted examination of the patient should include such details as:

- Orthostatic blood pressure, mental status, peripheral oedema
- Instantaneous leakage with single vigorous cough, when upright, relaxed with a full bladder
- Bladder palpable after voiding
- Pelvic: atrophic urethritis/vaginitis, uterine prolapse, cystocoele, masses, Bonney/Marshall test
- Rectal: anal wink/bulbocavernosus (sacral) reflexes, perineal sensation, sphincter resting tone and volitional control, faecal impaction
- Neurological: sensation/strength/tone/reflexes/plantar responses in lower extremities

Coupled with the above, patients should be encouraged to keep a voiding diary. A residual volume determination by portable bladder ultrasound or urethral catheterisation is obligatory if overflow incontinence is suspected. Culture and urinalysis should be performed. In selected cases, further laboratory investigations may need to be undertaken. If patients complain of pain or sterile haematuria is detected, urine cytology should be considered. Where polyuria occurs, a metabolic survey including blood glucose, calcium, urea and creatinine should be done. Urine flow studies and renal sonography are indicated when the post void residual volume exceeds 150ml and cystoscopy may be useful in selected cases.

Causes of established UI

The most frequent pathologies causing established UI include detrusor overactivity, stress incontinence, obstruction and an underactive detrusor muscle.

Detrusor overactivity

Overactivity of the detrusor muscle contributes to incontinence in 50 - 70% of older patients, regardless

TABLE I	
CONTRIBUTING FACTORS TO TRANSIENT URINARY INCONTINENCE	
D	Delirium
I	Infection (eg. symptomatic UTI)
A	Atrophic vaginitis/urethritis
P	Pharmaceuticals
	• Hypnotics/sedatives
	• Potent diuretics
	• Anticholinergics
	• Adrenergic agents
	• Calcium channel blockers
	• Ace inhibitors
P	Psychological
E	Excess urine output
R	Restricted mobility
S	Stool impaction

causes such as spinal cord lesions. Additionally, anatomical obstruction may precipitate an overactive detrusor muscle in 60% of cases.

Underactive detrusor

This condition is usually idiopathic, though neuropathy or outlet obstruction must be suspected and outruled. Sacral reflexes and sensation tend to be absent in most neuropathic cases. If bladder contraction is present, howsoever weak, and the patient strains to void, the residual urine volume may be low.

Treatment of UI

A general treatment plan augmented by treatment programmes for specific conditions is the mainstay of successful management for UI in older patients. Reversing transient precipitating factors for UI (DIAPPERS - table 1) is the first priority of treatment. Patients and carers must be trained regarding the correct toileting regimen based on their incontinence diary. Scrupulous perineal care remains a prerequisite. Where nocturnal incontinence is the predominant problem, the underlying cause (eg. excess excretion, insomnia or LUT dysfunction) must be satisfactorily ascertained and treated. The importance of avoiding culpable xanthines (tea, coffee) and alcohol must be emphasised. In all scenarios, the use of pads or diapers may prove helpful.

of cognitive function. 'Urge incontinence', where the abrupt flow of urine occurs with little or no warning, characterises this pathology. In addition, it is epitomised by frequent, periodic voiding with the patient remaining dry in between. Anal reflexes and perineal sensation are preserved and a low residual volume remains. Detrusor overactivity may be an early sign of other pathologies such as outlet obstruction.

Stress incontinence

This is predominantly (>90%) caused by urethral hypermobility with a small minority attributable to intrinsic sphincter deficiency. However, 25% of sufferers will also demonstrate detrusor overactivity. It is characterised by leakage occurring only when abdominal pressure is elevated. Leakage may then result instantaneously though generally only during the day. The bladder size remains normal. Unless uterine prolapse or pelvic muscle laxity is present, an examination will be normal. It must be emphasised that the presence of uterine prolapse or cystocoele is not always associated with stress incontinence.

Obstruction

Obstructive uropathy is rarely (<2%) found in elderly women, yet in men it may occur irrespective of past prostatectomy or palpated prostate size. Anatomical causes of obstruction, such as an enlarged prostate gland in men or a large prolapsing cystocoele in women, are much more common than neurological

Detrusor overactivity

All patients must aim to train their bladder, whether this is patient-orientated retraining for cognitively coherent patients or prompted voiding in a care scenario where cognitive function is impaired. Medications that may assist in this situation include anticholinergic drugs such as oxybutynin or tolterodine used alone or in combination with a muscle relaxant. The efficacy of a muscle relaxant such as flavoxate used on its own remains unproven. There is a role for the inclusion of tricyclic antidepressants such as imipramine or doxepin in selected cases. The risks of water retention and hyponatraemia may limit the use of desmopressin in older patients and further studies are required to clarify the role of calcium channel blockers.

Stress incontinence

Where incontinence is attributable to atrophic vaginitis, a simple regimen of an oral or vaginal oestrogen coupled with effective pelvic floor muscle exercises (Kegels) may alleviate symptoms.

TABLE 2 CAUSES OF ESTABLISHED UI		
Detrusor overactivity	Inappropriate contraction	Cortical insult eg. stroke, tumour, Alzheimer's or Parkinson's disease
		Local irritant eg. cystitis, bladder stone/cancer
Detrusor underactivity	Incomplete contraction	Neurogenic eg. neuropathy from diabetes, alcohol, pelvic surgery
		Obstruction
		Idiopathic
Stress incontinence	Outlet resistance too low	Childbirth trauma
		Post radical prostatectomy, distal TURP
Urethral/Outlet obstruction	Outlet resistance too high	Faecal impaction
		Pelvic mass
		Spinal cord compression/damage
		Prostate/urethral stricture

Biofeedback may augment the effect of Kegels exercises, though the efficacy of an electrostimulation approach requires further study. Where uterine prolapse exists, pessaries may work and, if not contraindicated in the older patient, both imipramine and phenylpropanolamine can be considered. If these fail to elicit a satisfactory response, a urodynamic evaluation may provide information indicating the potential benefit of pelvic floor surgery.

Obstruction

The appropriate management of obstructive uropathy is outlined in detail in the subsequent section on benign prostatic hyperplasia.

Underactive detrusor

The practical difficulty here is to eliminate the possibility of obstruction. The diagnosis of an underactive detrusor, therefore, involves the initial exclusion of medication-induced problems (attributable to anticholinergic or alpha-adrenergic drugs), faecal impaction or a large obstructing cystocoele. The bladder needs to decompress for up to 10 - 14 days, or longer if the post void residual volume is > 1000ml, and then a voiding trial must be undertaken. If the bladder subsequently fails to empty, it is often necessary to refer to a urologist or urogynaecologist with a view to excluding obstructive uropathy. In the absence of obstruction, palliative treatment may follow which includes augmented voiding, where voiding remains a possibility, following the Credé pattern of double voiding and then straining. This may be coupled as necessary with intermittent self-catheterisation, though permanent indwelling urethral catheterisation may be necessary in a minority of older patients.

Benign prostatic hyperplasia

Benign prostatic hyperplasia (BPH) describes the proliferation of glandular and stromal elements within the prostate gland found in 90% of the ageing male population. BPH always occurs within the central zone of the prostate gland and in 10% of patients may lead to the development of lower urinary tract symptoms secondary to bladder outflow obstruction at the level of the prostatic urethra. Hesitancy, poor urine flow rate and terminal dribbling are the cardinal symptoms of bladder outflow obstruction due to BPH and many patients also complain of a feeling of incomplete bladder emptying due to a failing detrusor muscle. In addition, up to 75% of males will develop symptoms of urge, nocturia and increased frequency of daytime voiding secondary to detrusor overactivity which develops in the face of bladder outflow obstruction.

Patients with untreated bladder outflow obstruction due to BPH may ultimately develop acute (painful) or chronic (painless) urine retention. Acute urinary retention is seldom misdiagnosed but chronic urinary retention may often go undiagnosed until other sequelae develop, such as chronic renal failure or enuresis due to overflow incontinence. Many patients with chronic urine retention will have biochemical and radiological evidence of obstructive uropathy at the time of diagnosis and management of fluid intake and output following initial catheterisation is critical in these patients.

Assessment

The diagnosis of bladder outflow obstruction secondary to BPH requires a detailed medical and drug history and careful clinical examination. Digital rectal examination is mandatory to assess the size and consistency of the prostate gland. In patients with acute or chronic urinary retention, digital rectal examination is best performed after full bladder decompression. The International Prostate Symptom Score may be used to assess symptom severity at baseline and can also be used as an objective determinant of treatment outcome. Urine flow rates (normal peak flow greater than 50mls per second) and ultrasound estimation of residual post micturition urine volume (normal <50mls) are now routine objective and reproducible non-invasive methods of assessing the severity of bladder outflow obstruction. The routine use of invasive simple cystometry for the diagnosis of bladder outflow obstruction secondary to BPH is not justified. It is a mandatory investigation, however, in patients with a history of previous bladder or prostatic surgery or when there is an associated suspected neurological problem, such as Parkinson's disease, multiple sclerosis or previous stroke.

Blood tests should include full blood count, urea and electrolytes and serum prostate specific antigen. The majority of patients with lower urinary tract symptoms due to BPH will not require specific radiological investigations. Patients with chronic retention, however, require renal ultrasonography to determine the presence and severity of secondary hydronephrosis and hydroureter. The majority of ageing males who present de novo with lower urinary tract symptoms will, on subsequent examination, be found to have symptoms secondary to BPH. In some instances however, the symptoms may be attributable to a previous or co-existing neurological illness. Patients with co-existing illnesses may also develop symptoms secondary to BPH which should be fully evaluated in their own right.

Treatment

Not all patients with bladder outflow obstruction due to BPH will demand or require treatment and watchful waiting is recommended in men with mild symptoms and those who do not perceive their symptoms to be particularly bothersome. The development of complications such as retention, persistent haematuria, bladder stones or obstructive uropathy, however, constitutes an absolute indication for treatment.

Bladder outflow obstruction reflects both mechanical obstruction secondary to the bulk of the prostate gland and dynamic obstruction due to alpha1-adrenoreceptor mediated smooth muscle fibre contraction causing constriction of the prostatic urethra.

Alpha1-adrenoreceptor antagonists reduce symptoms in men with moderate to severe BPH by promoting smooth muscle relaxation. Tamsulosin and alfuzosin are more selective antagonists for treating prostatic smooth muscle than agents which are also used to treat hypertension such as doxazosin, terazosin and prazosin. All alpha1-adrenoreceptor antagonists, however, can cause or exacerbate orthostatic hypotension. Patients should be advised that outflow obstructive symptoms such as poor flow, hesitancy and terminal dribbling will typically improve within two to four weeks of initiating alpha-blocker therapy. Irritable symptoms such as urgency, nocturia and increased frequency, however, may take weeks or months to improve, and may not respond at all in up to 25% of patients, irrespective of the treatment modality chosen.

5-alpha reductase inhibitors such as finasteride and dutasteride act by inhibiting the conversion of testosterone to dihydrotestosterone which stimulates prostate growth. These agents are most effective when the prostate volume is 40ml or greater but do not provide immediate symptom relief. Patients should be cautioned that approximately 6 months of therapy is required before clinical benefits become apparent. There is some evidence that combination therapy with an alpha-blocker and a 5-alpha reductase inhibitor may be more effective than monotherapy, but more work is needed in this area. Although 5-alpha reductase inhibitors may lower the overall risk of prostate cancer, there are some concerns that they may increase the risk of high-grade prostate cancer. Finasteride decreases PSA levels and, when screening for prostate cancer, the measured PSA level should be doubled to correct for this effect.

Transurethral prostatectomy under spinal or general anaesthesia has been the treatment of choice for decades when medical treatments fail. It may also be indicated for patients who develop refractory urinary

TABLE 3 INDICATIONS FOR THE INSERTION OF URINARY CATHETERS	TABLE 4 PROBLEMS ASSOCIATED WITH URINARY CATHETERISATION
DIAGNOSIS EVALUATION: • Accurate measurement of urine output in the critically ill • Cystography, cystourethrography, vesicoureteric reflux evaluation **THERAPEUTIC SHORT TO MEDIUM TERM (< WEEKS) INTERVENTION:** • Urologic, pelvic or lower abdominal surgery • Acute urinary retention **THERAPEUTIC LONG-TERM INTERVENTION:** • Non-correctable bladder outlet obstruction • Neurogenic bladder • Recalcitrant decubitus ulcers worsened or caused by incontinence • Palliative care – terminally ill or severely disabled – to avoid discomfort • Patient preference – not responding to continence measures	• Pain or discomfort • Trauma • Catheter associated urinary tract infections • Catheter obstruction • Bladder spasms & bladder contraction • Calculi formation • Bladder carcinoma • Problems resulting from damage to the catheter or balloon

retention, bladder stones or persistent haematuria. The procedure is well tolerated in the majority of patients, with an average hospital stay of 5 days and low morbidity. During the past two decades, however, there has been a decline of approximately 50% in the number of prostatectomies performed worldwide due to the increasing use of medical therapies. Complications of transurethral prostatectomy include haemorrhage, hyponatraemia, stricture and sexual dysfunction and a significant minority will require reoperation. A newer surgical technique, laser prostatectomy, is associated with reduced catheterisation time and hospital stay when compared with traditional transurethral prostatectomy and longer term outcome measures are similar. Other new therapies, such as transurethral needle ablation and microwave therapy, can be performed more cheaply and on an out-patient basis but have higher rates of treatment failure.

Urinary catheters

The main acute indication for the insertion of a urinary catheter is acute urinary retention which occurs predominantly in men and is usually related to prostatic enlargement. There are many other indications for catheter insertion (table 3) but they

should be removed as soon as possible to reduce the risk of potential complications that can arise (table 4). Urinary tract infections are a frequent complication and all efforts should be made to avoid such infections (table 5).

Urinary catheters can often become blocked leading to retention or bypassing of the catheter. Common reasons include a kinked tube, leg crossing, constipation, blockage of the catheter eye by bladder mucosa, downward displacement of the catheter and encrustation with calcium phosphate or struvite. The management of a blocked urinary catheter involves identifying and dealing with the underlying cause but replacement of the catheter is often required, especially if the likely cause is encrustation.

Different types of catheters are recommended depending on the individual needs of the patient (table 6). When long term catheterisation is required, intermittent self-catheterisation may be a better option rather than a long term indwelling catheter. This option reduces the need for catheterisation of patients post surgery and helps to avoid problems such as catheter obstruction, traction related trauma, encrustation, bladder calculi and bladder carcinoma. In addition, there are lower incidences of symptomatic urinary tract infections and urethral strictures. Bladder tone and capacity can also be maintained and there is no direct interference with sexual function. Intermittent self-catheterisation may not be a practical option, however, especially if the patient is infirm or very dependent.

Catheters should be removed under aseptic technique and ideally at midnight in hospital, as there is

TABLE 5
MEASURES TO REDUCE THE RISK OF CATHETER-ASSOCIATED URINARY TRACT INFECTIONS

GENERAL MEASURES:

- Avoidance of catheterisation as far as possible
- Consider alternative route to indwelling urinary catheter
- Aseptic insertion by trained personnel
- Remove as soon as no longer needed
- Maintain uncompromised closed drainage
- Ensure dependent drainage
- Minimise manipulation of the system
- Avoid cross infection between catheterised patients by separation and by adherence to universal precautions in handling, eg. good hand washing technique
- Adequate training of staff in the technique of urine sampling from catheter systems
- Separate clean container is used for each individual at the time of bag emptying
- Contact between drainage tap and container is avoided
- Gloves worn to empty drainage bags and changed after hand washing between each individual

SPECIFIC INTERVENTIONS:

- Use of antiseptic coated catheters (eg. silver alloy)
- Use of antibiotic coated catheters (eg. minocyclin + rifampicin impregnated)
- Anti infective lubricant
- Anti reflux valves*
- Sealed catheter – collecting tubing junction*

*Unproven benefit

TABLE 6
CATHETER MATERIAL AND RECOMMENDED USAGE

Catheter material	Recommended usage
Polyvinyl chloride (PVC)	Short term (≤7 days) or intermittent
Teflon coated with latex core	Short to medium term (≤28 days)
Silicone	Long term (≤12 weeks)
Hydrogel coated latex	Long term (≤12 weeks)
Silicone elastomer coated latex	Long term (≤12 weeks)
Hydrogel coated silicone	Long term (≤12 weeks)
*Antiseptic or **Antibiotic coated silicone or latex catheters	Short to medium term (< 28 days)

* Silver alloy/silver oxide

**Rifampicin & minocyclin

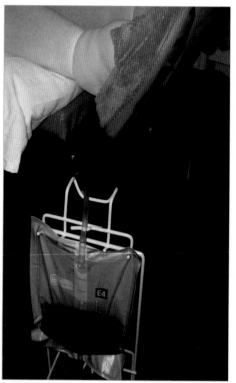

Figure 1: Urinary catheter

evidence that catheter removal at this time results in a reduction in length of stay. In addition, many studies have demonstrated a direct relationship between length of hospital stay and the duration of urethral catheterisation. While large studies are not available, there is little evidence for the use of intermittent clamping or alpha adrenergic blockers around the time of removal of urinary catheters.

Suggested further reading

- DuBeau CE, Resnick NM. Controversies in the diagnosis and treatment of benign prostatic hyperplasia. Adv Int Med 1992; 37: 55-83 (Review).
- Ouslander JG, Schnelle JF. Incontinence in the nursing home. ANN Int Med 1995; 122: 438-49.
- Resnick NM, Geriatric Medicine. In: Isselbacher K, Braunwald E, Wilson JD, et al. Harrison's Principles

of Internal Medicine (14th Ed). McGraw-hill, 1997; 37-46.

- Resnick NM. Urinary incontinence. Lancet 1995; 346: 94-99 (Review).
- Urinary incontinence Guideline Panel. Urinary Incontinence in Adults: Acute and Chronic Management. Clinical Practice Guideline, No.2, 1996 Update AHCPR Pub. No.96-0682 March 1996. Agency for Health Care Policy and Research, PHS, DHHS, 1996.
- Wagg A, Peel P, Lowe D, Potter J. National Audit of Continence Care for older people. London: Royal College of Physicians http:// continence audit. Rcplondon.ac.uk. November 2006.
- Niël – Weise BS and van den Broek PJ. Urinary catheter policies for short-term bladder drainage in adults. Cochrane Database of systematic reviews 2005, issue 3. Art. No.: CD004203. DOI: 10.1002/14651858. CD004203.pub2.
- Nicolle LE, Bradley S, Colgan R, et. al. Infectious Diseases Society of America guidelines for the diagnosis and treatment of asymptomatic bacteriuria in adults. Clin Infect Dis 2005; 40(5): 643-54.

Case Study 1

A 78 year old lady presents with a 4 day history of dysuria, urgency and urinary incontinence occurring several times during the day. She has a history of hypertension and osteoporosis. Her medication includes bendrofluazide, calcium/vitamin D and alendronate. She is a widow, living alone as her 5 children have emigrated. She had 2 assisted deliveries and 3 normal deliveries. Urinalysis reveals 300 pus cells and 250 red blood cells. The result of the urine culture is awaited.

This lady almost certainly has a urinary tract infection. However, close questioning reveals a tendency towards 'accidents' when she coughs or rushes about. She also complains of polyuria in the early part of the day which restricts her activities. Speculum examination confirms a cystocoele of moderate severity. Her infection should be treated and her anti-hypertensive (diuretic) therapy changed. If significant symptoms persist, urodynamic studies may be considered because detrusor overactivity remains a distinct possibility in this scenario. An alternative is a course of low dose anticholinergic therapy prescribed empirically while monitoring for side-effects. Pelvic floor exercises may be beneficial.

Gynaecological evaluation with a view to surgical repair of the cystocoele may, however, be required if symptoms remain problematic.

Case Study 2

An 80 year old man, who is chair-bound following a stroke 2 years previously complains of abdominal discomfort. Staff at the nursing home note that he is more restless than usual and his family report him as being less alert during visits. He has lost weight and low back pain, heretofore well-controlled with analgesia over a period of months has worsened during the last 2 days. Physical examination reveals a palpable mass consistent with a distended bladder. On rectal examination, a hard nodular prostate gland is accompanied by hard faeces but with no impaction. There is weakness of both legs with bilateral extensor plantar responses. It is not possible to confirm a sensory level due to dysphasia related to the previous stroke.

A urinary catheter inserted immediately drains 1100mls of urine. Radiographs of the spine confirm two sclerotic lesions at the level of T8 and T9 vertebrae and MRI scans reveal spinal cord compression at the T8 level. He is referred for urgent palliative radiotherapy, which results in relief of pain and temporary return of power in his legs.

The diagnosis is that of metastatic prostate cancer with cord compression. Most authorities would commence an LHRH analogue with an anti-androgen co-prescribed. His medium-term prognosis remains guarded.

Case Study 3

A 75 year old male presented with a 1 month history of diurnal and nocturnal incontinence as his primary presenting symptom. In the 12-month period prior to presentation he complained of nocturia 2-3 times per night, urgency and daytime voiding frequency of 10-12 times per day. In recent weeks, although his appetite had diminished he felt that his weight had increased and he noticed some puffiness of his ankles.

Physical examination revealed moderate abdominal distension and a palpable bladder indicating chronic urinary retention with a residual urine volume on catheterisation of 1100mls. The prostate gland was moderately enlarged post bladder decompression and felt benign. Blood urea was 24mmol/l and creatinine 310μmol/l and renal ultrasound confirmed mild hydronephrosis and hydroureter. Following catheterisation he had a sustained diuresis of 6 litres per day over a 3 day period requiring intravenous replacement therapy. Urea and creatinine levels both returned to normal levels after 5 days, following which he underwent a transurethral prostatectomy.

Three months post surgery, his renal function was normal, his hydronephrosis had resolved on ultrasound and, although still having to get up once per night to empty his bladder, he was continent with a normal urine flow rate and minimal residual urine volume. This man had chronic urinary retention secondary to BPH associated with renal failure due to hydronephrosis. He improved clinically following catheterisation and definitive surgical treatment.

Data Interpretation

Question 1

An 80 year old man is developing incontinence associated with poor stream and nocturnal frequency. He has an enlarged prostate on examination. Ultrasound of the abdomen reveals normal emptying of the bladder.

a.   What is the diagnosis?
b.   What is the correct initial management?
c.   What investigations may be necessary?

Question 2

A 74 year old lady with previously normal renal function becomes nauseated at home but does not seek help for a couple of days. She is admitted to hospital and noted to be oliguric. Her medication includes bendrofluazide and candesartan. Her urea level is 20.0mmol/l with a sodium of 163mmol/l, a potassium of 5.8mmol/l and a creatinine of 124μmol/l. Urine osmolarity is 515mosm/kg.

a.   What is the reason for her oliguria?
b.   What initial treatment does she need?
c.   What modifications may be necessary in her medications?

Best of five questions

Question 1

An 80 year old man has been noted to be increasingly disorientated. He has had a number of falls and also has complained of urinary incontinence. On examination he is very unsteady on his feet.

What is the most likely diagnosis?

a.   Alzheimer's disease
b.   Parkinson's disease
c.   Normal pressure hydro cephalus
d.   Hypothyroidism
e.   Benign prostatic hypertrophy

Question 2

A 70 year old woman complains of increased thirst and polyuria associated with frequency and occasional urge incontinence. She has a body mass index of 29 kg/m2 with a history of hypertension and dyslipidaemia. She has a history of a transient ischaemic attack and coronary artery stent insertion 5 years previously.

What is her likely new diagnosis?

a.   Hypercalcaemia
b.   Diabetes insipidus
c.   Type 2 diabetes mellitus
d.   Type I diabetes mellitus
e.   Urinary tract infection

Answers on page 311

Drugs and ageing

P Gallagher, H Hamilton, K O' Connor, D O' Mahony

Introduction

Older adults experience higher rates of chronic illness and dependency compared to the population at large. It is therefore not surprising that older patients are the major consumers of prescription and non-prescription medications in most developed nations. In Ireland, older people constitute 11.5% of the population but receive 47% of all prescribed medication on the General Medical Services scheme. In the United States, 12.5% of the population is over 65 years of age but consume 32% of all prescription medications and 30% of total healthcare expenditure. In Europe the value of healthcare consumed by people over the age of 65 years is, on average, about 2.3 times greater than those under 65 years. Prescribing decisions in older patients are often complex. There is marked heterogeneity in health status and functional capacity amongst older people, who range from fit, active, independent individuals to those who are physically and mentally frail with limited physiological reserve. Age-related changes in physiology affect drug pharmacokinetics and pharmacodynamics and together with various pathological processes, increase the risk of adverse drug events (ADEs). This risk is heightened by prescription of multiple medications to treat multiple co-morbidities. Prescription of multiple medications also results in difficulties with compliance, which in turn can lead to sub-optimal therapeutic efficacy. Balancing safety and quality of prescribing for older people with appropriate treatment of all co-morbidities can be challenging.

General principles of pharmacokinetics and ageing

Age-related changes in physiology and body composition can affect drug absorption, distribution, protein binding, metabolism and elimination of drugs. Such physiological changes are progressive and occur gradually over a lifetime, rather than abruptly at any given age (eg. 65 years of age). There is considerable variation in health status amongst older people, with chronological age not always reflecting 'functional' age. Such heterogeneity results in inter-individual variation in drug handling and drug-response.

Absorption

Age-related changes in the gastrointestinal tract include diminished gastric acid and pepsin secretion, reduced absorptive surface area and decreased splanchnic blood flow. Gastric emptying and intestinal motility remain relatively unchanged with age. In general, the rate and completeness of drug absorption is similar in older and younger patients. However, drugs that undergo first-pass metabolism in the liver (such as propranolol or nifedipine) may have an increased bioavailability because of a decline in hepatic mass and blood flow.

Distribution

With ageing, there is reduction in lean body mass and total body water with a relative increase in total body fat. Consequently, the volume of distribution of water-soluble drugs such as lithium, digoxin, theophylline and gentamicin is reduced in older adults and unadjusted dosing can lead to higher plasma concentrations. Conversely, lipid-soluble drugs such as long-acting benzodiazepines (eg. diazepam) have a greater volume of distribution, with consequent delays in maximal effect and accumulation with continued use.

Protein binding

Changes in serum albumin concentration with age are minimal unless there are associated disease states, poor nutrition or immobility. If serum albumin is decreased there will be an increase in the active unbound drug concentration for highly protein-bound drugs (eg. phenytoin, warfarin, sulphonylureas and salicylic acid). However, the clinical importance of this is questionable as the initial and transient effect of protein binding on free plasma concentration is rapidly counterbalanced by greater drug metabolism and excretion.

Hepatic metabolism

Advancing age is associated with a progressive reduction in hepatic mass and blood flow. Diminished hepatic blood flow of up to 40% in older people severely reduces the amount of drug delivered to the

TABLE I
MEDICATION TO BE AVOIDED OR USED WITH CAUTION IN RENAL IMPAIRMENT

Allopurinol
ACE inhibitors
Angiotensin II blockers
Aminoglycosides
Benzodiazepines
Bisphosphonates
Carbamazepine
Cephalosporins
Digoxin
Enoxaparin
Lithium
Metoclopromide
Metformin
Methotrexate
Nitrofurantoin
NSAIDs
Opioid analgesics
Spironolactone
Trimethoprim
Vancomycin

Renal elimination

Age-related changes in renal function arguably represent the single most important physiological factor predisposing to ADEs in older people. The glomerular filtration rate (GFR) may decrease by as much as 50% between the ages of 25 and 65 years, largely because of an age-related decrease in renal mass, loss of functional nephrons and diminished renal blood flow. However, significant elevations in serum creatinine do not occur until the majority of nephrons have been lost. Serum creatinine concentrations reflect a balance between creatinine production by muscle tissue and creatinine clearance by the kidney. Since creatinine production is decreased in older persons because of diminished muscle mass, 'normal' serum creatinine concentrations will not reflect a true decline in GFR and may not be a valid predictor of drug elimination. Creatinine clearance can be estimated using the Cockcroft and Gault formula in patients with stable renal function and without significant oedema or severe cachexia, as follows:

Creatinine clearance (male)

$$\frac{1.23 \times (140 - age) \times body\ weight\ (kg)}{plasma\ creatinine\ (\mu mol/l)}$$

Creatinine clearance (female)

$$\frac{1.03 \times (140 - age) \times body\ weight\ (kg)}{plasma\ creatinine\ (\mu mol/l)}$$

To avoid drug toxicity in older patients, dosages of renally excreted drugs (Table 1) must be adjusted if the creatinine clearance is less than 30ml/min. The clinical importance of such reductions of renal excretion is dependent on the likely toxicity of the drug. Drugs with a narrow therapeutic index such as digoxin, lithium and aminoglycosides are likely to have serious side effects if they accumulate only marginally more than intended.

liver. Drugs that have a first-pass effect in the liver eg. nifedipine, labetalol, verapamil and nitrates may have significantly higher bioavailability in older people and thus be effective at lower doses. Conversely, several angiotensin converting enzyme (ACE) inhibitors such as enalapril and perindopril are pro-drugs, which need to be metabolised to active drugs in the liver. Therefore, their first-pass activation might be slowed or reduced with advancing age. Elimination of compounds undergoing phase 1 metabolism (reduction, oxidation and hydroxylation) in the liver may be moderately reduced with age, though phase 2 metabolism (conjugation) does not change with ageing.

Drugs that are highly dependent on phase 1 hepatic metabolism eg. warfarin, opiates, phenytoin, carbamazepine, theophylline, macrolide antibiotics and statins may therefore have increased plasma concentrations in older people, thereby resulting in greater potential for ADEs and adverse drug interactions. However, there is considerable inter-individual variation in liver metabolism for any given drug and in most cases this may be more important than the changes associated with ageing.

General principles of pharmacodynamics and ageing

Ageing is associated with changes in drug pharmacodynamics, that is the end-organ responsiveness to drugs at the receptor or post-receptor level. Consequently, in older patients, the effects of similar drug concentrations at the site of action may be larger or smaller than those in younger patients. Older patients are more sensitive to drugs such as warfarin, benzodiazepines, neuroleptics, anticholinergics, levodopa and ACE inhibitors thereby increasing the risk of associated ADEs.

TABLE 2
COMMON NON-PRESCRIPTION DRUGS TAKEN BY OLDER ADULTS

Drug	Uses	Drug Interactions	Adverse Effects
NSAID eg. ibuprofen, aspirin	Pain, fever	Corticosteroids warfarin	Gastric and duodenal ulceration, acute kidney injury, fluid retention
Histamine H1 receptor antagonist	Allergy, urticaria, pruritus	Antidepressants (MAOIs and TCAs) Anxiolytics and hypnotics	↑ antimuscarinic and sedative effects
Histamine H2 receptor antagonist	Peptic ulcer disease Gastro-oesophageal reflux disease	Drugs metabolized by cytochrome p450 eg. warfarin, phenytoin, theophylline	↑ risk of bleeding, theophylline toxicity
Codeine	Pain, diarrhoea, cough suppression	Anxiolytics and hypnotics	Constipation, drowsiness, nausea, vomiting
Ginkgo biloba Tinnitus	Dementia	Aspirin, warfarin thiazide diuretics paracetamol	Bleeding, hypertension
St. John's Wort	Mild depression	Theophylline, warfarin digoxin, SSRIs	↓ drug absorption serotonin syndrome
Ginseng	Cure-all-herb	Warfarin Alcohol	↓ INR ↑ alcohol clearance
Senna, Cascara	Laxative	Interference with intestinally absorbed drug	↓ drug availability

This increased sensitivity may be due to changes in drug-receptor interaction, in post-receptor events or in adaptive homeostatic responses such as diminished baroreceptor responses and altered fluid and electrolyte regulation which increase the risk of orthostatic hypotension with vasodilator drugs. Some drugs whose effects are reduced with normal ageing eg. beta adrenergic blockers should also be used with caution because serious dose-related toxicity can occur, the signs of which may be delayed. Because of these pharmacokinetic and pharmacodynamic considerations, care must be taken when determining drug doses for older people. It is also important to note that changes in health status over time can cause medications that have been used long-term to become unsafe or ineffective.

Polypharmacy

Prescription medications

More than 85% of the ambulatory older population and 95% of nursing home residents are prescribed regular medication. Community-dwelling older people take an average of five prescription drugs and three non-prescription drugs concurrently. Nursing home residents take an average of eight prescription drugs reflecting a higher chronic disease burden. Though prescription of multiple drugs is necessary to treat multiple co-morbidities, polypharmacy is often problematic for older patients. Polypharmacy increases the risk of ADEs and geriatric syndromes including acute and chronic cognitive impairment, falls, fractures and urinary incontinence, all of which result in diminished functional status. Polypharmacy is associated with imprecise diagnoses, prescription of non-essential medicines and therapeutic duplication. One study reported that 59% of older outpatients were taking drugs without indication. Similarly, another study showed that 55% of older outpatients were taking non-essential drugs and 17% were taking drugs with therapeutic duplication. In a study of private nursing homes in the UK nearly half the patients were prescribed neuroleptics or benzodiazepines of whom only 12% had a clear indication for such therapy. Polypharmacy is linked with prescribing cascades i.e. where a new drug is prescribed to treat symptoms arising from unrecognized adverse effects of another drug, thereby increasing the potential for further ADEs and prescribing costs. Polypharmacy renders compliance with medications more difficult for older people. Non-compliance can result in sub-optimal therapeutic effectiveness and can have major clinical and economic consequences.

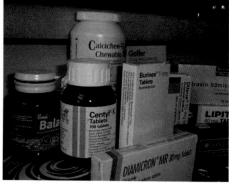

Figure 1: Polypharmacy

Older patients should have regular medication reviews to detect ineffective or non-essential drugs, therapeutic duplication and non-compliance. Careful review of medication can often result in benefit simply by stopping unnecessary medications. Medication reviews should also identify prescribing omissions i.e. non-prescription of medications that are indicated for treatment or prevention of disease.

Conditions such as hypertension, congestive cardiac failure (CCF), anticoagulation in those with atrial fibrillation and depression are often undertreated in older people.

Non-prescription medications

Two-thirds of community-dwelling older patients regularly self-medicate with non-prescription or over the counter products eg. non-steroidal anti-inflammatory drugs (NSAIDs), codeine, antacids, laxatives and herbal remedies. Unknown to many patients, concurrent use of such products may mimic,

TABLE 3
SELECTED SERIOUS DRUG INTERACTIONS

INTERACTION	POTENTIAL EFFECT	RECOMMENDATIONS
Carbamazepine plus cimetidine, erythromycin, clarithromycin or fluconazole	Increase carbamazepine levels	Monitor carbamazepine levels & neurotoxicity
Neuroleptic plus benzodiazepine, sedating antihistamine or opiate	Drowsiness, confusion, falls and fractures	Avoid combination if possible. Use lowest effective dose. Short or intermediate acting benzodiazepines only. Review need on a regular basis
NSAIDs plus ACE inhibitors or Angiotensin II receptor blockers	Renal failure	Avoid concomitant use
Opiates plus oral iron or anticholinergics	Severe constipation	Use of regular laxative with opiates. Regular review of analgesia requirements

magnify or oppose the effect of prescribed drugs (Table 2). Unfortunately, it is commonly perceived that non-prescription products are safe. However, both patients and doctors often overlook the use of such products when discussing medications. Older patients are also prone to potentially dangerous practices such as hoarding and borrowing of medicines. Therefore, self-medication in all its forms has to be actively sought when obtaining a detailed medication history from older patients.

ADEs occur three times more commonly in older than younger patients with up to 35% of community-dwelling older adults experiencing ADEs each year. ADEs can range from non-specific symptoms such as lethargy, confusion and light-headedness to falls with resultant injury such as hip fracture or even death. Drug related morbidity accounts for 20 – 30% of admissions in older people, though it represents only 2% - 6% of medical admissions in the younger population. One half of drug-related deaths occur in persons over the age of 60 years. A recent prospective study of 18,820 patients admitted to two hospitals in the UK reported that ADEs imposed a heavy financial burden on the National Health Service, mainly because of higher morbidity and mortality rates. Other data from community-dwelling older populations indicate that between 13% and 28% of ADEs are avoidable, whereas in nursing home populations up to 50% of all ADEs may be avoidable. Polypharmacy, inappropriate prescribing and inadequate monitoring of medications are amongst the principal causes of ADEs in older people. The most common drug-drug interactions involve digoxin, ß-blockers, oral hypoglycaemics, diuretics and NSAIDs (Table 3). The use of sedative drugs is particularly common in older patients and results in a high incidence of over-sedation, confusion and falls.

Guiding principles of prescribing for older patients

Appropriateness of drug therapy
Appropriate prescribing refers to the use of clinically indicated potentially beneficial medications at an appropriate dose and for an appropriate duration of time. The therapeutic benefits must outweigh potential risks and consideration should always be given to the possibility of drug-drug and drug-disease interactions. Older patients often have multiple co-morbidities for which they are prescribed numerous medications, thereby increasing the risk of ADEs.

TABLE 4
CLINICALLY SIGNIFICANT DRUG INTERACTIONS WITH WARFARIN

DRUGS THAT INCREASE THE INR

Allopurinol
Amiodarone
Cimetidine
Ciprofloxacin
Erythromycin
Ethanol (acute)
Fluconazole
Ketoconazole
Metronidazole
Moxifloxacin
Omeprazole
Ofloxacin

DRUGS THAT DECREASE THE INR

Carbamazepine
Cholestyramine
Oestrogens
Griseofulvin
Rifampicin
Vitamin K

DRUGS THAT INCREASE THE RISK OF BLEEDING WHEN PRESCRIBED WITH WARFARIN

Aspirin
Clopidogrel
NSAIDs
Dipyridamole

Other factors complicating prescribing decisions in older patients include age–related changes in drug handling and response and the heterogeneity of health and functional status between individuals. The most important aspects of medication use in the elderly include optimisation of drug therapy to meet the individual patient's needs and avoidance of and vigilance for, ADEs. Review of the patient's drug therapy should be performed at each consultation. Guidelines for healthy prescribing in the older patient are listed in Table 5.

Starting medication
The well-known recommendation to 'start low and go slow' has been a guiding principle of prescribing in geriatric practice. It is important to bear in mind that this can only be the start of the therapeutic process. This principle is often overstated and may lead to

inappropriately low doses of drugs and slow escalation of dosage. Older people as a group are heterogeneous and significant variability occurs in their rate of decline in hepatic and renal function. In those older patients with a 'younger' functional age 'start low and go slow' would be inappropriate. The emphasis on avoidance of adverse reactions can be so great that many old people receive paediatric or homeopathic doses of drugs that fail to have the desired effect. In general, this principle of 'start low and go slow' applies to a small but important list of drugs, such as medications with a narrow therapeutic index (warfarin, lithium, digoxin) or those with an increased pharmacodynamic effect in old age eg. atenolol, oxybutynin and lisinopril. Medications that predispose to bleeding (NSAIDs and warfarin), to geriatric syndromes such as falls (benzodiazepines, neuroleptics, antihypertensives) or to confusion (anticholinergics, benzodiazepines, neuroleptics and opiates) should also be avoided where possible. There are often alternatives to many of these drugs, including more appropriate non-pharmacological strategies.

Compliance

Non-compliance with regular medication is very common. Over half of the prescriptions written annually are taken incorrectly and 30 – 50% of prescribed medications fail to produce their intended results. Noncompliance exists in many forms including: (i) failure to fill the original prescription; (ii) failure to refill the prescription and (iii) failure to take the dose as prescribed. Older patients are more likely to have problems that affect their ability to comply with a prescribed medication regime. Visual impairment can result in difficulties identifying tablets or reading finely printed administration instructions. Impaired cognition can result in poor adherence with a prescribed regime. Opening childproof containers and handling small pills may also cause difficulty for patients with poor manual dexterity. The more complex a therapeutic regime, the less likely a patient is to be fully compliant. Older patients tend to have lower incomes and spend relatively more on prescription medication. This financial burden of paying for prescription medicines may be prohibitive and result in attempts to make a prescription last longer by reducing the dose or frequency of a medication or even discontinuing therapy altogether. It is important to consider drug compliance when patients fail to respond to treatment, when patients present with new symptoms after a recent change in medication or when drug regimens are being reviewed. A standardised assessment of the ability of the older patient to take medications does not exist but several indicators have been identified (Table 6). In general, the barriers to compliance are polypharmacy, complex regimens, miscommunication and unresolved patient concerns about therapy.

A number of methods can be used to enhance compliance.
- Educate the patient (and caregiver when needed) about intended therapeutic effect, potential adverse effects and signs of toxicity
- Give written instructions with the drug name, indication and dosage with the table or capsule attached if possible. Use of a simple drug card is helpful (Figure 2)
- Ensure that the drug formulation is manageable and practical for the patient eg. would a syrup or liquid formulation be more palatable?
- Ensure drug-frequency is appropriate i.e. give drugs periodically if possible eg. six-monthly vitamin D injection instead of daily tablet

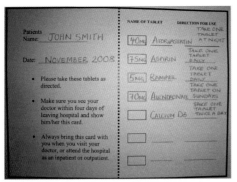

Figure 2: Simple drug card

• Use dosset boxes to optimise compliance with long-term prescriptions

Cost-effective prescribing

Although older patients are at an increased risk for inappropriate drug prescription, adverse drug reactions and drug-drug interactions, they may also be undertreated when effective therapies are not used or are used in suboptimal doses. In order to avoid adverse drug events and polypharmacy, older adults are sometimes not prescribed drugs that are beneficial in the treatment or prevention of serious diseases. Under-representation of older patients in clinical trials has resulted in a knowledge gap regarding dosage requirements and the effects of medication in older people. Medications commonly not prescribed in older patients despite evidence for their use include angiotensin-converting enzyme inhibitors for heart failure and anticoagulants for non-valvular atrial fibrillation. For some treatments, such as β-blockers post-myocardial infarction, most benefit is found in those older than 65 years. Treatment with expensive drugs may be cost-effective in the long-term by preventing disease progression and resulting in fewer hospitalisations.

Conversely, certain drugs are used excessively and inappropriately where cheaper and more cost-effective alternatives are available. In the treatment of hypertension any reduction in blood pressure appears to confer benefit; treatment of hypertension reduces the risk of stroke, CHD, myocardial infarction and mortality. The Joint National Committee VII recommends initiating pharmacotherapy for hypertension where blood pressure goals are not achieved through lifestyle modification. Thiazide type diuretics should be instituted at low dose as initial therapy for most patients with hypertension, unless they are contraindicated or unless a compelling indication requires the use of a specific antihypertensive agent as first line therapy (for example angiotensin converting enzyme inhibitors in the setting of chronic kidney disease or diabetes). Despite these guidelines, the more costly calcium channel antagonists and ACE inhibitors are often inappropriately used as first line agents. Other examples of drugs that are often used inappropriately and excessively when cheaper more appropriate alternatives are available are proton pump inhibitors, NSAIDs, tramadol, clopidogrel and imidazopyridine hypnotics (zolpidem). The major factors contributing to increased state expenditure on medicines include the prescription of new and more expensive medications and growth in the number of prescription items and in the number of tablets per prescription. The fact that 24% of all drugs prescribed to the elderly act on the central nervous system should also be a cause for concern. Cost-effective prescribing in older people requires the use of proven therapies at therapeutic doses and the avoidance of expensive newer products when older and cheaper products are just as effective.

Potentially inappropriate prescribing

Inappropriate prescribing (IP) encompasses the use of medicines that pose more risk than benefit to patients, particularly where safer alternatives exist. IP also includes the use of medicines that have clinically significant drug-drug and drug-disease

TABLE 7

STOPP - SCREENING TOOL OF OLDER PEOPLE'S POTENTIALLY INAPPROPRIATE PRESCRIPTIONS

The following prescriptions are potentially inappropriate in persons aged ≥ 65 years of age

A. Cardiovascular System

1. Digoxin at a long-term dose > 125µg/day with impaired renal function* (increased risk of toxicity).
2. Loop diuretic for dependent ankle oedema only i.e. no clinical signs of heart failure (no evidence of efficacy, compression hosiery usually more appropriate).
3. Loop diuretic as first-line monotherapy for hypertension (safer, more effective alternatives available).
4. Thiazide diuretic with a history of gout (may exacerbate gout).
5. Non-cardioselective beta-blocker with Chronic Obstructive Pulmonary Disease (COPD) (risk of bronchospasm).
6. Beta-blocker in combination with verapamil (risk of symptomatic heart block).
7. Use of diltiazem or verapamil with NYHA Class III or IV heart failure (may worsen heart failure).
8. Calcium channel blockers with chronic constipation (may exacerbate constipation).
9. Use of aspirin and warfarin in combination without histamine H2 receptor antagonist (except cimetidine because of interaction with warfarin) or proton pump inhibitor (high risk of gastrointestinal bleeding).
10. Dipyridamole as monotherapy for cardiovascular secondary prevention (no evidence for efficacy).
11. Aspirin with a past history of peptic ulcer disease without histamine H2 receptor antagonist or Proton Pump Inhibitor (risk of bleeding).
12. Aspirin at dose > 150mg day (increased bleeding risk, no evidence for increased efficacy).
13. Aspirin with no history of coronary, cerebral or peripheral arterial symptoms or occlusive arterial event (not indicated).
14. Aspirin to treat dizziness not clearly attributable to cerebrovascular disease (not indicated).
15. Warfarin for first, uncomplicated deep venous thrombosis for longer than 6 months duration (no proven added benefit).
16. Warfarin for first uncomplicated pulmonary embolus for longer than 12 months duration (no proven benefit).
17. Aspirin, clopidogrel, dipyridamole or warfarin with concurrent bleeding disorder (high risk of bleeding).
    * estimated GFR <50ml/min.

B. Central Nervous System and Psychotropic Drugs

1. Tricyclic antidepressants (TCAs) with dementia (risk of worsening cognitive impairment).
2. TCAs with glaucoma (likely to exacerbate glaucoma).
3. TCAs with cardiac conductive abnormalities (pro-arrhythmic effects).
4. TCAs with constipation (likely to worsen constipation).
5. TCAs with an opiate or calcium channel blocker (risk of severe constipation).
6. TCAs with prostatism or prior history of urinary retention (risk of urinary retention).
7. Long-term (i.e. > 1 month), long-acting benzodiazepines eg. chlordiazepoxide, fluazepam, nitrazepam, chlorazepate and benzodiazepines with long-acting metabolites e.g. diazepam (risk of prolonged sedation, confusion, impaired balance, falls).
8. Long-term (i.e. > 1 month) neuroleptics as long-term hypnotics (risk of confusion, hypotension, extra-pyramidal side effects, falls).
9. Long-term neuroleptics (> 1 month) in those with parkinsonism (likely to worsen extra-pyramidal symptoms).
10. Phenothiazines in patients with epilepsy (may lower seizure threshold).
11. Anticholinergics to treat extra-pyramidal side-effects of neuroleptic medications (risk of anticholinergic toxicity).
12. Selective serotonin re-uptake inhibitors (SSRIs) with a history of clinically significant hyponatraemia (non-iatrogenic hyponatraemia <130mmol/l within the previous 2 months).
13. Prolonged use (> 1 week) of first generation antihistamines i.e. diphenydramine, chlorpheniramine, cyclizine, promethazine (risk of sedation and anti-cholinergic side effects).

C. Gastrointestinal System

1. Diphenoxylate, loperamide or codeine phosphate for treatment of diarrhoea of unknown cause (risk of delayed diagnosis, may exacerbate constipation with overflow diarrhoea, may precipitate toxic megacolon in inflammatory bowel disease, may delay recovery in unrecognised gastroenteritis).

2. Diphenoxylate, loperamide or codeine phosphate for treatment of severe infective gastroenteritis ie. bloody diarrhoea, high fever or severe systemic toxicity (risk of exacerbation or protraction of infection).
3. Prochlorperazine (Stemetil) or metoclopramide with Parkinsonism (risk of exacerbating Parkinsonism).
4. PPI for peptic ulcer disease at full therapeutic dosage for > 8 weeks (earlier discontinuation or dose reduction for maintenance/ prophylactic treatment of peptic ulcer disease, oesophagitis or GORD indicated).
5. Anticholinergic antispasmodic drugs with chronic constipation (risk of exacerbation of constipation).

D. Respiratory System.
1. Theophylline as monotherapy for COPD. (safer, more effective alternative; risk of adverse effects due to narrow therapeutic index).
2. Systemic corticosteroids instead of inhaled corticosteroids for maintenance therapy in moderate-severe COPD (unnecessary exposure to long-term side-effects of systemic steroids).
3. Nebulised ipratropium with glaucoma (may exacerbate glaucoma).

E. Musculoskeletal System
1. Non-steroidal anti-inflammatory drug (NSAID) with history of peptic ulcer disease or gastrointestinal bleeding, unless with concurrent histamine H2 receptor antagonist, PPI or misoprostol (risk of peptic ulcer relapse).
2. NSAID with moderate-severe hypertension (moderate: 160/100mmHg – 179/109mmHg; severe: ≥180/110mmHg) (risk of exacerbation of hypertension).
3. NSAID with heart failure (risk of exacerbation of heart failure).
4. Long-term use of NSAID (>3 months) for relief of mild joint pain in osteoarthtitis (simple analgesics preferable and usually as effective for pain relief).
5. Warfarin and NSAID together (risk of gastrointestinal bleeding).
6. NSAID with chronic renal failure (risk of deterioration in renal function).
7. Long-term corticosteroids (>3 months) as monotherapy for rheumatoid arthrtitis or osterarthritis (risk of major systemic corticosteroid side-effects).
8. Long-term NSAID or colchicine for chronic treatment of gout where there is no contraindication to allopurinol (allopurinol first choice prophylactic drug in gout).

F. Urogenital System
1. Bladder antimuscarinic drugs with dementia (risk of increased confusion, agitation).
2. Bladder antimuscarinic drugs with chronic glaucoma (risk of acute exacerbation of glaucoma).
3. Bladder antimuscarinic drugs with chronic constipation (risk of exacerbation of constipation).
4. Bladder antimuscarinic drugs with chronic prostatism (risk of urinary retention).
5. Alpha-blockers in males with frequent incontinence i.e. one or more episodes of incontinence daily (risk of urinary frequency and worsening of incontinence).
6. Alpha-blockers with long-term urinary catheter in situ i.e. more than 2 months (drug not indicated).

G. Endocrine System
1. Glibenclamide or chlorpropamide with type 2 diabetes mellitus (risk of prolonged hypoglycaemia).
2. Beta-blockers in those with diabetes mellitus and frequent hypoglycaemic episodes i.e. ≥ 1 episode per month (risk of masking hypoglycaemic symptoms).
3. Oestrogens with a history of breast cancer or venous thromboembolism (increased risk of recurrence).
4. Oestrogens without progestogen in patients with intact uterus (risk of endometrial cancer).

H. Drugs that adversely affect those prone to falls (≥ 1 fall in past three months)
1. Benzodiazepines (sedative, may cause reduced sensorium, impair balance).

2. Neuroleptic drugs (may cause gait dyspraxia, Parkinsonism).
3. First generation antihistamines (sedative, may impair sensorium).
4. Vasodilator drugs known to cause hypotension in those with persistent postural hypotension i.e. recurrent > 20mmHg drop in systolic blood pressure (risk of syncope, falls).
5. Long-term opiates in those with recurrent falls (risk of drowsiness, postural hypotension, vertigo).

I. Analgesic Drugs

1. Use of long-term powerful opiates eg. morphine or fentanyl as first line therapy for mild-moderate pain (WHO analgesic ladder not observed).
2. Regular opiates for more than 2 weeks in those with chronic constipation without concurrent use of laxatives (risk of severe constipation).
3. Long-term opiates in those with dementia unless indicated for palliative care or management of moderate/severe chronic pain syndrome (risk of exacerbation of cognitive impairment).

J. Duplicate Drug Classes

Any regular duplicate drug class prescription eg. two concurrent opiates, NSAID's, SSRIs, loop diuretics, ACE inhibitors (optimisation of monotherapy within a single drug class should be observed prior to considering a new class of drug). This excludes duplicate prescribing of drugs that may be required on a prn basis eg. inhaled beta2 agonists (long and short acting) for asthma or COPD, and opiates for management of breakthrough pain.

---

interactions and importantly, the under-use of potentially beneficial medicines that are clinically indicated. IP is highly prevalent in older people with up to 25% of community dwelling older people, 35% of hospitalised older people and over 40% of nursing home residents regularly receiving at least one potentially inappropriate prescription. IP is associated with increased morbidity, mortality and healthcare cost, largely because of an increased prevalence of associated ADEs.

STOPP (Screening Tool of Older Persons' Prescriptions) is a new physiological systems-based screening tool which incorporates 65 instances of potentially inappropriate prescribing in older people including drug-drug and drug-disease interactions, drugs which adversely affect older patients at risk of falls and duplicate drug-class prescriptions (Table 7). Each criterion is accompanied by a concise explanation as to why the prescription is potentially inappropriate. START (Screening Tool to Alert doctors to Right Treatment) is an evidence-based screening tool comprising 22 prescribing indicators that highlight prescribing omissions in older people (Table 8). STOPP/START criteria were validated by a panel of 18 experts in geriatric pharmacotherapy from Ireland and the United Kingdom and inter-rater reliability is excellent. The criteria are arranged

according to physiological systems for ease of use in everyday clinical practice. Juxtaposition of potential errors of prescribing commission with potential errors of omission provides a comprehensive assessment of prescribing appropriateness.

In a recent prospective study of 715 non-selected acute admissions of older patients to a university teaching hospital in Ireland, application of STOPP criteria showed that 35% of patients were receiving at least one potentially inappropriate prescription, with one third of these patients presenting with symptoms that were attributable to the inappropriately prescribed drug. START criteria have been applied in 600 older patients admitted to hospital with acute illness. At least one indicated medication was omitted in 57% of patients, without contraindication. The main prescribing omissions were statins for cardiovascular disease, ACE inhibitors for congestive cardiac failure, aspirin for symptomatic arterial disease and calcium supplementation for osteoporosis. The probability of omission was significantly related to age, with the highest incidence of omission in those older than 85 years.

Drug-induced falls

There are a number of ways in which drugs might

TABLE 8
START- SCREENING TOOL TO ALERT DOCTORS TO RIGHT IE. APPROPRIATE, INDICATED TREATMENTS

These medications should be considered for people ≥ 65 years of age with the following conditions, where no contraindication to prescription exists.

A. Cardiovascular System
1. Warfarin in the presence of chronic atrial fibrillation.
2. Aspirin in the presence of chronic atrial fibrillation, where warfarin is contraindicated, but not aspirin.
3. Aspirin or clopidogrel with a documented history of atherosclerotic coronary, cerebral or peripheral vascular disease in patients with sinus rhythm.
4. Antihypertensive therapy where systolic blood pressure consistently > 160 mmHg.
5. Statin therapy with a documented history of coronary, cerebral or peripheral vascular disease, where the patient's functional status remains independent for activities of daily living and life expectancy is > 5 years.
6. Angiotensin Converting Enzyme (ACE) inhibitor with chronic heart failure.
7. ACE inhibitor following acute myocardial infarction.
8. Beta-blocker with chronic stable angina.

B. Respiratory System
1. Regular inhaled beta 2 agonist or anticholinergic agent for mild to moderate asthma or COPD.
2. Regular inhaled corticosteroid for moderate-severe asthma or COPD, where predicted FEV_1 <50%.
3. Home continuous oxygen with documented chronic type 1 respiratory failure (pO_2 < 8.0kPa, pCO_2 <6.5kPa) or type 2 respiratory failure (pO_2 < 8.0kPa, pCO_2 > 6.5kPa).

C. Central Nervous System
1. L-DOPA in idiopathic Parkinson's disease with definite functional impairment and resultant disability.
2. Antidepressant drug in the presence of moderate-severe depressive symptoms lasting at least three months.

D. Gastrointestinal System
1. Proton Pump Inhibitor with severe gastro-oesophageal acid reflux disease or peptic stricture requiring dilatation.
2. Fibre supplement for chronic, symptomatic diverticular disease with constipation.

E. Musculoskeletal System
1. Disease-modifying anti-rheumatic drug (DMARD) with active moderate-severe rheumatoid disease lasting > 12 weeks.
2. Bisphosphonates in patients taking maintenance oral corticosteroid therapy.
3. Calcium and Vitamin D supplement in patients with known osteoporosis (radiological evidence or previous fragility fracture or acquired dorsal kyphosis).

F. Endocrine System
1. Metformin with type 2 diabetes +/- metabolic syndrome (in the absence of renal impairment).
2. ACE inhibitor or Angiotensin Receptor Blocker in diabetes with nephropathy i.e. overt urinalysis proteinuria or micoralbuminuria (>30mg/24 hours) +/- serum biochemical renal impairment*.
3. Antiplatelet therapy in diabetes mellitus if one or more co-existing major cardiovascular risk factor present (hypertension, hypercholesterolaemia, smoking history).
4. Statin therapy in diabetes mellitus if one or more co-existing major cardiovascular risk factor present.

* estimated GFR <50ml/min.

TABLE 9
COMMON CAUSES OF DRUG-INDUCED CONFUSION IN THE ELDERLY

ANALGESICS
* NSAIDs
* All strong opiates – morphine, fentanyl, oxycodone
* Dihydrocodeine

SEDATIVES AND ANTIDEPRESSANTS
* Benzodiazepines – both long-acting benzodiazepines (eg., nitrazepam, flurazepam) and short-acting benzodiazepines (eg., triazolam)
* Tricyclic antidepressants
* Selective Serotonin Reuptake Inhibitors

NEUROLEPTICS

MEDICATIONS USED TO TREAT PD
* Anti-cholinergics (eg. benztropine)
* Dopamine agonists
* Levodopa
* Selegiline

OTHERS
* Corticosteroids
* Antihistamines
* Digoxin
* Diuretics
* Oxybutynin
* Cimetidine

TABLE 10
MEDICATIONS COMMONLY IMPLICATED IN FALLS IN OLDER PATIENTS

Anticonvulsants
Antihypertensives, particularly alpha-blockers and vasodilators in those with postural hypotension
Benzodiazepines
Diuretics
Neuroleptic agents
Sulphonylureas and insulin – inducing hypoglycaemia
Selective Serotonin Reuptake Inhibitors
Tricyclic antidepressants

increase the risk of falls in older people. The most important of these are sedation, impaired balance and reaction time, hypotension and drug-induced parkinsonism. Falls in older people are usually multifactorial and a thorough assessment of predisposing medical and environmental factors is necessary. The commonest drugs associated with falling are listed in Table 10. There is also a clear association between falling and polypharmacy. Even medication that is appropriately recommended and prescribed for the treatment of a disease can lead to falls. All medications, including over-the-counter medications, should be thoroughly reviewed and considered for possible elimination or dose reduction. Psychotropic medications warrant particular attention, since there is very strong evidence that these medications are linked to recurrent falls. Reducing the total number of medications to four or fewer, if feasible, has also been demonstrated to reduce the risk of falling.

Suggested further reading

* Barry P, Gallagher P, Ryan C, O'Mahony D. START Screening Tool to Alert doctors to Right Treatment. An evidence-based screening tool to detect prescribing omissions in elderly patients. Age Ageing 2007; 36: 628-631.
* Field TS, Gurwitz JH, Avorn J, et al. Risk factors for adverse drug events among nursing home residents. Arch Intern Med 2001; 161: 1629-1634.
* Fu AZ, Liu GG, Christensen DB. Inappropriate medication use and health outcomes in the elderly. J Am Geriatr Soc 2004; 52: 1934-39.
* Gallagher P, Barry P, Ryan C, Hartigan I, O'Mahony D. Inappropriate prescribing in an acutely ill population of elderly patients as determined by Beers' criteria. Age Ageing 2008; 37(1): 96-101.
* Gallagher P, O'Mahony D. Inappropriate prescribing in older people. 2008 Cambridge University Press doi: 10.1017/SO95925980800261X.
* Gallagher P, O'Mahony D. STOPP (Screening Tool of Older Persons' potentially inappropriate Prescriptions): Comparison with Beers' Criteria. Age Ageing 2008; 37: 673–679.
* Gallagher P, Ryan C, Byrne S, Kennedy J, O'Mahony D. STOPP (Screening Tool of Older Persons' Prescriptions) and START (Screening Tool to Alert Doctors to Right Treatment): Consensus Validation. Int J Clin Pharm Ther 2008; 46(2): 72-83.
* Gurwitz JH, Field TS, Harrold LR, et al. Incidence and preventability of adverse drug events in nursing homes. Am J Med 2000; 109: 87–94.
* Hanlon JT, Schmader KE, Ruby CM, Weinberger M. Suboptimal prescribing in older inpatients and

TABLE 11 DRUGS WHICH CAN INDUCE CONGESTIVE HEART FAILURE IN THE ELDERLY	TABLE 12 DRUGS THAT AFFECT GLUCOSE CONTROL IN OLDER PATIENTS
Expansion of Plasma Volume NSAIDs Corticosteroids Drugs with high sodium content **Negatively Inotropic Agents** β-blockers Calcium channel blockers (amlodipine has the least effect) Flecanide Quinidine **Direct Cardiotoxins** Doxorubicin	**Drugs that can Induce Hypoglycaemia** Alcohol β -blockers (↓ warning signs, ↓ glycogenolysis) Insulin Salicylates (high doses) Sulphonlyureas **Drugs with Diabetogenic Properties** Thiazide diuretics Glucocorticoids

outpatients. J Am Geriatr Soc 2001; 49: 200-09.
- Juurlink DN, Mamdami M, Kopp A et al. Drug-drug interactions among elderly patients hospitalised for drug toxicity. JAMA 2003; 289: 1652.
- Klarin I, Wimo A, Fastbom J: The association of inappropriate drug use with hospitalisation and mortality: a population based study of the very old. Drugs Aging. 2005; 22(1): 69-82.
- Lau DT, Kasper JD, Potter DE, Lyles A, Bennett RG. Hospitalization and death associated with potentially inappropriate medication prescriptions among elderly nursing home residents. Arch Intern Med 2005; 165: 68-74.
- Leipzig RM, Cumming RG, Tinetti ME. Drugs and falls in older people: a systematic review and meta-analysis. I. Psychotropic drugs. J Am Geriatr Soc 1999;47:30-39.
- Mangoni AA, Jackson SH. Age-related changes in pharamcokinetics and pharmacodynamics: basic principles and practical applications. Br J Clin Pharmacol 2004; 57: 6-14.
- Pirmohamed M, James S, Meakin S, et al. Adverse drug reactions as a cause of admission to hospital: prospective analysis of 18820 patients. BMJ 2004: 329: 15 – 9.
- Ravio MM, Laurila JV, Strandberg TE, Tilvis RS, Pitkala KH. Use of inappropriate medications and their prognostic significance among in-hospital and nursing home patients with and without Dementia in Finland. Drugs Aging 2006; 23: 333-43.
- Rochon PA, Gurwitz JH. Optimising drug treatment for elderly people: the prescribing cascade. BMJ 1997; 315: 1096-9.
- Spinewine A, Schmader KE, Barber N et al. Appropriate prescribing in elderly people: how well can it be measured and optimised? Lancet 2007; 370: 173-84.
- Tinetti ME. Preventing Falls in Elderly Persons. N Engl J Med 2003; 348: 42-49.

📁 Case Study 1

J.M., an 82 year old man, has resided in a nursing home for the past 14 months. His medical records show the following diagnoses: 1) Osteoarthritis, 2) Cardiomegaly and 'mild' CCF, 3) Hypertension, 4) Constipation, 5) Depression, 6) Dizziness, 7) 'Organic Brain Syndrome' with progressive confusion. His admission weight was 66 kg, blood pressure 108/66mmHg and pulse rate was regular at 74 beats/min. There was no systematic recording of vital signs since admission to the nursing home but occasional recordings in the nursing notes show little variation. His current medications are: bendrofluazide 2.5mg daily, methyldopa 250mg BD, aspirin 75mg daily, haloperidol 0.5mg tds, betahistine 16mg daily, amitriptyline 50mg daily, ibuprofen 400mg six-hourly PRN for pain, lactulose 10ml six-hourly PRN and gaviscon 10ml eight-hourly PRN. He is in no acute distress. Nursing staff report that J.M. is often confused. J.M. himself reports lassitude and dizziness when walking, and complains of intermittent joint pains.

This case demonstrates some of the problems with drug prescribing and polypharmacy in the elderly. 'Organic brain syndrome, cardiomegaly and dizziness' are imprecise diagnoses and are therefore difficult to treat. Many of his symptoms may actually be adverse effects of prescribed medications (eg. constipation, dizziness, confusion and depression) and it is unclear whether this possibility has been considered. The history of 'organic brain syndrome' needs to be clarified. The cognitive impairment of a degenerative dementia can be exacerbated by flurazepam, haloperidol, betahistine and amitriptyline. Careful evaluation of the indications for these medications is needed. Flurazepam is a long-acting benzodiazepine and its use is not recommended in older people. There are numerous alternatives to amitriptyline, which lack its anticholinergic side-effects. In view of J.M's confusion, the doses of all his psychotropic medication should be gradually reduced and eventually discontinued. A baseline cognitive function and psychiatric state should be recorded. If psychotic behavioural disturbances or depression are manifest then each disorder should be managed and monitored. Chronic prescription of NSAIDs for treatment of mild osteoarthritic pain in older people is inappropriate because safer alternatives such as regular paracetamol are equally effective. In this case, ibuprofen is prescribed on a PRN basis, but is not adequately controlling the pain. The combination of ibuprofen and aspirin puts J.M. at increased risk of upper gastrointestinal bleeding. His use of Gaviscon may indicate the presence of NSAID-related upper gastrointestinal symptoms. Ibuprofen should be discontinued and the indication for aspirin reviewed. The use of simple analgesia e.g. regular paracetamol, is indicated in this case with regular assessment for pain and analgesic requirements.

J.M. has a diagnosis of hypertension for which goal-directed treatment is required. Though this necessitates regular recording of blood pressure, there is poor documentation of his vital signs since admission to the nursing home. His current borderline low blood pressure may indicate that his hypertension is being over-treated and his intermittent dizziness could be a symptom of orthostatic hypotension. In this case, the use of methyldopa is questionable as it can exacerbate both depression and confusion. The potential hazard of hypokalaemia should be considered in patients taking a thiazide diuretic and complaining of lassitude. If his blood pressure remains low both antihypertensive medications should be discontinued and his blood pressure observed. If hypertension recurs, bendrofluazide could be re-introduced at 1.25mg daily with periodic monitoring of serum potassium concentration.

📂 Case Study 2

J.K., a 77 year old man with osteoarthritis and congestive heart failure presents with anorexia, nausea and vomiting. His medications are aspirin 75mg daily, frusemide 80mg daily, ramipril 2.5mg daily, digoxin 0.25mg daily and ibuprofen 400mg TDS. Laboratory results include: Na 136mmol/l (normal 134 – 144 mmol/l), K 2.8mmol/l (normal 3.5 – 5.2 mmol/l), Urea 16.6 mmol/l (normal 2.5 – 7.0 mmol/l) and creatinine 210 μmol/l. He was dehydrated. He weighed 56kg having lost 2kg in the previous week.

This case shows how one patient can present with multiple adverse drug events (ADEs) and drug-drug interactions. J.K. is prescribed a NSAID for osteoarthritis. NSAIDs can cause fluid retention (exacerbating his heart failure), increase upper gastrointestinal problems (particularly with concomitant use of aspirin) and cause renal failure (particularly with the concomitant use of an ACE inhibitor). He may also have digoxin toxicity as suggested by the symptoms of nausea, anorexia and palpitations. Digoxin toxicity can present with many symptoms including nausea, vomiting, lethargy, visual disturbance, confusion and cardiac rhythm disturbances. Digoxin is a renally excreted drug. However, the estimated GFR in this case is only 20ml/min. It is recommended that digoxin be prescribed at a dose of not greater than 125mcg per day when GFR is less than 50ml/min because of the risk of digoxin toxicity with higher doses. Hypokalaemia is also a major contributor to digoxin toxicity. Twice as much digoxin is required to produce toxicity in patients with potassium of 5.0mmol/l as compared to a serum level of 3.0mmol/l. All diuretics, with the exception of potassium-sparing diuretics, may cause hypokalaemia. Vomiting usually intensifies hypokalaemia. The indication for digoxin in this case needs to be reviewed and the severity of heart failure classified. Treatment of patients with chronic heart failure and normal sinus rhythm with digoxin impacts positively on morbidity but not mortality. This effect, however, occurs in New York Heart Association (NYHA) Class II and III rather than NYHA Class I ('Mild CHF') and this effect was found only when digoxin was co-prescribed with ACE inhibitors and diuretics.

ACE inhibitors and NSAIDs are associated with renal failure particularly in the setting of dehydration and vomiting. ACE inhibitors cause efferent glomerular arterioles to vasodilate thereby removing the beneficial compensatory mechanism to compromised renal blood flow. NSAIDs inhibit prostaglandin E2 and I2 which dilate afferent renal arterioles when renal blood flow is compromised. Therefore, J.K. had a blunted compensatory mechanism to respond to dehydration and vomiting and developed acute renal failure. Concomitant use of NSAIDs and ACE inhibitors is contra-indicated. Patients need to be warned to discontinue ACE inhibitors when vomiting or diarrhoea occurs. J. K. had his digoxin withheld. He had intravenous fluid and potassium replacement. All his medications were temporarily stopped. A gastroscopy revealed severe gastritis. He was discharged 10 days later with a serum creatinine concentration of 86 μmol/l. His discharge prescription included frusemide 40mg daily, ramipril 2.5mg daily, lanzoprazole 30mg daily and paracetamol 1g bd. He will have a repeat serum creatinine concentration measurement in a week. He will remain on his proton pump inhibitor for one month to allow gastric mucosal healing.

📁 Case Study 3

L.M. is a 79 year old man with prosthetic aortic and mitral valve replacements, who was commenced on amiodarone for atrial fibrillation with a rapid ventricular response. One week later, he developed a lower respiratory tract infection and was commenced on erythromycin (penicillin avoided because of a penicillin allergy). Other drug therapy included frusemide, allopurinol, perindopril, amiloride, and warfarin. The INR had been stable ranging between 2.5 and 4.0. However, following commencement of erythromycin the INR increased to a peak of 10.7 and remained elevated for 4 days despite discontinuation of warfarin.

Many drugs have clinically significant drug interactions with warfarin (Table 4). In this case, amiodarone, allopurinol or erythromycin may have potentiated the anti-coagulant effect of warfarin. However, the allopurinol was a long-standing prescription without previous disturbance of coagulation status, and the amiodarone was prescribed for one week without adverse effects on the INR until erythromycin was added. Amiodarone may inhibit the hepatic metabolism of warfarin, resulting in 50% to 100% increases in the INR in patients previously stabilised on warfarin. Elevations in the INR typically occur within one week and stabilize after approximately one month of combination therapy. Erythromycin, like many antibiotics, may inhibit the metabolism of warfarin

and can cause an increase in the INR. For L.M., the best choice would be to discontinue the erythromycin and consider a cephalosporin or tetracycline instead. Careful INR monitoring should continue since the introduction of any change in treatment, as well as acute illness, may alter the patient's response to warfarin therapy. Following adjustment of his medications, L.M makes a full recovery from his acute illness and his INR is subsequently maintained within the therapeutic range. Three months later, he develops severe pain and swelling in his left first metatarsophalyngeal joint. He is diagnosed with acute gout and a regular non-steroidal anti-inflammatory medication is prescribed.

The subsequent diagnosis of acute gout presents a therapeutic dilemma, as warfarin therapy is a relative contraindication to NSAID use. In patients over 65 years of age the risk of hospitalization from bleeding peptic ulcer disease is 3 times higher for patients taking concurrent warfarin and NSAIDs compared to either drug alone and 13 times higher than in patients not taking warfarin or an NSAID. Although all NSAIDs may cause bleeding, ibuprofen and the COX-II selective drugs carry the lowest risk. Older patients are also at higher risk of other adverse reactions from NSAIDs, such as hypokalaemia, fluid retention and nephrotoxicity. Where possible, alternative treatments to oral NSAIDs should be sought, including simple analgesics, local or topical treatments and physiotherapy. If combination treatment with an NSAID and warfarin is required, one of the lower risk NSAIDs should be used for the shortest period possible and the patient followed closely, with frequent stool testing for traces of blood loss. Gastric protection with concurrent proton pump inhibitor drugs is recommended, should combination therapy be unavoidable.

📁 Case Study 4

MO'L, a 78 year old woman, is brought to her General Practitioner for evaluation by her daughter with whom she has been living for the past 18 months. Her daughter reports that MO'L had been in good health until 4 months ago when she began showing little interest in her usual activities. She has lost 4kg in weight in these 4 months, has been irritable and has trouble sleeping. Her physical examination is normal apart from being a thin, nervous woman. On mini-mental state examination (MMSE) she scores 26/30 with a number of 'I don't know' answers. A biochemistry profile and full blood count are within

normal limits. She is on no medication except for a stool softener.

A decision is made to treat her with one of the selective serotonin reputake inhibitors (SSRI's) – sertraline 50mg o.d. – for possible depression. The following week MO'L returns complaining of nausea and difficulty sleeping at night. Cimetidine is prescribed for her upper gastrointestinal symptoms and a two-week course of diazepam 2mg at night is given to control her irritability and insomnia while her SSRI has time to take effect. Ten days later she is reviewed at home on the request of her daughter following a fall. She has become increasingly confused and drowsy over the preceding week. Her MMSE is now 14/30 and laboratory results reveal a sodium level of 122 mmol/l (normal 134 - 144 mmol/l).

Depression in later life typically is more difficult to recognize compared to younger adults. Dementia can present with inability to concentrate, loss of usual interests and loss of memory. Therefore, depressed individuals with secondary cognitive disturbances can be difficult to distinguish from those with a true dementia. A therapeutic trial of an antidepressant in the depressed patient with cognitive impairment, such as MO' L, may reverse the cognitive symptoms. After one week the patient is experiencing typical adverse effects of an SSRI. The adverse effects of SSRI's include nausea, vomiting, diarrhoea, insomnia, headache, confusion, dizziness and sedation. Elderly people are more prone to adverse effects of SSRIs and therefore a lower starting dose may be appropriate even though comparable doses to younger patients may be needed for full therapeutic effect. All SSRIs are associated with hyponatraemia, which commonly results in confusion. Confusion is characteristic of toxicity with many drugs in old age (Table 9). In one study 17% of patients over 70 years of age admitted to a general medical unit with a confusional state were on drugs that either definitely or possibly contributed to the condition. Instead of reviewing the medication MO' L was already on when she represented with new symptoms one week after starting a SSRI, she was erroneously prescribed two further drugs to treat the side effects of the SSRI. Both of the new drugs prescribed could have contributed to her increased confusion. Older patients are more likely than younger patients to develop cognitive impairment as a result of taking medications. This reflects age- and disease-associated changes in brain neurochemistry and drug handling. Almost any drug can cause delirium, especially in a vulnerable patient. Anticholinergic

medications, in particular, are important causes of acute and chronic confusional states in the elderly. Despite this, polypharmacy with anticholinergic compounds is common, especially in nursing home residents. Psychoactive drugs are important causes of delirium in the elderly. Opiates are among the most important drug causes of delirium in postoperative patients but when used in appropriate doses in the postoperative period or in terminal care will reduce the risk of confusion by achieving effective relief from pain and anxiety. Special care is needed when prescribing for people with dementia as such patients are at greatest risk of a drug-induced deterioration in their cognitive state. Early diagnosis of drug-induced confusion, and withdrawal of the offending agent or agents is essential to prevent morbidity, falls, fractures, hospitalization and even death.

🗁 Case Study 5

WM, an 80 year old man, presents with a 6-month history of worsening shortness of breath, ankle oedema and 10 kg weight gain. He is now short of breath after walking just 20 metres. His other medical problems include hypertension, peptic ulcer disease and rheumatoid arthritis. His current medications are bisoprolol 5mg daily, ibuprofen 400mg tds; nifedipine slow release 20mg bd and ranitidine 150mg daily. Physical examination reveals a BP of 156/88mmHg, pulse 70 beats / minute and a respiratory rate of 26 breaths / minute. His neck veins are distended and he has 3+ pitting oedema of his lower limbs and sacral oedema. Respiratory examination reveals basal crackles.

W M's age and poorly controlled hypertension make him vulnerable to the development of congestive heart failure (CHF), one of the most common clinical disorders in older patients. The mean age of patients with CHF in the community is 74 years. There are a number of drugs that may precipitate or aggravate systolic CHF (Table 11). Drug-induced CHF is mediated via two basic mechanisms - i.e, inhibition of myocardial contractility (negatively inotropic agents) or expansion of plasma volume. All β-blockers decrease myocardial contractility and slow the heart rate compromising the heart's ability to empty effectively. Even topically applied β-blockers (eg. timolol eye drops for glaucoma) can cause systemic effects in sensitive individuals. Beta-blockers should not be used in acute heart failure, but there is evidence to support their use in chronic stable CHF. All NSAIDs have sodium-retaining properties resulting in increased intravascular fluid volume. Ibuprofen may have contributed to fluid overload and hypertension in this case.

🗁 Case Study 6

HM is a 76 year old lady with a 15-year history of Type II Diabetes Mellitus and a 4-year history of diabetic nephropathy. Her diabetes has been well controlled over the past two years (HbA$_1$C 5.9% two months ago). She has impaired eyesight secondary to cataracts, osteoarthritis of her hips and knees and had a transient ischaemic attack 4 years previously. She has had 4 falls in the previous 3 weeks and reports constant lethargy. She had a flu-like illness 6 weeks ago and has developed anorexia and nausea since then. Her medications are paracetamol 1g tds, aspirin 75mg daily and glibenclamide 10mg daily. Laboratory results reveal: glucose 2.8mmol/l; urea 15.7mmol/l and creatinine 288 μmol/l.

HM has developed hypoglycaemia secondary to her sulphonylurea – glibenclamide. Sulphonylureas and insulin account for almost all the cases of drug-induced hypoglycaemia in the elderly. A number of other drugs can, however, interact with glycaemic control in the elderly (Table 12). Sulphonylureas are metabolized in the liver and the metabolites are excreted via the kidneys. For this reason both hepatic and renal impairment increase the likelihood of sulphonylurea-induced hypoglycaemia. Hypoglycaemia induced by glibenclamide may be more pronounced than that with other sulphonylureas because it concentrates within islet cells and its metabolites retain some hypoglycaemic activity. Most sulphonylureas can cause fatal hypoglycaemia, although it has been most often associated with chlorpropamide and glibenclamide. Therefore, agents with a shorter half-life such as gliclizide and glimepiride are more appropriate sulphonylureas in older people.

HM probably had progressive accumulation of her glibenclamide secondary to her progressive renal impairment; her HbA$_1$C result from two months earlier was suggestive of tight glycaemic control. Her flu-like illness may have caused a further acute decline in her renal function with the symptoms of nausea and anorexia likely to be secondary to uraemia. Despite nausea, anorexia and reduced oral intake, she continued to take her drugs including glibenclamide. Her decreased intake probably led to dehydration and further compromised her renal function. Since glibenclamide has a long duration of action, associated hypoglycaemia may last for days. Therefore, as well as stopping the glibenclamide, HM needs to be hospitalized and treated with an intravenous glucose infusion until good oral intake resumes. In older patients hypoglycaemia can be mistaken for transient neurological or cardiac events. Hypoglycaemia in older patients has a worse outcome than in younger patients, with a mortality of up to 10%. Falls are one of the possible presentations of hypoglycaemia in the elderly. HM had other risk factors for falling – osteoarthritis and impaired vision. Given her history of diabetes with nephropathy, an ACE inhibitor should be considered once her acute illness has resolved and GFR has returned to baseline. Similarly, given her history of cerebrovascular disease and diabetes, she should be commenced on statin therapy as appropriate secondary prevention.

Data Interpretation

Question 1

A 74 year old woman with a history of hypertension and atrial fibrillation presents with dysphasia and right upper limb weakness of 10 minutes duration with complete resolution. Her medications are aspirin 75mg daily, digoxin 125μg daily and indapamide 1.5mg daily. Her average blood pressure measurement was 154/88mmHg. Investigations are as follows:

Full blood count	normal
Urea	8.6mmol/l
Creatinine	124 μmol/l
Na⁺	138 mmol/l

Full blood count normal
Urea 8.6mmol/l
Creatinine 124 μmol/l
Na⁺ 138 mmol/l
K⁺ 3.8mmol/l
Fasting glucose 11mol/l
HbA₁C 8.1%
Fasting cholesterol 6.8mmol/l
Urinalysis ++protein, +++glucose
CT brain scan microvascular ischaemic changes, no evidence of recent infarct, no haemorrhage

a.   What is the likely diagnosis?
b.   What abnormalities are evident on laboratory tests?
c.   What new medications would you consider?

Question 2

A 72 year old man presents with a two-week history of fatigue, anorexia, nausea, progressively worsening confusion. Laboratory investigations were normal two months ago. His medications include bendrofluazide for dependent lower limb oedema, low-dose prednisolone for polymyalgia rheumatica diagnosed 8 years ago, ibuprofen and tramadol for low back pain of four weeks duration. Investigations are as follows:

Hb 8.4g/dl
MCV 72fl
MCHC 30 g/dl
Urea 14.6mmoll
Creatinine 168μmol/l
Na⁺ 128mmol/l
K⁺ 3.5mmol/l
Faecal occult blood positive
Lumbosacral x-ray Compression fractures of 5th lumbar vertebrae
Bone densitometry Consistent with osteoporosis

a.   Describe the laboratory abnormalities
b.   What medications are potentially responsible for this presentation?
c.   What changes would you make to the medication regime?

Question 3

A 75 year old woman presents with lethargy and general malaise. She has a 3 year history of ischaemic heart disease and ventricular tachycardia for which she has been taking amiodarone. Her laboratory investigations are as follows:

Full blood count: normal
Urea and electrolytes: normal
T4:   4pmol/l
TSH: 46mU/l

a.   What is the diagnosis?
b.   What new medication would you consider?

Best of five questions

Question 1

Adverse drug events in older people are associated with:

A.   Polypharmacy
B.   Inappropriate prescribing of medications
C.   Inadequate monitoring of prescribed medication
D.   10 - 20% of all hospital admissions of older people
E.   All of the above

Question 2

Which of the following is most likely to improve drug compliance in older people?

A.   Reduced drug dosage
B.   Simplifying drug regimens and avoiding polypharmacy
C.   Written instructions for drug administration
D.   Regular medication review
E.   Reduced drug cost

Question 3

Which of the following prescriptions are potentially inappropriate?

a.   Beta-blockers with chronic stable heart failure
b.   Warfarin with chronic atrial fibrillation in patients aged >80 years
c.   Alpha-adrenergic blocker with postural hypotension
d.   Calcium and vitamin D supplementation with known osteoporosis
e.   Donepezil in moderate Alzheimers disease

Answers are on page 311

Movement disorders

R Lannon, T J Counihan, E C Mulkerrin

This chapter describes some of the commoner movement disorders affecting older patients. However the emphasis will be on Parkinson's disease (PD) which is the commonest treatable disorder found in this age group.

Parkinson's disease

Parkinson's disease is the only neurodegenerative disease for which adequate symptomatic therapy is available. The onset of symptoms is insidious, and many patients are unaware of the degree of disability produced by rigidity and bradykinesia. Patients may erroneously ascribe their ponderous movements, stooped posture and deteriorating gait to 'old age' and it is only when such symptoms are alleviated, sometimes dramatically, by medication that the full extent of their disability becomes apparent.

The first step in the assessment of patients in whom PD is suspected is to try to verify that the patient does, in fact, have idiopathic PD. The triad of rest tremor, rigidity and bradykinesia, when present, makes the diagnosis relatively straightforward. The *sine qua non*, however, is the presence of bradykinesia, which occurs in all patients even in the absence of a rest tremor. Manifestations of bradykinesia include a masked face, hypophonia, micrographia and a slowness of gait and movements in general. A tremor that is truly present at rest (best appreciated during gait testing when the forearm muscles are relaxed) is highly suggestive of PD but it must be remembered that 30% of patients with PD do not develop rest tremor. Disturbances in postural reflexes occur later in PD, and the presence of falls early in the course of the disease should prompt a reappraisal of the diagnosis. Bilateral onset and rapid progression of symptoms early in the course of the disease also supports a diagnosis of a PD–plus syndrome rather than true PD, discussed later in this chapter.

Medication for PD

Existing knowledge does not permit the adoption of a standardised treatment algorithm for PD, although several attempts have been made. The natural history of the disease, the predominant symptom, and the response to treatment is highly variable from patient to patient. Very few have identical drug regimens. A variety of treatment options are available for patients newly diagnosed with PD:

- •. Low-potency drugs, such as amantadine (Symmetrel), selegiline (Eldepryl), rasagiline (Azilect) and the anticholinergic agents trihexyphenidyl [benzhexol] (Artane – withdrawn from Irish market), benztropine (Cogentin), procyclidine (Kemadrin), and biperidin (Akineton)
- •. Intermediate potency drugs include the direct-acting dopamine agonists bromocriptine, pergolide, ropinirole and pramipexole
- •. High potency drugs: levodopa, administered in combination with a dopa decarboxylase inhibitor, either benserazide (Madopar) or carbidopa (Sinemet). Apomorphine has equivalent potency to levodopa, but must be administered parenterally, making it unsuitable for patients with mild disease

It is noteworthy that, given the variety of drugs available for the treatment of PD, levodopa remains the most potent and effective medication. Perhaps this should not be too much of a surprise when one considers that the symptomatic treatment of PD is aimed primarily at reversing the deficiency

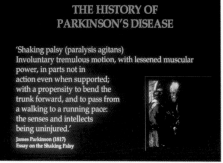

THE HISTORY OF
PARKINSON'S DISEASE

'Shaking palsy (paralysis agitans)
Involuntary tremulous motion, with lessened muscular power, in parts not in
action even when supported;
with a propensity to bend the
trunk forward, and to pass from
a walking to a running pace:
the senses and intellects
being uninjured.'

James Parkinson (1817)
Essay on the Shaking Palsy

Figure I: The original description of Parkinson's Disease

TABLE I

DOPA DECARBOXYLASE INHIBITOR (DDI)/LEVODOPA PREPARATIONS

Formulation	DDI/Levodopa (mg)	Colour
Cocarbidopa 62.5 tablets	12.5/50	Yellow
Cocarbidopa 110 tablets	10/100	Blue
Cocarbidopa tablets	25/100	Yellow
Cocarbidopa 275 tablets	25/250	Blue
Cocarbidopa CR tablets	25/100	Pink
Cocarbidopa CR tablets	50/200	Peach
Cobeneldopa Dispersible 62.5 tablets	12.5/50	
Cobeneldopa Dispersible 125 tablets	25/100	
Cobeneldopa 62.5 capsules	12.5/50	Blue/grey
Cobeneldopa 125	25/100	Blue/pink
Cobeneldopa 250	50/200	Blue/caramel
Cobeneldopa CR	25/100	Green/blue

of dopamine induced by degeneration of the nigrostriatal dopaminergic neurons. If levodopa is the most potent drug, then why not give it to all patients requiring treatment? The principle argument for deferring levodopa therapy relates to the well-recognised complications of long-term therapy, namely the development of motor fluctuations (wearing off, delayed time to 'on', 'on-off' phenomenon) and dyskinesias (drug-induced choreiform or dystonic movements). Dopamine agonists have a much lower incidence of motor fluctuations and dyskinesias. Recent clinical trials comparing dopamine agonist therapy with levodopa have confirmed the greater effectiveness of levodopa in alleviating motor symptoms as well as improving quality of life, albeit at the greater risk of producing dyskinesias. Some authorities advocate that dopamine agonists are the treatment of choice for patients with early PD. However, it must be recognised that less than a quarter of patients will be able to be effectively treated using dopamine agonist monotherapy at five years. In addition, there are other important potential side effects of dopamine agonists, particularly in older people, including hallucinations and sudden onset of sleep, both of which have also been described with levodopa therapy but are more common in patients treated with dopamine agonists.

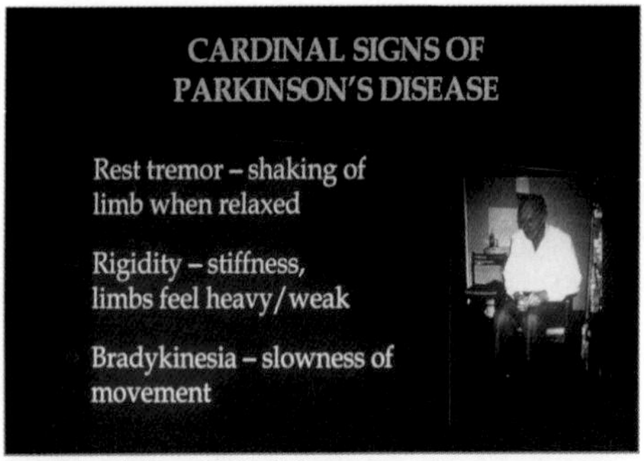

Initial therapy with low-potency drugs

In patients with minimal symptoms, it is reasonable to start therapy with selegiline, amantadine or an anticholinergic drug. However, all of these drugs may be poorly tolerated in older patients. Selegiline blocks one of the main dopamine degradation pathways by inhibiting the B isoform of monoamine oxidase (MAO-B). Rasagiline, a newer agent in this group, has mild symptomatic effects but is promising in early disease and is best given as a single morning dose of 1 mg. Suggestions that rasagiline may have neuroprotective effects are as yet unsubstantiated but studies in this area are ongoing. The Tempo study suggested an advantage from early initiation of rasagiline with those patients given delayed therapy failing to achieve similar responses to therapy. Interactions between MAO-B inhibitors and selective serotonin reuptake inhibitors (SSRIs), tricyclic antidepressants (TCADs) and non-selective MAO inhibitors are theoretically possible but rarely encountered in clinical practice. No special diet is required. Important side effects

CARDINAL SIGNS OF PARKINSON'S DISEASE

Rest tremor – shaking of limb when relaxed

Rigidity – stiffness, limbs feel heavy/weak

Bradykinesia – slowness of movement

Figure 2: The cardinal signs of Parkinson's Disease

TABLE 2
DOPAMINE AGONIST PREPARATIONS

Drug	Formulations (mg)	Starting Dose (mg)	Maintenance dose (mg)
Bromocriptine (Parlodel)	2.5, 5, 10	1.25 daily	5 tds
Pergolide (Celance)	0.05, 0.25, 1.0	0.05 daily	0.5 tds
Lisuride	0.2	0.2 daily	0.2 tds
Cabergoline (Cabaser)	1, 2, 4	1 daily	2 once daily
Pramipexole (Mirapexin)	0.088, 0.180, 0.7	0.088 tds	0.36 tds
Ropinirole (Requip)	0.25, 1, 2, 5	0.25 tds	3 tds or OD (extended release)
Rotigotine patch (Neupro)	2,4,6,8	2mg daily	2-8mg daily

of selegiline include orthostatic hypotension and insomnia.

Amantadine has mild symptomatic effects at the usual maintenance dose of 100mg tds. It may cause pedal oedema, is associated with livedo reticularis and should be used with caution in patients with renal impairment. Short courses are often useful to get patients through special occasions such as weddings, but its effectiveness rapidly wears off. Anticholinergic drugs are especially useful for treating tremor, although they are associated with a substantial risk of serious side effects in older patients, including confusion, memory impairment, blurred vision, urinary retention and constipation, and are seldom used by Geriatricians.

Using levodopa as initial treatment

For the majority of patients over the age of sixty, the most appropriate initial therapy is a levodopa preparation. A favourable response to levodopa is highly suggestive of idiopathic PD. The drug is administered with an inhibitor of the enzyme dopa decarboxylase (cocarbidopa; Sinemet or cobeneldopa; Madopar) in order to prevent conversion of levodopa to dopamine in the peripheral circulation. Both Sinemet and Madopar are available as immediate-release or controlled-release preparations (table 1), with a bewildering number of options available for monotherapy in early PD.

The usual maintenance levodopa dose for initial therapy is 25/100mg tds of an immediate release preparation. The dispersible preparation of cobeneldopa instead of the tablet form is best avoided in early disease due to its short half-life. Cocarbidopa 110mg (Sinemet 110) is less commonly used than Cocarbidopa 125mg (Sinemet Plus) as the latter offers a carbidopa:levodopa optimal ratio of 1:4 and ensures

a minimum daily carbidopa dose of 75mg. However, cocarbidopa 110 it is still used in older patients, the rationale being that ageing is associated with less gastric acid production resulting in decreased enteral breakdown of levodopa. Controlled-release preparations of levodopa are also best avoided as initial therapy, as their bioavailability is less than that of the immediate-release preparations. It is often difficult to ascertain whether sub-optimal responses in patients are due to subtherapeutic doses of levodopa or resistance to levodopa therapy, suggesting that the underlying diagnosis is not idiopathic PD. Pre-treating patients with domperidone (Motilium) 10mg tds for the first three days of treatment can offset the risk of transient nausea from levodopa. For patients with severe nausea, the dosage escalation phase of levodopa may need to be much slower, perhaps starting with domperidone 20mg tds for three days, and then slowly introducing levodopa in 50mg increments. It is important to remember that nausea is almost universally transient, and the physician should not conclude that the patient is 'allergic' to the drug on the basis of initial gastrointestinal upset. Metoclopramide (Maxolon) and prochlorperazine

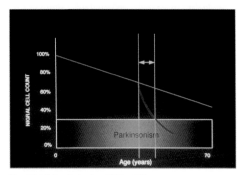

Figure 3: Striatal dopamine in ageing and Parkinson's Disease

(Stemetil) are dopamine antagonists and must be avoided in PD due to their potential for extrapyramidal side effects. Once nausea subsides, patients should be instructed to take the medication on an empty stomach, preferably one hour before meals. This is necessary as levodopa is absorbed in the intestine via a saturable transport system that is shared with other large neutral amino acids. Large amounts of dietary protein, therefore, will inhibit absorption of levodopa. Taking levodopa on an empty stomach is probably less important for patients with early PD, but becomes critical for patients who have developed motor fluctuations who experience 'dose failures'. In many of these cases, the apparent failure of levodopa is attributable to inadequate absorption.

The main goal of therapy is to restore a patient's normal function using the smallest possible dose of levodopa. Clinical effects of levodopa may take several weeks to become apparent, and the temptation to increase either the frequency or strength of the daily dose too soon should be resisted, especially in younger patients who carry the greatest risk of developing motor fluctuations and dyskinesias. This risk appears to be substantially less in older patients who may require larger initial doses for a clinical effect to become apparent. Most patients will show a clear response to a total daily levodopa dose of 600 mg. Patients who show no clinical improvement at a dose of 1000mg/day almost certainly do not have idiopathic PD, and other causes of parkinsonism should be considered.

Dopamine agonists as initial treatment

There are seven dopamine agonists available for the treatment of early PD (table 2), four of which are ergot derivatives; bromocriptine (Parlodel), pergolide (Celance), lisuride and cabergoline (Cabaser). The two latest non-ergot preparations, pramipexole (Mirapexin) and ropinirole (Requip) have largely replaced the older agents on account of the rare but serious potential for retroperitoneal fibrosis. Pergolide, pramipexole and ropinirole are probably equally efficacious, with bromocriptine less potent. Ropinirole (ER) and cabergoline have the advantage of once daily dosing, although the latter drug is extremely expensive. The dopamine agonist rotigotine is available in a patch formulation, though experience with its use in older patients is limited at present.

The principle argument in favour of using a dopamine agonist as initial monotherapy in early PD

is to delay the point at which a patient will require levodopa, and by extension, delay the development of motor fluctuations and dyskinesias. There is a clear indication for use of these drugs in patients with young-onset PD (<40 years old) who have the greatest propensity to develop disabling motor fluctuations and dyskinesias over time. The indications for use of a dopamine agonist become less clear with older patients for the following reasons:

- Dopamine agonists are less effective at reducing motor symptoms and improving activities of daily living than levodopa
- Motor fluctuations and dyskinesias are less frequent in older patients and often not disabling
- Dopamine agonists have frequent adverse side effects including sleep attacks, nausea, orthostatic hypotension, impulsivity and hallucinations. Patients should be specifically cautioned about the risk of sudden 'sleep attacks', particularly during the titration phase. Some authorities advocate suspension of driving during the initial weeks of treatment
- Dopamine agonists have complicated dose escalation regimens requiring months of treatment to reach a therapeutic dose
- Dopamine agonists are considerably more expensive than standard levodopa preparations
- Ergot derived agents eg pergolide, cabergoline are associated with valvular fibrosis and regurgitation as well as pulmonary fibrosis

Recent studies using functional neuroimaging techniques with both ropinirole and pramipexole have suggested that these drugs may exert a neuroprotective effect on dopamine neurons. Unfortunately, several technical and methodological issues have arisen as a result of these studies, as outlined in an excellent review of the evidence by Ahlskog.

Non-pharmacological therapy

For patients whose activity level is curtailed by motor symptoms, an evaluation by a physiotherapist with experience in treating PD is invaluable, particularly when the patient is starting drug therapy. Indeed, with advancing age the emphasis of treatment often shifts away from drugs which may only be tolerated in low to moderate dosage. Speech and language therapy provides valuable help to patients who develop problems with speech and swallowing. Home exercise programmes and aquatherapy may also be beneficial. Patients should be encouraged to remain informed about the disease and any therapeutic developments, possibly through involvement in a support group. It must be emphasised that support groups are not for everyone, and, while many patients feel empowered and better informed through such groups, other patients become despondent seeing fellow patients with advanced disease. It is useful to educate patients about the spectrum of disease, and that it is not incompatible with a long and fulfilling life in many cases. The skills of social workers and specialist nurses in PD help to enhance the essential liaison between primary and secondary care and improve quality of life.

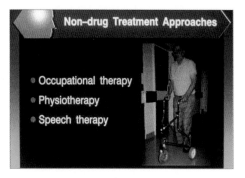

Figure 4: Multidisciplinary management of Parkinson's Disease

Treatment of advanced disease

It should be expected that the majority of patients will not clinically deteriorate as a result of disease progression within the first 3 to 5 years of treatment. If a patient and their family return to the physician complaining of deteriorating symptoms before this time, a careful search should be made for alternative explanations. The patient should be questioned about the following:

Medications
• Are they spaced adequately throughout the day
• Taken with or without meals
• Compliance
• Side-effects especially confusion and hallucinations

Motor fluctuations and dyskinesias
• 'Wearing off' phenomenon
• 'On-off' phenomenon

Sleep
• Daytime somnolence, often related to dopamine agonist treatment
• Nocturnal akinesia which may be improved by adding controlled release preparations of levodopa at bedtime
• Other causes of poor sleep such as pain, nocturia, parasomnia or depression

Mood
• Is there evidence of psychomotor retardation?

Comorbid conditions
• Arthritis
• Infection

Most causes of worsening symptoms can be attributed to one or a combination of the above factors. Teasing out the details of a complicated medication regimen requires patience on behalf of both patient and physician. It is helpful to use a medication chart and to record any changes for the patient to take home. An hourly diary completed by the patient, detailing whether they are 'on', or 'off' completed for a day or two prior to the clinic appointment gives useful information regarding the possible development of motor complications and how to treat them. It cannot be overemphasized that a multidisciplinary team is required to deliver optimal care to older patients with advanced PD.

Treatment of motor fluctuations

One of the early signs of the development of motor fluctuations is the 'wearing off' phenomenon. 'Wearing off' can be elicited by asking patients whether or not they feel the first tablet of the day has 'kicked in'. If not this implies that there has been some decrement in the response to levodopa overnight, often with resulting nocturnal akinesia. This is best treated by the addition of a controlled release preparation of levodopa at bedtime. For patients with more frequent 'wearing off' between doses, the addition of entacapone, an inhibitor of one of the degradative enzymes of dopamine, catechol-o-methyl transferase (COMT) may be effective. This compound was originally available in 200mg tablets and administered in conjunction with each dose of levodopa to prolong its duration of action. However a combination tablet containing levodopa, decarboxylase inhibitor and COMT inhibitor (Stalevo) is now the formulation of choice in clinical practice. Occasionally the dose of levodopa may need to be reduced to counteract the emergence of dyskinesias or nausea. The addition of a dopamine agonist is an alternative strategy, mindful of the extensive side effect profile of these drugs. Freezing of gait is a common symptom in patients with advancing disease, and a frequent cause of falling forwards. Freezing is often manifested as difficulty initiating walking or getting stuck in doorways. Patients may describe their feet as being like they are stuck in wet cement. It is important to ascertain whether the freezing is a manifestation of being 'off', or whether it is occurring regardless of the state of the patient's motor function. The latter is notoriously difficult to treat and usually refractory to medication. It may respond transiently to the use of visual cues, such as placing taped lines on the floor, or using a modified cane. For 'wearing off' and 'off' related freezing, the treatment is to augment the amount of dopamine available using the following options:

- Increase the amount of levodopa using controlled release levodopa
- Increase the frequency of levodopa administration to qid dosing
- Add entacapone (using combined medication)
- Add a dopamine agonist
- Liquid levodopa

Occasionally, patients with unpredictable 'off' periods benefit from liquid levodopa which has a faster onset of action but a shorter duration. This is made up daily by dissolving the total daily levodopa dose in the equivalent millilitre volume of water (eg. if a patient is taking 800mg of sinemet/day, dissolve 8 x 25/100 tablets in 800ml water), and dividing into the required number of doses for the day. A vitamin C tablet added to the solution will act as a preservative for overnight storage in a fridge. Enternal infusion of levodopa/carbidopa via a PEG/jejunostomy is sometimes utilised in advanced cases with variable results.

Treatment of dyskinesias

Dyskinesias typically occur as the plasma levels of levodopa reach a peak between doses. The movements are choreiform and random. Less common are dyskinesias which occur at the beginning of a dose interval or at the end, known as biphasic dyskinesias or dyskinesia-improvement-dyskinesia [D.I.D]. This type of dyskinesia tends to be more dystonic in nature, with sustained posturing of an extremity. Unlike peak-dose dyskinesias, which are often not distressing to the patient, biphasic dyskinesias may be painful. For peak dose dyskinesias, the following treatment strategy may be adopted:

- Initiate a dopamine agonist, gradually increasing the dose
- Begin to lower the dose of levodopa by 25mg per dose decrements
- Add amantadine which has an anti-dyskinetic effect in doses of 300mg/day, although its effect may take up to 6 weeks to become apparent

Treatment of refractory motor fluctuations/ dyskinesias

It is widely believed that motor fluctuations and dyskinesias are the result of pulsatile stimulation of dopamine receptors in the striatum. This theory is supported by the experimental finding that motor fluctuations do not develop during continuous dopaminergic stimulation with intravenous levodopa infusions. Unfortunately, it has been difficult to provide a form of continuous dopaminergic stimulation that might be useful in the clinical setting. For patients with refractory motor fluctuations, the parenterally-administered short-acting dopamine agonist apomorphine is a useful option. This can be given by subcutaneous injection as a rescue remedy for severe off episodes (Britaject) or as a continuous infusion via a subcutaneous pump. Typically, patients are hospitalized overnight and pre-treated with domperidone prior to an apomorphine challenge.

Falls

Falls are common and often preventable, particularly in older patients with advanced disease. There are several possible causes including freezing and sudden 'off' periods, orthostatic hypotension and postural instability. The history may help determine the cause. Backward falls are most often the result of postural instability, which is a symptom of relatively advanced PD. If backward falls occur within the first year or two of the diagnosis of PD, an atypical form of parkinsonism such as progressive supranuclear palsy (PSP) or multisystem atrophy (MSA) must be considered. Serious consideration should be given to the use of a wheelchair in patients with backward falls. Orthostatic hypotension may result from the disease process itself or from medications, particularly selegiline and dopamine agonists. Falls due to freezing and 'off' periods may respond to adjustment of the levodopa regimen as discussed above. Physiotherapy and a home assessment by an occupational therapist are especially important for older patients with frequent falls.

Surgical therapy for advanced PD

Surgical treatments for PD are not a new concept.

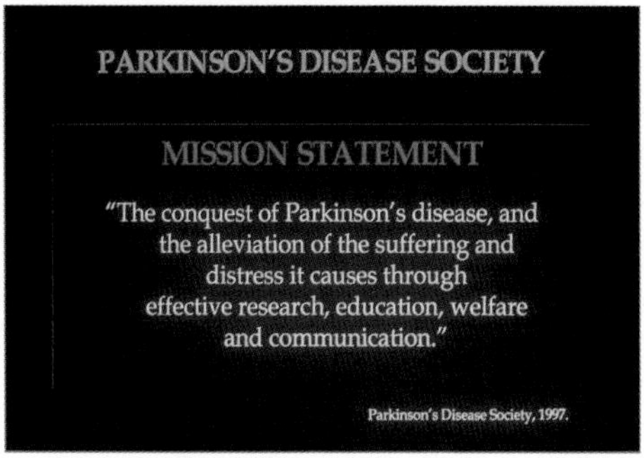

Figure 5: The role of voluntary organisations

TABLE 3
DIFFERENTIAL DIAGNOSIS OF PARKINSONISM

Drug induced parkinsonism
Metoclopramide
Prochlorperazine
Chlorpromazine
Risperidone
Olanzapine
Haloperidol
Betahistine

Frontal lobe syndromes
Normal Pressure Hydrocephalus

Parkinson's "plus" syndromes
Multiple System Atrophy
Striatonigral Degeneration
Olivopontocerebelar Atrophy
Shy-Drager syndrome
Progressive Supranuclear Palsy

Depression (Pseudoparkinsonism)
Wilson's Disease
Vascular Pseudoparkinsonism

Effective surgical interventions were available in the 1960s in the pre-levodopa era. It was found that placing lesions in the thalamus (thalamotomy) or globus pallidus (pallidotomy) reversed many of the symptoms of PD, especially tremor and bradykinesia. This form of treatment was largely abandoned following the discovery of levodopa, but re-emerged in the 1990s once the long-term complications of levodopa therapy became apparent. More recently, surgical therapies have centred on electrically stimulating the thalamus, globus pallidus or subthalamus using deep brain stimulation (DBS). DBS works by inactivating those areas of the basal ganglia which are overactive in PD, possibly by overriding the normal neuronal electrical activity within those structures. Simplistically speaking, DBS replaces chemical treatments (drugs) with electrical impulses. DBS has several advantages over pallidotomy, including the ability to alter the amount and location of stimulation, as well as the ability to remove the device or stop stimulation if there are adverse effects. As a general rule, DBS only improves symptoms that formerly responded well to levodopa therapy. The ideal patient for surgery will have:
• A clear diagnosis of levodopa-responsive idiopathic PD
• Medically refractory motor fluctuations and dyskinesia
• No history of dementia or significant psychiatric disease
• Good insight into the expectations of surgery

It will be clear from the above that surgery is only suitable for a minority of PD patients. However, surgery must not be perceived as a last resort therapy. DBS only improves symptoms that result from dopaminergic dysfunction. PD also affects non-dopaminergic pathways, for instance cholinergic and noradrenergic pathways and symptoms such as orthostatic hypotension and postural instability may not be improved. It is also tempting to refer patients for surgery who are levodopa resistant, but these patients, by definition, do not have idiopathic PD and almost uniformly do poorly. Other factors to be considered include the patient's general medical health and the availability of trained programmers for the post-operative and long-term management of DBS devices. In carefully selected patients, however, DBS can be a highly effective therapy and allows for a reduction in medication by about 70%.

Non-motor manifestations of PD

Constipation
Constipation due to gut hypomotility as a result of autonomic dysfunction is almost universal in PD, but may also be exacerbated by medications, especially anticholinergics. The following approaches may be helpful:
• Increase bulk of diet with prune juice, linseeds, bran, psyllium or methylcellulose
• Increase fluid intake
• Increase fruit and vegetable intake

- Exercise
- Avoid constipating medications such as anticholinergics, and TCADs
- Use a stool softener such as docusate
- Use osmotic laxatives such as Movicol

Orthostatic hypotension
Patients complain of light-headedness, dizziness or 'fogginess'. The following approach may be helpful:
- Stop offending drugs such as anti-hypertensives, selegiline and dopamine agonists
- Increase daytime fluid intake
- Liberalise salt intake
- Use compression stockings
- Recommend small regular meals
- Fludrocortisone
- Midodrine

Depression and anxiety
Depression affects at least 30% of PD patients. Psychomotor symptoms may be difficult to differentiate from bradykinesia. It remains unclear to what extent depression represents part of the symptom complex of PD or whether it is a reactive disorder in the presence of debilitating disease. Patients often complain of anxiety during 'off' periods which are rapidly reversed when they turn 'on', suggesting a direct effect of dopamine on mood. Whatever the cause, depression should be treated aggressively. Patients may need professional help from a psychiatrist or psychotherapist, to allow the patient re-establish a sense of worth in the face of declining physical function. SSRIs may be useful, although there are reports of fluoxetine exacerbating motor symptoms in some patients. The SSRI of choice may be sertraline (Lustral). Non-selective MAO inhibitors may be particularly effective for refractory cases, but should only be prescribed by physicians familiar with the potential interactions of these drugs. Electroconvulsive therapy is also an effective modality in selected cases and may transiently improve motor function.

Psychosis
The development of psychotic symptoms in a patient with PD presents a major management problem. The most common cause is medication. Patients typically present with mild, non-threatening visual hallucinations, which over time become associated with paranoid features and a gradual loss of insight. In these cases, all medications with the exception of levodopa should be withdrawn with particular attention paid to anticholinergics which need to be tapered slowly. Levodopa should be reduced to the lowest acceptable dose. Night time dosing should be minimised, preferably using controlled release preparations. If an antipsychotic is required, quetiapine (Seroquel) is associated with the fewest extrapyramidal side-effects. Half a 25mg tablet at night may be a sufficient initial dose. Risperidone and olanzepine should be avoided if possible as they may worsen motor symptoms. Clozapine is the only proven medication for treatment of psychotic symptoms in PD, but requires regular blood monitoring due to the risk of agranulocytosis. Nonetheless, in refractory cases, this agent may be effective and prevent unnecessary nursing home placement.

Cognitive decline and dementia
It is important to remember that cognitive disturbance in PD may not be related to the disease itself, but arise from infection, organ failure, medications, subdural haematoma, depression, Lewy body dementia or coincident Alzheimer's disease. Up to 30% of PD patients will however eventually develop dementia. Every effort needs to be made to eliminate potentially reversible causes by appropriate use of CT scanning and haematological and biochemical evaluation following clinical assessment. A proportion of patients with parkinsonism who develop dementia or psychotic symptoms within a year of diagnosis will turn out to have Lewy body dementia. Often these patients have prominent visual hallucinations and marked sensitivity to neuroleptics which should be avoided if the condition is suspected. Acetylcholinesterase inhibitors, such as donepezil (Aricept) or rivastigmine (Exelon) may be helpful although they are associated with increased drooling and urinary incontinence in some patients.

Sleep disturbances
Sleep disturbance in PD may result from a variety of causes, including nocturnal akinesia, nocturia, depression, drug-induced insomnia (especially selegiline), or hallucinations. Parasomnias, including REM sleep-behaviour disorder are also common as is restless legs syndrome. Patients with advanced PD may nap more during the day with ultimately inversion of the normal sleep pattern. Low doses of clonazepam (0.5mg nocte) are particularly effective for patients with REM sleep-behaviour disturbance.

Vascular gait dyspraxia
Many patients with multi-infarct disease, including

TABLE 4
POSSIBLE SYNONYMS AND OVER-LAPPING SYNDROMES OF GAIT DYSPRAXIA

No.	Disorder
1	Frontal ataxia
2	Frontal ataxia and dysequilibrium
3	Gait apraxia
4	Marche à petit pas
5	Arteriosclerotic parkinsonism
6	Lower body parkinsonism
7	Vascular pseudoparkinsonism
8	Gait disorder of Binswanger's disease
9	Gait disorder of normal pressure hydrocephalus
10	Idiopathic gait disorder of the elderly

those with severe periventricular white matter disease and lacunar infarctions, may have significant gait abnormalities in the absence of obvious mental decline or neurological impairment. These gaits have been poorly described in the literature and have been variously labelled as vascular pseudoparkinsonism, arteriosclerotic parkinsonism or lower body parkinsonism. Other authors have used the term *'gait apraxia'* to describe what is essentially the same gait disorder with prominent features of gait ignition failure, shuffling, freezing, difficulty making turns and dysequilibrium. These gait disorders are not however sufficiently explained by the sensory or motor disturbances that may be present and as such are *'out of proportion'* to any neurological deficits. Other clinical features of multiple infarct disease include abrupt episodes and step-wise progression, weakness, reduction in spontaneous activity and emotional lability. There have been few attempts to formulate unifying theories regarding these gait disorders, borne out by the large number of synonyms used to describe what are essentially the same or very similar gait disorders. A list of possible overlapping syndromes is shown in table 4.

It has recently been suggested that these gait disorders could be condensed into three major types: Ignition apraxia where gait ignition failure and freezing predominate; Equilibrium apraxia where poor balance predominates and Mixed gait apraxia with features of both. These three clinical descriptions correlate to putative sites of damage in the frontal lobes such as supplementary motor area and premotor area and their connections, through the periventricular white matter, to the basal ganglia. Pathological mechanisms may include athero-embolic stroke, cardiogenic embolic stroke, small vessel disease due to hypertension and hypoperfusion due to hypotension. When these mechanisms affect the deep penetrating arteries supplying watershed areas of the brain, they lead to lacunar infarction and periventricular white matter changes resulting in 'cortico-cortico disconnections' disrupting critical pathways involved in the motor programming of normal gait, leading to dyspraxic gait disorders. The risk factors for the development of these vascular dyspraxic disorders are largely similar to those for vascular disease in general. Of these, hypertension appears to be the most important. It would seem sensible to control these risk factors in patients with dyspraxic gait disorders but there are no large scale clinical trials to support this approach. The importance of vascular dyspraxic gait disorders lies in the comparatively long life expectancy of patients with multiple infarct disease since approximately 50% of patients survive 6 years from the onset of symptoms. Immobility is a major reason for institutionalisation and nursing home care and falls are a substantial cause of morbidity.

Restless leg syndrome

Restless leg syndrome (RLS) is characterised by abnormal unpleasant sensations which are relieved by movement of the legs. The irresistible urge to move the legs results from a variety of sensory symptoms such as a creeping or crawling sensations or simply a feeling of restlessness. The relief of the symptoms by movement is a very important point, which must be elicited specifically on history taking. The symptoms are often severe and are a common cause of sleep disturbance as well as chronic sleep deprivation and daytime somnolence in older patients. Formerly known as Ekbom's syndrome, RLS occurs in approximately 10% of the population with a well-described age-related increase in prevalence. Symptoms can be very mild but often become progressively more problematic over time. All patients with RLS should be screened for deficiencies in iron, vitamin B12, folic acid and hypothyroidism. Evidence of renal impairment should also be out-ruled and many patients experience significant improvement in symptoms following correction and management of the above deficiency states.

Drug management of RLS is often necessary with variable tolerance and success, particularly in older patients. Traditionally, low dose levodopa therapy at night was the most effective treatment but many patients failed to respond or tolerate this treatment. Newer dopamine agonists, particularly pramipexole seem very effective in this condition, usually given as a single night-time dose so that some of the aforementioned side-effects are less problematic. Cabergoline may be effective although the long half-life of this agent may not be an advantage in RLS, since there are rarely daytime symptoms. Ropinirole has also been shown to be effective. Other agents such as gabapentin, other anti-convulsants and clonazepam appear to be effective though they can cause sedative side-effects even in low dose in older patients.

Suggested further reading
- Chapus S, Ouchchane L, Metz, Gerbund L, Durif F. Impact of the motor complications of Parkinson's disease on the quality of life. Mov Disord 2005, 20: 224–230.
- Fan S, Oakes D, Shoulson I, et al. Levodopa and the progression of Parkinson's disease. N Engl J Med 2004; 351: 2498–2508.
- Rascol O, Brooks DJ, Melamed E, et al. Rasagiline as an adjunct to levodopa in patients with Parkinson's disease and motor fluctuations (LARGO, Lasting effect in Adjunct therapy with Rasagiline given once daily, study) a randomised, double-blind, parallel-group trial. Lancet 2005; 365: 947–954.
- Fenelon G, Gimenez-Roldan S, Montastruc JL, et al. Efficacy and tolerability of entacapone in patients with Parkinson's disease treated with levodopa plus a dopamine agonist and experiencing wearing-off motor fluctuations. A randomised, double-blind, multicentre study. J Neural Transm 2003; 110: 239–251.
- Visser-Vandewalle V, Temel Y, van der Linden C, Ackermans L, Beuls E. Deep brain stimulation in movement disorders. The applications reconsidered. Acta Neurol Beig 2004; 104: 33–36.
- Pahwa R, Factor SA, Lyons KE, et al. Practice Parameter: Treatment of parkinson disease with motor fluctuations and dyskinesia (an evidence-based review); report of the quality standards subcommittee of the American Academy of Neurology. Neurology 2006; 983–995.
- Schade R, Anderson F, Suissa S, Haverkamp W, Garbe E, Dopamine Agonists and the Risk of Cardiac–Valve Regurgitation. N Engl J Med 2007; 356: 29–38.
- Transdermal Delivery of Dopaminergic Agents. Neurology 2005; 65, 2(Suppl 1): 51–14.
- Parkinson Study Group-A controlled, Randomized, Delayed – Start Study of Rasagiline in Early Parkinson Disease. Arch Neurol. 2004; 61: 561–566.
- Schrang A. Entacapone in the treatment of Parkinson's disease Lancet Neurol 2005; 4: 366–70.
- Olanon CW, Rascol O and ADAGI0 investigators. Early Rasagiline treatment slows UPDRS decline in the ADAGI0 delayed start study. Annals Neurol 2008. 64(suppl 12): 568.

Case Study 1

A 65 year old recently retired carpenter is referred by his GP for assessment of a tremor. His wife had noticed the tremor while her husband was watching television. There are no other symptoms although his wife says his posture has become stooped and his handwriting has deteriorated. He remains very active with golf and woodwork; he has not noticed any difficulty using his tools. His examination demonstrates a rest tremor and mild slowing of rapid alternating movements of the right hand. There is an absent arm swing on the right with gait testing. The patient and his wife are concerned about the possibility of Parkinson's disease and, if so, are there any treatments that might delay the progression of the disease.

In this case the diagnosis is clearly that of idiopathic PD, given the presence of a rest tremor and the finding of bradykinesia. The asymmetry of signs is entirely consistent with idiopathic PD. Based on the available history, there is no apparent functional disability. The patient should be told that he has mild PD and that, for now, there is no need for specific symptomatic therapy. With regard to the question concerning any neuroprotective or neurorestorative therapies for PD, it is reasonable to tell the patient that there currently are no proven treatments that delay the progression of the disease. It is important to emphasize that the prognosis for PD is highly variable with many patients living full and active lives, wherein the symptoms of PD may only remain as nuisance problems. Patients may be disappointed at the end of the evaluation not to have received a treatment, so it is equally important to reiterate that there are many useful treatments for the symptoms but that at present the patient's disease is so mild as to not warrant intervention.

Case Study 2

A 70 year old retired teacher is referred for assessment of a tremor which she has had for the previous two years. She admits to finding the tremor socially embarrassing and prefers not to dine out, as she finds the tremor increases when she is in public. She was a keen bridge player but recently gave this up. On directed questioning she reports difficulty getting comfortable in bed and consequently poor sleep. She is unable to write letters on account of poor penmanship. On examination she was soft spoken and her writing was almost illegible. There was an obvious rest and postural tremor of both hands, right more than left, with some rigidity. Her gait was slow.

The goal for the physician is to keep patients in the mainstream of life. Patients with definite functional impairment, such as the patient above, clearly need to be treated. What precisely constitutes functional impairment will vary from patient to patient. Patients who lead a sedentary life and who have a mild resting tremor may not require specific symptomatic therapy, whereas those who lead active lives may find even a mild tremor distressing. The patient, therefore, must take part in the decision process. It is important to enquire about patients' routine work and leisure practices when coming to a decision regarding initiation of treatment. It may be useful to ask 'Are there any activities that you used to do which you have had to give up?' Patients may have been keen card players but discontinued because of difficulty holding them or because of embarrassment at the presence of tremor. Many patients will not volunteer this kind of information unless it is specifically sought after. If there is a suggestion that the patient is withdrawing from society, either as a direct result of their parkinsonism or as a result of secondary depression, this must be taken as evidence of serious disability, and treated aggressively. On the other hand, it is important to emphasise to patients that delaying treatment will not lead to a faster rate of progression of the disease.

Case Study 3

A 75 year old man who has had PD for 8 years returns for review. He has noticed a progressive deterioration in his walking to the point where he has had several falls, one of which resulted in a fractured wrist. He says Sinemet, which he takes 4 times a day, is no longer working, particularly in the afternoons, when he is virtually confined to the chair. His son is concerned about involuntary fidgeting movements which the patient has not noticed. On examination, there is severe bradykinesia, the patient having to lever himself out of the chair, after which there is a period of hesitation before he is able to walk. There are frequent freezing spells during gait testing. There is retropulsion on the pull test. By the end of the evaluation, the examiner notices involuntary dyskinetic movements of the head and trunk, in conjunction with some increase in mobility.

Treatment with apomorphine continuous infusion subcutaneously may be very useful in this case. If this fails, enteral infusion of cocarbidopa via PEG/jejunostomy is having promising results.

Case Study 4

A 65 year old woman is referred for a second opinion regarding her Parkinson's disease, which was diagnosed 2 years ago. There is a history of progressive slowing of walking with multiple falls. She also complains of dysphasia and double vision when reading. She has been treated with Sinemet in doses up to 600mg/day. On examination, there is marked rigidity, which is symmetric, and prominent at the neck. Her voice has a "strangled" quality. Saccadic eye movements are impaired, particular with vertical gaze. The posture is lordotic and there is prominent postural instability.

Several aspects of this case suggest that the diagnosis is not idiopathic PD:
• The relatively rapid progression of symptoms
• The absence of tremor and the symmetry of signs
• The absence of a response to levodopa
• The prominence of axial symptoms (neck rigidity, abnormal eye movements and early postural instability)

The most likely diagnosis is progressive supranuclear palsy (PSP). Other parkinsonian syndromes include multiple systems atrophy (MSA) where the signs may be mostly extrapyramidal (striatonigral degeneration), cerebellar (olivopontocerebellar degeneration – OPCA) or autonomic (Shy-Drager syndrome). Patients with so-called 'lower extremity Parkinsonism' may have underlying subcortical vascular disease or normal pressure hydrocephalus (NPH). The latter diagnosis should always be suspected in patients with a subacute deterioration in gait, with associated urinary incontinence and cognitive decline.

Case Study 5

A sixty six year old mechanic is referred for possible Parkinson's disease. He reports having a tremor of both hands, which is now interfering with his work. He has difficulty using a spanner and a drill on account of shaking. He has to drink from a cup using both hands, and he is no longer able to write cheques because of poor writing. His brother and mother also suffer from tremors. On examination his writing is tremulous but not micrographic. There is a prominent postural and action tremor, with cogwheeling, but no rigidity at proximal joints. His voice is strong but tremulous. His gait is normal.

This patient does not have PD. He has a history of tremor, which is not present at rest, and, importantly, there is no bradykinesia. The family history suggests the possibility of familial essential tremor (ET). Cogwheeling may be present at the wrist in patients with ET and is not specific for PD.

Data Interpretation

Question 1

A 75 year old man has a history of falls. His mobility has become restricted and examination reveals a coarse tremor of his right hand. He has evidence of bruising over the left hip but good range of movement in the hip joint. His gait is slow to start and festinant. Cogwheel rigidity is prominent at the right elbow and the left knee. He has a stooped posture.

a.   What is the likely diagnosis?
b.   What is the initial optimal management?
c.   What investigations are essential?

Question 2

An 80 year old man complains of problems with sensation in his legs. He has symptoms mainly at night with an urge to move the legs. When he is moving about the symptoms recede. He also complains of day-time somnolence.

a.   What is the diagnosis?
b.   What investigations are essential?
c.   What is the best initial management?

Question 3

A 70 year old man attends the OPD with a tremor which has been present for 10 years. He has had no response to levodopa therapy. The tremor is coarse and symmetrically affects both arms.

a.   What is the likely diagnosis?
b.   What historical features would help make the diagnosis?
c.   What test might help with making the diagnosis?

Question 4

An 80 year old woman presents with excessive involuntary movements which preceded the recent prescription of levodopa by her doctor. Examination reveals an MMSE of 18/30 and choreiform movements affecting all limbs.

a.   What is the diagnosis?
b.   Describe the management
c.   What is the initial treatment of the abnormal movements?

Best of five questions

Question 1

A 70 year old woman is becoming increasingly stiff. She was commenced on treatment for vertigo and tinnitus 6 months ago. On examination there is symmetrical increased tone in all 4 limbs. She has a slow, short stepping gait.

What is the most likely diagnosis?

a.   Idiopathic parkinsons disease
b.   Lewy Body dementia
c.   Restless leg syndrome
d.   Drug induced parkinsons disease
e.   Alzheimers disease

Question 2

A 68 year old man has been noted to be increasingly disoriented by his family for 9 months. There are behavioural problems and significant vivid visual hallucinations. This seems to fluctuate from day to day. He has a parkinsonian appearance.

What is the likely diagnosis?

a.   Cerebral tumour
b.   Alzheimers disease
c.   Lewy Body dementia

d.   Fronotemporal dementia

e.   Endogenous depression

Question 3

A 70 year old man has been recently diagnosed with PD although his symptoms are confined to a tremor of his left hand which is not a major problem since he is right handed. However it is clumsy when he is dressing himself.

The best initial drug therapy is?

a.   Levodopa/dopadecarboylase inhibitor (DDI) in moderate dose

b.   Levodopa /DDI/ entacapone in lowest dose

c.   Observe the patient

d.   Selegeline/rasagiline therapy

e.   Apomorphine therapy

Question 4

A 75 year old patient with longstanding PD is developing severe 'off' periods and this is despite treatment with ropinirole ER and cocarbidopa 125mg TID. These periods occurs 30 minutes prior to her next dose of levodopa.

The best initial management is?

a.   Change ropinirole to subcutaneous apomorphine

b.   Double the dose of cocarbidopa to 250mg TID

c.   Add rasagiline

d.   Add amantadine

e.   Increase frequency of cocarbidopa to 125mg QID

Answers are on page 311

Ethical issues

S T O'Keeffe

Principles of ethical reasoning

Ethical issues and problems commonly arise when caring for older people. One approach to thinking about these issues is to consider the fundamental ethical principles of medicine. In general, problems arise when there is a conflict, or apparent conflict, between opposing principles. The key principles are:
• Autonomy (What does the patient want?)
• Beneficence (What can be done to help the patient?)
• Maleficence (Are there risks associated with a proposed treatment?)
• Justice (Is the proposed treatment fair to the patient and to all other patients?)

Autonomy

The competent patient has the right to refuse any treatment however beneficial. Hence, consideration of competence and mental capacity is often important when considering the weight to give patients' views. This is particularly important when dealing with older people where there is an increased prevalence of cognitive impairment. Autonomy is also at the root of ideas such as informed consent, disclosure of bad news and patient confidentiality.

Beneficence & maleficence

The primary goal of medical care is to improve the patient's well-being and health while avoiding harm. This refers back to the Hippocratic principle of 'primum non nocere' ('above all, do no harm'). Balancing the benefits and risks of treatment options is the traditional main role of clinicians. While making decisions in the best interests of our patients may seem straightforward and uncontroversial, patients' views of what constitutes an important benefit or harm may not be the same as that of their doctors.

Justice

It is important to be fair to the individual patient but, when caring for older people, one must also strive to be fair to hard-pressed carers. In addition, when resources are restricted, there is an argument that one may need to consider whether it is fair to other patients if, for example, a proposed course of action would consume a lot of resources and deprive other patients of what they require.

Changing cultural norms

A transition from a culture of medical paternalism – the view that doctor knows best - to one where respect for patient autonomy is paramount has occurred in Western countries in recent decades. Difficulties may arise when different generations of doctors and patients have assimilated this change to different degrees. There is no evidence that older people are less likely than younger people to want their preferences heard, although they may be less assertive in making this clear.

Although an over-simplistic analysis, there is some truth in the suggestion that tension between the demands of autonomy and beneficence underlies many current ethical issues (Figure 1). In the following sections, some of the problems that commonly arise when caring for elderly people will be discussed. The list is not intended to be exhaustive, but the principles illustrated can be applied to other scenarios.

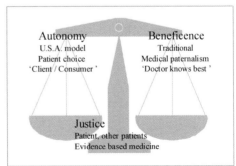

Figure 1: A parody of bioethics – with some element of truth

End-of-life decisions

Do-not-resuscitate orders

The proportion of patients receiving cardiopulmonary resuscitation (CPR) who survive to discharge is about 15 - 20%. Survival rates are even lower in older people. However, this reflects the effects of comorbid illness more than that of age itself, and selected older people have an excellent chance of survival. CPR is an undignified and violent way to die if death is inevitable. It has been proposed that do-not-resuscitate (DNR) orders should be considered:

- Where the patient's condition indicates that CPR is unlikely to be successful
- Where CPR is not in accord with the wishes of a mentally competent patient
- Where successful CPR is likely to be followed by a length and quality of life that would not be in the best interests of the patient to sustain

The first criterion requires some judgement as to the likely success of CPR. Certain conditions, such as metastatic carcinoma, renal failure and stroke, are consistently associated with poor survival. Conversely, patients who arrest after a myocardial infarction tend to do very well. The circumstances and nature of the cardiac arrest are also important determinants of outcome. Death, often preceded by a long stay in an intensive care unit, and survival with neurological or cognitive deficits are most likely in patients whose arrest is unwitnessed, who have a rhythm other than a ventricular tachyarrhythmia or who require prolonged resuscitation.

If you believe that the patient's chances of survival are very low, does it follow that writing a DNR order without discussing it with him or her or their relatives is acceptable? In the USA, agreement by the patient or surrogate decision maker or an advance directive are required before a DNR order can be written. The more paternalistic approach previously common in European countries may no longer be acceptable to patients. The recent revision of resuscitation guidelines from the British Royal College of Physicians effectively eliminates the unilateral writing of DNR orders. Some authors have recommended that CPR may be withheld if the clinician judges that it would be 'futile'. However, there is considerable controversy about how to define 'futility' and about the validity of the concept.

If DNR orders are to be discussed, with whom and how should this be performed? Studies in Britain and Ireland show that many patients have clear preferences regarding CPR, and that relatives, like doctors, are not very good at predicting those preferences. It is also now clear that the individual is the best judge of his or her own quality of life. Many doctors are uncomfortable about discussing CPR with patients and feel that it may give rise to unnecessary distress or lead to unrealistic demands. There are difficulties when discussing such issues with acutely ill or anxious patients or when there is cognitive impairment, but many patients are able to participate in decision-making. Patients' views, while initially influenced by unrealistic survival rates on television shows, change with education about the likely success rate.

Open discussion of end-of-life issues does not have to involve an explicit offer of a choice that one believes to be illusory. While most patients want their doctors to discuss plans for resuscitation with them, they do not necessarily wish to make the final decision themselves, and it is important that doctors offer active guidance in this matter.

Tube feeding in end-stage dementia

End-of-life issues become important in patients with advanced dementia. Poor oral intake, perhaps related to swallowing problems and aspiration, and weight loss become increasingly common. This may lead to consideration of tube feeding. Although this might seem to have the potential to be a major ethical problem, the existing evidence is that tube feeding is not effective in achieving its aims in patients with severe dementia. Thus, there is no evidence that tube feeding prolongs life, decreases aspiration pneumonia, improves functional status, decreases infections or pressure sores, or increases comfort. Instead, it may increase discomfort, result in complications (including death), decrease enjoyment of food and lead to increased restraint use. Hence a decision to withhold such interventions is a medical rather than an ethical decision.

Truth disclosure

Surveys have found that most patients in Western countries wish to know about a diagnosis of cancer, although there is considerable within- and between-culture diversity. More recently recognised as a significant issue in this regard is the disclosure of a diagnosis of Alzheimer's disease, a more difficult decision because of the presence, by definition, of cognitive deficits.

A recent Irish study was consistent with previous studies in showing that older people want to be told about a diagnosis such as cancer even though their relatives often wish the diagnosis to be withheld. While the intentions of relatives who ask doctors not to tell patients they have cancer are undoubtedly good, the detrimental consequences of the subsequent 'conspiracy of silence' are well known. Moreover, advance consultation with the relatives of competent patients violates the patients' rights to confidentiality. Almost a quarter of patients in the Irish study did not want relatives told automatically of the diagnosis by the doctor.

A significant minority of patients in many studies report that they would not like to be told about bad news such as cancer. It is important to attempt to identify patients who do not want bad news, but it is unacceptable that the desire to protect such patients should lead to a lack of candour with the majority who do want to know. One approach may be to ascertain patient preferences regarding bad news before investigations are performed, although preferences may change with the clinical situation. A common approach to this problem is to wait until patients ask about cancer before revealing the diagnosis. However, it is not always true that patients who want more information will ask for it.

These arguments do not eliminate the need for sensitivity when discussing bad news with patients. Special care is often needed in older patients, because the high prevalence of cognitive and communication disorders may make the transmission and processing of information more difficult. However, while it is appropriate to allow people to explore and assimilate information at their own pace, truth-telling should be the usual practice with older as well as younger patients.

Consent and competence

Some of the most difficult ethical problems in clinical practice arise from a conflict between patients' wishes (autonomy) and what is deemed to be in their best interests (beneficence). One critical issue in such cases is whether the patient is truly autonomous, that is whether they possess the competence (or decision-making capacity) to make decisions about their own care. Similar concerns may arise when considering the validity of informed consent, for example prior to surgical interventions.

'Competence' can be defined as a state in which a patient's decision-making capacity is sufficiently intact for their decisions to be respected. There are a

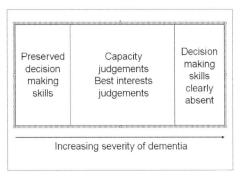

Figure 2: A schematic representation of the relationship between dementia severity and decision-making capacity

number of general legal and ethical maxims that are widely accepted in Western societies:
- Incompetence is related to but not the same as impaired mental status. The latter should not create an automatic presumption of incompetence
- Incompetence refers to functional deficits. Thus, cognitive deficits are only important if they interfere with decision-making
- Incompetence is situation-dependent. It depends not only on a person's abilities but also on the match or mismatch between the patients' abilities and the decision making demands of the situation that the patient faces
- Competence depends on the consequences of a decision. If a patient refuses a treatment that is very beneficial and carries little risk, the threshold for declaring him or her incompetent would be relatively low
- A person's level of competence can change even over a short period of time, for example in those with delirium due to acute illness

Abilities that are critically related to competence include: the ability to express a choice; the ability to understand information relevant to treatment choice; the ability to appreciate the significance of this information for one's own situation; and the ability to reason with relevant information in order to weigh up different treatment options.

It is important not to label decisions that you disagree with as due to faulty reasoning when they may simply arise from different priorities. Many clearly competent older people state that they would rather die than go into a home. For example, in a recent study, 80% of elderly women surveyed would rather be dead than experience the loss of independence and quality of life that results from a bad hip fracture and subsequent admission to a nursing home. This view reflects personal factors such as whether one is a risk taker or risk averse.

It is important to try to view the situation and the benefits and risks of a given course of action from the perspective of the patient. Health care professionals often regard safety and duration of life as synonymous with welfare. This is not true. Quality of life is as important to many people as duration of life. It is unlikely that admitting someone to extended nursing care against their wishes will enhance their quality of life, particularly, as often happens, if the change in environment leads to worsening of cognitive function and to use of sedative medications.

Elder abuse

Elder abuse can be defined as a single or repeated act or lack of appropriate action occurring within any relationship where there is an expectation of trust which causes harm or distress to an older person. Although there has been an increasing awareness in recent decades that a significant minority of older people are sometimes abused, neglected or mistreated, much abuse remains hidden whether in the home or in care settings. Forms of abuse include:
• Physical abuse (infliction of physical pain or injury, physical coercion)
• Physical (or chemical) restraint
• Psychological abuse (infliction of mental anguish)
• Material or financial abuse (the illegal or improper exploitation and/or use of funds or resources)
• Sexual abuse
• Neglect (refusal or failure to undertake a caretaking obligation)

Abused older people commonly suffer from physical or mental frailty. It is generally accepted that the poor and women are more vulnerable to elder abuse. Risk factors for abuse among carers include mental illness, social isolation and misuse of alcohol. However, people of all socio-economic, ethnic and religious backgrounds are vulnerable to abuse. Recognition of abuse is often difficult, and a high index of suspicion is needed when there are unexplained physical, psychological or financial problems.

In Ireland, there has been a major advertising campaign to highlight the issue of elder abuse, and investigation and intervention in this area has been greatly improved by the appointment of elder abuse officers in most parts of the country in recent years.

Irish considerations

There are major gaps at present in how Irish law deals with people who have limited capacity. Patients with early dementia often have sufficient competence to make a valid Enduring Power of Attorney (EPA). This allows patients to determine who they would prefer to administer their affairs when they become incapable themselves. However, an EPA does not deal with health care decisions. If there is no EPA and an incompetent patient has significant assets, it may be necessary to make the patient a Ward of Court. This is a sometimes costly and slow process and again is unsuitable for dealing with most healthcare decisions.

The Law Reform Commission (LRC) issued an important report on this subject in 2006 (Figure 3), and it seems likely that their recommendations will be enshrined in law within the near future. The LRC recognises several important principles discussed earlier: a presumption of capacity, even if there is a diagnosis of dementia; the need for a statutory definition of capacity that focuses on respecting remaining cognitive abilities and on a 'functional' test of a person's ability to deal with particular decisions; and that adults are free to make what others regard as poor or eccentric decisions provided that they understand the nature of the decision they are making.

The Irish Medical Council has an important regulatory and advisory role in guiding ethics and professional conduct in Ireland. The current Ethical Guide strongly supports the principles of respecting patient autonomy.

Making decisions in real life

Dealing with ethical problems is often more demanding and stressful for doctors and patients than dealing with medical problems. Adequate time should be allowed for discussions and to give people a chance to consider often complex information and to seek clarification if necessary. All relevant details of a case should be sought and considered before reaching a decision. Seeking a second opinion from an experienced colleague is often helpful when you are uncertain about the best course of action and is also invaluable when there is serious conflict with patients or relatives. Careful documentation of discussions and of the reasons and reasoning behind any decisions is also needed in such cases.

This chapter has emphasised the principles-based approach to ethical reasoning. This approach to ethics is extremely useful, but it may give rise to the illusion that a simplistic cookbook approach (a generous helping of autonomy, a sprinkling of beneficence, etc) will suffice when making ethical decisions. We all decide and discuss ethical issues in our daily life without any special jargon like 'autonomy' and 'beneficence'. Thus, while looking at principles sometimes helps with analysis of dilemmas, their use will not necessarily improve our ethical reasoning. It is also always important to take individual circumstances into account. Deciding that 'autonomy' trumps all other considerations in all circumstances is not a satisfactory or realistic approach. Instead, these principles merely serve as a starting point for consideration of the individual case and individual circumstances. Others have noted the importance of moral virtues, including compassion, honesty and trustworthiness, to the proper practice of medicine. Cultivation of such virtues will also help us to reach the right decisions in difficult cases.

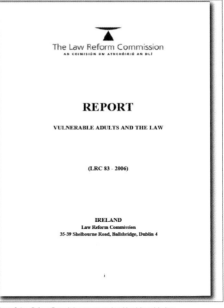

Figure 3. Law Reform Commission report on vulnerable adults and the law

Suggested further reading

- Law Reform Commission. Vulnerable adults and the law. http://www.lawreform.ie/VulnerableAdultsReport FinalDec2006
- Medical Council. A Guide to Ethical Conduct and Behaviour 6th Edition http://www.medicalcouncil.ie/_fileupload/standards/Ethical_Guide_6th_Edition
- A joint statement from the British Medical Association, the Resuscitation Council (UK) and the Royal College of Nursing. Decisions relating to cardiopulmonary resuscitation. October 2007 http://www.bma.org.uk/ap.nsf/AttachmentsByTitle/PDFCPRDecisions07/$FILE/DecisionsRelatingResusReport
- Keating DT, Nayeem K, Gilmartin JJ, O'Keeffe ST. Advance directives for truth disclosure. Chest 2005 http://www.chestjournal.org/cgi/content/full/128/2/1037
- Hoffer et al. Tube feeding in advanced dementia: the metabolic perspective. BMJ 2006 http://www.bmj.com/cgi/content/full/333/7580/1214
- Flegel KM, MacDonald N. Decision-making capacity in an age of control. CMAJ. 2008 http://www.cmaj.ca/cgi/content/full/178/2/127
- Doyal L. Informed consent: moral necessity or illusion? Qual Health Care. 2001 http://qshc.bmj.com/cgi/content/full/10/suppl_1/i29

Case Study 1

Mrs W is an 83 year old woman who has been admitted for the third time in 6 months with a chest infection and an exacerbation of her severe chronic airways disease. Even at her best, she is short of breath at rest and struggles to manage at home alone. The nurses ask you to write a do-not-resuscitate order.

Because of her acute illness, general frailty and significant comorbidity, it is judged that Mrs W has a low chance of surviving to discharge in the event of a cardiac arrest. It is also felt that it might prove difficult to get her off a ventilator if this intervention were required. Mrs W is a competent adult, and the issue of resuscitation is discussed with her. She regards her own quality of life as satisfactory despite her limitations and would prefer to live than to die but would not like to end up receiving prolonged ventilation. It is agreed that a limited DNR order is appropriate in which she would be defibrillated if she had a witnessed arrest due to ventricular tachycardia or fibrillation, but that intubation would not be performed in any circumstances.

Case Study 2

Mr S has severe Alzheimer's disease and is bedridden. Nurses on the long-stay unit where he has lived for the last 3 years report that he has lost a lot of weight in recent weeks and that he tends to cough and choke when taking fluids. Bedside swallow assessment confirms that he is prone to aspirating fluids. He looks cachectic. The issue of inserting a percutaneous gastrostomy (PEG) feeding tube is raised.

Based on the absence of evidence of any benefit associated with parenteral feeding in patients with late stage dementia, it was decided that PEG insertion would not be indicated. The family were informed that life expectancy would be very limited and it was agreed that CPR should not be attempted and that antibiotic therapy should be withheld unless judged necessary for patient comfort.

Case Study 3

Mrs F has lost a lot of weight in recent months. She is a heavy smoker and a chest X-ray shows a suspicious mass. You are on your way to discuss bronchoscopy with her when you are waylaid by her daughters who insist that she should not be informed about your suspicion of cancer. They state that she has always been an anxious person and this knowledge would inevitably cause her unnecessary distress.

You politely explain to the relatives the general principle that you cannot discuss their mother's care with them without her permission. You thank them for informing you about her tendency to anxiety and note that you will ask her whether she would wish to hear of bad or worrying news and, if so, whether she would like her daughters present during any such discussions. Mrs F does indeed want to know the results of her tests and asks that her daughters are present. They, despite continued unhappiness about your management of this issue, prove helpful during discussions of the pros and cons of chemotherapy for the lung cancer that is eventually diagnosed.

Case Study 4

Mr S, an 82 year old man with mild cognitive impairment and severe disability from arthritis wishes to go home to live alone after a recent admission following a fall. Family and community health staff believe he cannot cope and that they will not be able to provide the level of support he requires. A home visit confirms that he will be at great risk of falling again, with the potential for serious injury.

The undoubted risks of living alone were discussed with Mr S. He clearly appreciated and accepted that he would be at risk of falling and having a long lie on the floor before help would arrive. He was not willing to consider extended nursing home care because he was 'a very private person' and because of his experiences with nursing homes as a visitor on many occasions. He agreed to get a personal alarm and to make the changes to his home recommended by the hospital therapists. It was decided that he was competent to make his own decision, and that, in any event, this seemed the best management option for Mr S given his personal views.

Data Interpretation

Question 1

An 80 year old man with known advanced Alzheimer's disease is unable to swallow food and only takes sips of water. He refuses to take fluids with thickeners added and has had several pneumonias.

a. How should this situation be addressed with the patient and his family?
b. What is the appropriate management?

Question 2

An 85-year-old lady has a metastatic breast neoplasm and has been informed by her oncologist that further chemotherapy will provide no benefit in terms of survival or improving her symptoms. She develops severe heart failure which is unresponsive to treatment. She is bedbound and hoist dependent. She is well orientated and wants no further treatment if she develops a pneumonia or other intercurrent illnesses.

a. How should this situation be assessed with the patient?
b. What is the appropriate management?

Best of five questions

Question 1

You perform a preoperative assessment on a 75-year-old woman with a fractured hip. She was diagnosed with early Alzheimer's disease a few months earlier. Cognitive function seems unchanged since then with a MMSE of 22 and good insight into her current problem. She is medically well and was independent prior to her fall. A few hours later, the surgeon contacts you for advice because the hip surgery is now due to begin but the patient's daughter will not sign the consent form. You advise:

a. The surgeon should seek another member of family to sign the consent form
b. The patient should be made a Ward of Court before the operation can proceed
c. The operation should be cancelled indefinitely, under protest
d. The patient's consent to proceed should be sought
e. The operation should proceed irrespective of the patient's or of the daughter's view

Question 2

An 80-year-old man with severe Alzheimer's disease has had several admissions to hospital with chest infections and dehydration in the last few months. He has a history of COPD and does not seem to be aspirating. When well, he potters around the unit and seems cheerful although he does not communicate verbally. Staff in the long-stay unit where he resides suggest that his quality of life is poor and that he should not be admitted to hospital when he gets the next chest infection. When you raise the subject with them, three of his children agree, and one is adamantly opposed to this proposal. The best approach is:

a. The views of the nursing staff and of the majority of his family should apply and a do-not-hospitalise order should be written
b. In view of the family disagreement, the patient should be made a Ward of Court and the Court should determine the appropriate response
c. A quiet arrangement not to admit the patient to hospital should be made with the nursing staff
d. Make no decision, and arrange to have further discussions when and if future illness arises, depending on the patient's condition at that time
e. Arrange a further meeting with the dissenting family member, and offer to obtain a second binding medical opinion

Question 3

An 80-year-old man presents with haematemesis, weight loss and anaemia. He has no cognitive impairment. He is told that gastroscopy is required, and a simple explanation of the risks, benefits and alternatives to the procedure is provided. When approached on the morning of the procedure, he obviously understands the information provided and agrees to have the gastroscopy. However, he refuses to sign the 'consent form', stating that he does not like signing things. You decide to:

a. Document your discussion and his refusal to sign the form and ask the endoscopist to proceed with the gastroscopy
b. Cancel the gastroscopy and book a barium meal
c. Defer the gastroscopy and seek a psychiatric opinion regarding his capacity
d. Contact a family member and ask them to sign the consent form instead
e. Contact the hospital solicitors for advice

Answers on page 311

Infectious diseases

F McSweeney, M Horgan

Introduction

In view of the significant morbidity and mortality associated with infectious diseases in older people, prompt recognition and appropriate initiation of antimicrobial therapy is critical. Frequently, however, there may be a failure to recognise the presence of infection in this group due to an absence of the classic symptoms and signs of infection. There is often blunting of the febrile response and an absence of localising signs. As a result, infections may present with non-specific symptoms such as acute confusional states, behavioural changes, incontinence and falls. Failure to recognise these subtle clinical manifestations can lead to crucial delays in intervention and worse overall outcomes.

There is a natural decline in immune function with ageing and this is further compounded by reduced mobility, malnutrition, polypharmacy, institutionalisation and an increased frequency of admissions to hospital. The risks of infection are increased due to underlying comorbidities such as stroke, diabetes and malignancies and older people are particularly vulnerable to the rising incidence of nosocomial infections.

This chapter will discuss the changes that occur in the immune system with age, common infections in older people and the treatment challenges that these present. Issues relating to nosocomial infections, vaccinations and the increasingly pertinent issue of human immunodeficiency virus infection in the ageing population will also be addressed.

Immunosenescence

Immunosenescence refers to the decline in the immune system that occurs with age. This manifests as an increased incidence of both bacterial and viral infections, poorer outcomes from infection with respiratory viruses such as influenza and an increased incidence of malignancy.

The innate immune system is made up of local barriers, secretions, cytokines, complement and cellular components that have no antigen specificity. Important alterations in this system occur with advancing age that can enhance susceptibility to infection. An impaired swallow reflex and defective mucociliary clearance mechanisms may contribute to the risk of pneumonia and intestinal mucosal changes have been implicated in the development of infectious diarrhoea.

Changes also occur in adaptive immunity with T cells and B cells most affected by ageing. Aged T cells produce less interleukin-2, express lower levels of interleukin-2 receptors and proliferate less than young T cells. There is a shift from naïve to memory T cells resulting in a poorer response to certain antigens. Further age-related changes in adaptive immunity include thymic involution, decreased generation of naïve T cells, a reduced T cell repertoire for foreign antigens, altered peripheral blood T cell subsets and the distortion of repertoire antigen driven oligoclonal expansion.

There is an increased incidence in the reactivation of infections in older people, including varicella zoster virus (in the form of shingles) and tuberculosis, which is possibly attributable to a decline in the production of tumour necrosis factor by macrophages.

Vaccination in older people

Immunisation forms an important part of the strategy for the prevention of infection in older people. It is recommended that the annual influenza vaccine should be administered to all persons over the age of 50 years and their carers and healthcare workers. Several studies have observed that repeated vaccinations increase the protective levels of antibody and the development of cellular immunity to the influenza virus. The pneumococcal vaccine is recommended every five years in those over the age of 65 years but should be repeated if the patient was less than 65 on the last occasion it was administered. Alterations in formulations of certain pneumococcal vaccines are thought to overcome the age-related decline in responsiveness.

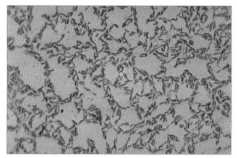

Figure 1: Bacteroides

Indwelling catheter use

The use of indwelling urinary catheters is the leading cause of complicated urinary tract infections and gram-negative bacteraemias in older patients. Uro-sepsis accounts for about 40% of life-threatening septicaemias. A progressive increase in mortality has been shown to be independently associated with the duration of catheterisation. Polymicrobial bacteriuria is common. Urease-producing bacteria lead to encrusted and blocked catheters. The routine use of indwelling catheters should be avoided and healthcare workers should remove catheters when no longer needed and endeavour to develop alternative methods for care of incontinence. Non-invasive methods should be employed to measure urine output and improve urine drainage systems.

Microbial colonisation in the elderly

Older patients residing in long term care facilities are more often colonised with resistant gram-negative organisms. Poor dentition and sub-optimal oral hygiene increase bacterial load and the potential for colonisation of the oral cavity. Particular attention should be paid to oral hygiene in older patients to decrease this bacterial load. Substance P is increased by oral care and has been shown to have a role in both cough and swallow mechanisms.

Skin and soft tissue infections

The integrity and physiology of the skin change with age, conferring additional predisposition to skin infections such as cellulitis, erysipelas and scabies. There is a loss of collagen and the dermo-epidermal junction is flattened making it easier to break the integrity of skin barriers. The epidermal renewal time increases from twenty days in younger people to thirty days in older people and this, coupled with the reduction in collagen synthesis, leads to impaired wound healing. Drying of the stratum corneum can cause older patients to scratch their skin, once again predisposing to infections.

Extrinsic factors in combination with the aforementioned skin changes may lead to the development of pressure ulcers in older people. Common complications of pressure ulcers include cellulitis of the surrounding area, contiguous osteomyelitis of the nearest bony prominences and bacteraemia. Organisms that are frequently implicated include Proteus mirabilis (19%), Staphylococcus aureus (16%), Bacteroides fragilis (16%) and Group A streptococci (10%). It is vital to suspect concomitant underlying osteomyelitis, especially with deeper pressure sores, as the management differs. Staphylococcus aureus is commonly found in extremity ulcers and faecal flora, such as Bacteroides fragilis, may be found in sacral and perianal ulcers in addition to Staphylococcus aureus. Plain x-rays, MRI and radioisotope bone scans can be used to investigate possible underlying osteomyelitis. Infected pressure ulcers are usually polymicrobial and swabs should be sent for culture and sensitivity along with sterile blood cultures. Antibiotic therapy should cover gram positive, gram negative and anaerobic organisms.

Pyrexia of unknown origin

Petersdorf and Beeson defined pyrexia of unknown origin (PUO) in 1961 according to the following criteria:
- A temperature greater than 38.3°C on several occasions
- Accompanied by more than 3 weeks of illness
- Failure to reach a diagnosis after 1 week of inpatient investigation

Studies of adults estimate the overall prevalence of PUO in hospitalised patients to be 2.9% but distinct data is lacking on the aetiology of PUO in patients over 65 years. Numerous studies confirm that approximately 20% to 30% of older patients will not mount a robust fever response to infection. A definition of PUO that includes a temperature of 38.3°C may not, therefore, be applicable to older patients and it has been suggested, that the definition of pyrexia in this group should be changed. As baseline temperatures have been found to be lower in frail nursing home patients, a fever may be considered to be present if there is a change in temperature over baseline of 1.3°C or more.

A precise diagnosis can be made in most (over 70%) older persons with PUO, whereas up to 51%

TABLE I	
AETIOLOGY OF PYREXIA OF UNKNOWN ORIGIN	
Endocarditis	Inflammatory
Intra-abdominal/pelvic abscess	Carcinoma
Tuberculosis	Lymphoma
Epstein Barr virus	Alcoholic cirrhosis
Cytomegalovirus	Drug fever
Brucellosis	Crohn's disease
Q fever	Subacute thyroiditis
Whipple's disease	Venous
	thromboembolism

TABLE 2
INVESTIGATIONS TO CONSIDER FOR PUO
Full blood count
Liver/renal function tests
Thyroid function tests
Erythrocyte sedimentation rate, C reactive protein
Rheumatoid factor, antinuclear and anti-neutrophil
cytoplasmic antibodies
Viral/atypical pneumonia screen
Monospot
Human immunodeficiency virus antibody test
Tumour markers
Urine, sputum, stool, blood, CSF cultures
Chest x-ray
Mantoux test, sputum and gastric aspirate staining for
tuberculosis
Ultrasound
Echocardiography
Computerised tomography
Magnetic resonance imaging
Labeled white cell scan
Temporal artery biopsy
Liver biopsy
Bone marrow aspirate/biopsy
Skin biopsy
Fluorodeoxyglucose Positron Emission Tomography
(FDG-PET)

of adults of all ages with PUO remain undiagnosed despite extensive work-up. The aetiology of PUO (table 1) differs considerably with advancing age. Older patents are more likely to have infectious (such as tuberculosis or abscess), inflammatory non-infectious (such as polymyalgia rheumatica) and neoplastic causes than younger people.

Tuberculosis is more common in older patients with fever. Although the classic presentation with fever, haemoptysis and a positive response to a Mantoux test may not be evident in frail older patients, they are more likely to have disseminated disease. A new or changing murmur should raise suspicion regarding the possibility of infective endocarditis and multiple blood cultures and transoesophageal echocardiography should be considered. It is also important to consider human immunodeficiency virus infection in older people as 10% of cases occur in patients over the age of fifty.

Important inflammatory causes of fever that are more pertinent in the older patient include polymyalgia rheumatica, temporal arteritis, rheumatoid arthritis and polyarteritis nodosa. Patients with a thickened temporal artery, an erythrocyte sedimentation rate >50mm/hour or suggestive symptoms should be considered for prompt temporal artery biopsy.

Drug fevers are a frequently overlooked cause of PUO and should be suspected when patients are on potentially sensitising medications, such as sulfa-containing diuretics or stool softeners, anti-arrhythmics, hypnotics, analgesics, antipsychotics, anticonvulsants and narcotics. Antibiotics commonly associated with drug fever include the beta-lactams and the antimicrobials with a sulfa component.

Drug fever is a diagnosis of exclusion. PUO patients with an elevated erythrocyte sedimentation rate, relative bradycardia, mildly elevated serum transaminases and eosinophils or atypical lymphocytes in the peripheral smear are likely to have drug fever. The diagnosis is confirmed by discontinuing the sensitising medication.

The diagnostic approach to PUO should begin with a thorough history with particular attention paid to the following;
• Recent subtle clinical or functional changes
• Detailed medication history
• Animal or occupational exposures
• Travel history
• Implanted devices eg. valve replacements, pacemakers

Physical examinations should be repeated at regular intervals with particular attention paid to dentition, temporal arteries, skin integrity and the cardiovascular examination.

Investigations that may be of use for patients with PUO are outlined in table 2. Empirical treatment with antibiotics is not advised if the patient is stable but if the clinical suspicion for temporal arteritis is high, steroid treatment should be considered even before histological confirmation.

Clostridium difficile associated diarrhoea

Clostridium difficile associated diarrhoea is the most common cause of diarrhoea following antibiotic treatment. It has been implicated as the causative organism in 10 - 15% of patients with antibiotic associated diarrhoea , 50-75% of those with antibiotic associated colitis and 90 - 100% of those with pseudomembranous colitis. Clostridium difficile is a gram positive, spore-forming rod that is an obligate anaerobe. It is a commensal bacterium in 3 - 5% of the healthy adult population but the carriage in hospital in-patients reaches 16 - 35%. The percentage is proportional to the duration of hospital stay and increases with exposure to antibiotics.

Antibiotics cause disruption of normal flora leading to proliferation of Clostridium difficile while toxin A, toxin B and the binary toxin may contribute to diarrhoea. The main risk factors for infection are:

• Antibiotic use
• Older age
• Co-morbidities
• Hospitalisation
• Immunosuppression
• Chemotherapy
• Proton Pump Inhibitor use within preceding 8 weeks

The antibiotics most commonly associated with Clostridium difficile are outlined in table 3. Historically the most frequently implicated antibiotics were ampicillin, cephalosporins and clindamycin. Currently, a higher risk is associated with the third generation cephalosporins and quinolones than with penicillins and beta lactamase inhibitor combinations. Interestingly, there have been cases of Clostridium difficile associated diarrhoea associated with vancomycin and metronidazole that are used to treat the infection.

Symptoms vary with the severity of the disease with mild infections manifested by cramping lower abdominal pain. Moderate to severe colitis can present with profuse diarrhoea, abdominal distension and occult colonic bleeding. Patients often have systemic upset with fever, nausea and anorexia. When the disease primarily affects the right colon and caecum there may be an absence of diarrhoea. Fulminant colitis has been reported in 1% to 3% of patients, leading to ileus, toxic megacolon, perforation, and death. Chronic diarrhoea and hypoalbuminaemia with anasarca can occur while polyarticular reactive arthritis has also been described. As a result, Clostridium difficile associated diarrhea is associated with substantial mortality, being nearly 20% in the first month after diagnosis and 27% after 3 months.

Although early reports advocated simple cessation of the offending antibiotic, sufferers today tend to be more debilitated and to have received more intensive antibiotic therapy than in the past, suggesting that an even smaller proportion than originally reported might respond to this measure alone. In the hospital setting, delaying the initiation of antibiotic therapy for Clostridium difficile associated diarrhoea prolongs the period of contagion. Traditionally, the infection is treated with oral metronidazole or oral vancomycin. Initial therapy with ten days of oral

TABLE 3
ANTIBIOTICS MOST COMMONLY ASSOCIATED WITH CLOSTRIDIUM DIFFICILE

Common	Less common	Rare
Clindamycin	Sulphonamides	Aminoglycosides
Ampicillin	Trimethoprim	Metronidazole
Cephalosporins	Co-trimoxazole	Teicoplanin
Amoxycillin	Quinolones	Rifampicin

metronidazole was previously recommended with subsequent switch to vancomycin if there was a failure or recurrence of diarrhoea. Metronidazole was initially favoured because of the lower cost and due to concerns regarding the emergence of vancomycin resistant enterococcus. It has been recently recognised, however, that there is a lower success rate with metronidazole with 25% failing to respond to two weeks of treatment and a further 25% relapsing within two months. As a result, oral vancomycin is now favoured in moderate to severe cases. Early surgical review is recommended if there is clinical suspicion of ileus.

Nitazoxanide (an antiprotozoal agent), rifaximin, or OPT-80 may become acceptable alternatives if approved for such use, and might be preferred because of the desire to avoid vancomycin in the hospital environment. Intravenous immunoglobulin contains Clostridium difficile antitoxin and has been used in some patients with relapsing or severe colitis.

Probiotic preparations with lactobacilli, bifidobacteria, and streptococcus species have been evaluated for the prevention or treatment of diarrhoea associated with antibiotic use and found to be safe. Several reviews support benefit but still call for large placebo-controlled trials to determine species and dose effectiveness for prevention, to show effectiveness in preventing diarrhoea caused by Clostridium difficile, and to establish cost effectiveness and the effect on length of hospital stay. A Cochrane review has concluded that as yet there is still insufficient evidence to recommend probiotic therapy as an adjunct to antibiotic therapy for Clostridium difficile colitis or to support the use of probiotics alone.

Gastric anti-secretory drugs have been associated with other forms of gastroenteritis such as Salmonella and Campylobacter infection. There has been a huge rise in the community prescription of proton pump inhibitors in older patients in recent years and proton pump inhibitor use within the preceding 8 weeks is associated with an increased risk of developing Clostridium difficile diarrhoea. Primary prevention with the judicious use of antibiotics and proton pump inhibitors in older people may help to reduce infection rates. In addition, as alcohol based hand gels are ineffective on Clostridium difficile spores, hand washing with soap and water and strict adherence to infection control measures are important.

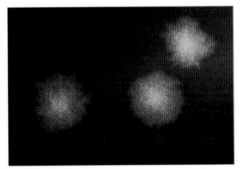

Figure 2. Clostridium difficile toxin

Viral gastroenteritis

Most cases of infectious diarrhoea in older patients are caused by viruses with norovirus, rotavirus and astrovirus identified as the main pathogens. Epidemic norovirus outbreaks occur frequently in institutions such as hospitals and long term care facilities. Norovirus is spread by the faeco-oral route and they are highly transmissible particles with an incubation period of 24 - 48 hours. Although norovirus infection has traditionally been referred to as the 'winter vomiting bug', there is no seasonal predilection for the transmission of this illness. Treatment is supportive with fluids to prevent volume depletion and monitoring for electrolyte disturbances.

Varicella zoster Infection

Primary infection with Varicella causes chicken pox in susceptible hosts and is usually a disease of childhood. Older age, immunocompromise and pregnancy are risk factors associated with a greater severity of primary infection, with mortality being highest in infants and in older people. Although infection may be more severe in immunocompromised patients, most cases of severe morbidity and mortality are seen in healthy people. Following recovery from the primary infection, latent infection is then established in the dorsal root ganglion.

Reactivation of the Varicella zoster virus is predominantly a disease of older individuals, with people over 60 years having an eight to ten-fold increased risk of infection. Waning cell-mediated immunity is thought to be a major factor in the increased incidence of herpes zoster in older people, given that antibody titres remain unchanged or may even increase with age.

Reactivation in later life presents with what is commonly termed 'shingles', derived from the

Latin word 'girdle'. Any level of the neuroaxis can be affected, but it tends to involve the cutaneous sites where the highest burden of lesions containing viral particles was present during chickenpox. In immunocompetent individuals, herpes zoster usually presents as a single episode and more than three recurrences is extremely rare. Infection usually manifests with a vesicular eruption occurring in a unilateral dermatome with crusting of the lesions within five days. Once the lesions are crusted over they are no longer infectious. Seventy five percent of patients experience prodromal pain and itching and post herpetic neuralgia is a distressing but usually self-limiting disorder. Occasionally there is an absence of skin signs but a rise in antibody titres, a condition known as zoster sine herpete.

Reactivation of the Varicella zoster virus may also be associated with central nervous system complications such as encephalitis, myelitis and focal vasculopathies. Zoster associated encephalitis typically presents with delerium within days following the vesicular eruption but occasionally it can precede the dermatological eruption and has also been described six months after an episode of shingles. The main risk factors for the development of zoster encephalitis include cranial or cervical dermatomal involvement and recurrent or disseminated reactivation. Myelitis is a rare complication and may present with paraparesis, impaired sensation at a level compatible with the dermatome of reactivation, and sphincter dysfunction. However, in most patients involvement of the spinal cord is subtle and asymptomatic and complete recovery is the norm.

Two clinicopathological entities have been delineated on the basis of the size of blood vessels that may be involved: large vessel unifocal granulomatous arteritis and small vessel multi-focal vasculopathy. The large vessel variety is mainly a disorder of older individuals where brain infarction may develop weeks to months following ipsilateral trigeminal zoster and is associated with a mortality of up to 25%. The cerebrospinal fluid may show mild lymphocytic pleocytosis, elevated protein, and occasionally oligoclonal bands. PCR is positive for Varicella zoster nucleic acid. Small vessel multifocal vasculopathy usually occurs in immunocompromised patients. Typically, it occurs without any skin lesions and consists of subacute multifocal neurological deficits accompanied by headache, fever, mental changes and seizures.

The risk of post herpetic neuralgia increases with age, and almost half of patients over 60 years who experience shingles will develop it, with immunocompromised patients being more susceptible.

Human Immunodeficiency Virus (HIV) infection in older patients

The term 'older patient with HIV' has traditionally described persons aged over fifty years. By the late 1980's approximately 10% of people with HIV were 50 years or older but the number of older adults with HIV is steadily rising. The United States Senate Special Committee on Ageing predicts that 50% of patients with HIV/AIDS will be over fifty years old by the year 2015. This trend is due to an improved survival rate with advances in treatment coupled with an increased pick up rate in this demographic group. Patients with HIV are living longer and older patients with HIV constitute a new treatment challenge in terms of the cumulative effects of ageing and antiretroviral therapy.

As with many other illnesses in older patients, the presentation of HIV may be subtle with flu-like symptoms, fatigue, weight loss and night sweats. Older patients may have symptoms similar to those of younger patients but are less likely to report their symptoms. More particularly, one large study found that they are less likely to report diarrhoea, white oral patches or sinus trouble compared with younger adults but more inclined to complain of neuropathic symptoms and weight loss. There is a similar spectrum of AIDS defining illnesses in older HIV infected patients with the five most common opportunistic infections being Pneumocystis jiroveci pneumonia, tuberculosis, Mycobacterium avium complex, Herpes zoster, and Cytomegalovirus. Some studies have observed an increased incidence of HIV encephalopathy and HIV wasting syndrome.

Although older patients may have similar opportunistic infections, in general, their prognosis is much worse, particularly when suffering from Pneumocystis jiroveci pneumonia or tuberculosis. This higher morbidity and mortality may be due to more rapid disease progression, a higher risk for systemic progression and the presence of co-morbidities.

Older adults have less HIV-1 replication that is independent of highly active retroviral therapy, drug compliance and disease stage. In addition, the duration of infection and age at sero-conversion are independently associated with a reduction in CD4 cell counts. Moreover, Centres for Disease Control surveillance data from 1996 to 2001 shows that people who are older at the time of HIV diagnosis are more likely to develop AIDS within 1 to 3 years than younger patients, possibly due to an impaired ability to replace functional T cells after T cell death.

Older patients have similar indications for the initiation of antiretroviral therapy, choices of antiretroviral medication, and goals of treatment to younger groups. Greater attention should be paid to the risks of adverse drug events and the potential for interactions and toxicity when in combination with other medications. Depressive symptoms and non-adherence to medications are each independent predictors of disease progression and mortality.

Suggested further reading

- Cohen and Powderly, Infectious Diseases Second Edition. Elsevier Publishers 2003. ISBN 9780323024075
- Robert M. Coleman, William E. Paul. Fundamental Immunology, Fifth Edition. 2004, Blackwell Publishing.
- Immunisation Guidelines for Ireland, National Immunisation Advisory Committee, Royal College of Physicians. 2008. (www.rcpi.ie.collegestructure/Pages/NationalImmunisationAdvisoryCommittee.aspx)
- Norman DC, Wong MB, Yoshikawa TT. Fever of Unknown Origin in Older Persons. Infectious Diseases Clinics of North America. 2007: 21; 937-945.
- Cluff LE, Johnson JE. Drug fever. Progr Allergy. 1969: 168; 41-51.
- Bartlett JG. Clostridium Difficile: clinical consideration. Rev Infect Dis. 1990: 12pp; S243 S251.
- Bartlett JG. Clinical Practise: Antibiotic associated diarrhoea. NEngl J Med 2002: 346; 334-3.
- Settle CD, Wilcox MH, Fawley WN, Corrado OJ, Hawkey PM. Prospective study of the risk of Clostridium difficile diarrhoea in elderly patients following treatment with cefotaxime or piperacillin-tazobactam. Aliment Pharmacol Ther. 1998; 1217-1223.
- Kelly CP, LaMont JT. Clostridium difficile infection. Ann Rev Med. 1998: 49; 375-390.
- Jacobs A, Barnard K, Fishel R et al. Extracolonic manifestations of Clostridium difficile infections. Presentation of 2 cases and review of the literature. Medicine (Baltimore). 2001: 80(2); 88-101.
- Veillard E, Guggenbuhl P, Bello S et al. Reactive oligoarthritis in a patient with Clostridium difficile pseudomembranous colitis. Review of the literature. Rev

Rhum Engl 1998: 65(12); 795-798.
- Musher DM, Aslam S. Treatment of Clostridium Difficile Colitis in the Critical Care Setting, Critical care Clinics- Volume 24, issue 2, 2008.
- Hickson M, D'Souza AL, Muthu N et al. Use of probiotic Lactobacillus preparation to prevent diarrhoea associated with antibiotics: randomised double blind placebo controlled trial. BMJ. 2007: 335: 80-83.
- Pillai A, Nelson RL. Probiotics for treatment of Clostridium difficile-associated colitis in adults. Cochrane Database of Systematic Reviews 2008, Issue 1. Art. No.: CD004611. DOI: 10.1002/14651858.CD004611.pub2
- Steiner I, Kennedy PGE, Pachner AR. The neurotropic herpes viruses: herpes simplex and varicella-zoster. Lancet Neurology. 2007: 6; 1015-1028.
- Soriano V, Castilla J, Gomez-Cano M et al. The decline in CD4+ T lymphocytes as a function of the duration of HIV infection, age at seroconversion, and viral load. J Infect 1998: 36; 307-311.

🗁 **Case Study 1**

A 78 year old man with hypertension and hypercholesterolaemia who was previously well presents with a five-day history of a painful vesicular eruption over his right temple. He takes Atenolol 50 mg and atorvastatin 10mg once daily. He is noted to be drowsy, confused and disoriented. On examination, the skin on the affected eye is erythematous with mild swelling. The lesions have begun to crust over. There is chemosis of the conjunctiva and an ipsilateral third nerve palsy. An abbreviated mental test score is 6 out of 10.

This man has herpes zoster ophthalmicus and his level of consciousness and mental state strongly suggest a complicating viral encephalitis. He should have a formal ophthalmology review and a CT or MRI scan of brain. If there is no contraindication, a lumbar puncture should be performed and cerebrospinal fluid sent for culture, cell counts, protein, glucose and viral PCR. Findings in cerebrospinal fluid suggestive of the diagnosis include a lymphocytosis, negative culture, elevated protein, normal glucose and a positive viral PCR for varicella. An electroencephalogram may show encephalopathic features. Treatment should be commenced with an intravenous antiviral agent such as acyclovir.

An 83 year old previously healthy woman presented to her general practitioner with symptoms consistent with an infective exacerbation of chronic obstructive pulmonary disease. She was commenced on a seven-day course of co-amoxiclav with good resolution of her respiratory symptoms. Three days after completing her antibiotic therapy, she complained of cramping lower abdominal pain and developed foul smelling diarrhoea a further two days later. The diarrhoea persisted despite the use of anti-diarrhoeal agents and she became progressively more debilitated, and dehydrated and was admitted to hospital.

The acute onset of diarrhoea in conjunction with a history of recent antibiotic use should raise suspicion of an antibiotic-related colitis. She should be isolated and commenced on intravenous fluids. Stool samples should be sent for Clostridium difficile toxin and culture for other bacterial pathogens. She should initially be treated with oral metronidazole 500mg three times daily for ten to fourteen days, but oral vancomycin 125mg four times daily can be considered an initial alternative for severe cases. Relapse or failure of primary treatment can be treated with oral vancomycin, with the option of doubling the dose or continuing extended therapy for 21 days. Intravenous immunoglobulin could be considered in resistant cases. Although solid evidence for efficacy is lacking, probiotic therapies are safe and could be considered.

Case Study 3

A 79 year old woman with a background of aortic and mitral valve replacements five years previously presents to her local casualty department with fever, chills, weight loss, arthralgia and myalgia. Two years previously she was diagnosed with infective endocarditis and treated successfully. Investigations included a normal chest radiograph, an elevated white cell count at 15.67x10⁹/l with 90% polymorphs, ESR of 88mm/hr and a c-reactive protein of 220. Six sets of blood cultures were taken in the first 48 hours of admission, three of which grew coagulase negative staphylococci of differing species. Trans-thoracic echocardiography was technically difficult due to her large body habitus and she declined a transoesophageal echocardiogram. Although no vegetations were seen, she was treated presumptively with Linezolid. After two weeks she

had failed to respond to treatment and throughout her stay she had a persistent low-grade pyrexia. She continued to complain of generalised aches and pains in the neck and shoulders but there was no synovitis and plain radiographs were normal.

The fact that three sets of blood cultures grew coagulase negative staphylococci of different species makes the likelihood of contamination high. Although a high index of suspicion needs to be maintained for bacterial endocarditis in this lady, alternative diagnoses should be sought for her symptoms and laboratory findings. Her presentation is consistent with a non-infectious inflammatory disorder and she should be questioned specifically regarding headache, jaw claudication and visual disturbances and her temporal arteries palpated to exclude temporal arteritis. Consideration should be given to a temporal artery biopsy. Even in the absence of findings suggestive of temporal arteritis, her presentation is compatible with polymyalgia rheumatica and consideration should be given to a trial of steroid therapy.

Data Interpretation

Question 1
A 72 year old lady with a background of alcohol dependency is brought by ambulance to hospital. Her public health nurse reports she has had a productive cough with copious amounts of dark green sputum for the past month. She has refused admission to hospital on numerous occasions. On examination she has clubbing, poor dentition and

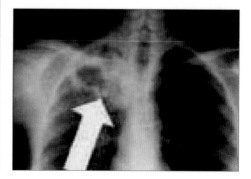

foul smelling breath. Lung examination reveals bronchial breathing in the right upper lobe.

a. Describe the abnormality on this chest radiograph
b. List the possible causes
c. How would you investigate the patient?

Question 2

A 66 year old retired Dutch gentleman presents to the Emergency Department following an episode of collapse with loss of consciousness. On further questioning he shows the admitting doctor that he has an unusual rash on his calf for the past three weeks. He also complains of sore throat, fevers, chills and arthralgia. He has conjunctivitis. On further history taking, he spends a lot of time hunting in the countryside. The rash is macular with central clearing. His blood test results are as follows:

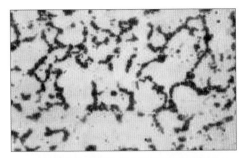

HB 11.2g/dl   Complement c3 and c4 normal
WCC 12.3x10⁹/l   Autoantibody screen negative
Lymphocytes 0.5x10⁹/l
ESR 67mm/hr
Urea 5 mmol/l
Creatinine 77umol/l
Alt 56U/l

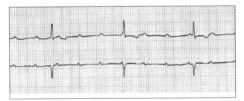

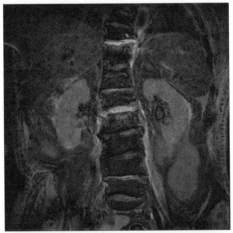

a. What is the name of the rash described?
b. Interpret the rhythm strip above
c. What is the unifying diagnosis?
d. What treatment would you give?
e. List three other potential complications

Question 3

A 79 year old gentleman with a background of severe rheumatoid arthritis and bilateral hip prostheses presents to his general practitioner with general malaise and hip and lower back pain. He is on long-term steroids but not taking any immuno-modulatory therapy. His doctor refers him immediately to the local hospital for treatment. On examination he is pyrexial with a temperature of 38°C. His blood white cell count is 26x10⁹/l, c-reactive protein 198 and ESR 99mm/hr. Blood cultures were performed and aerobic and anaerobic bottles grow the following organism:

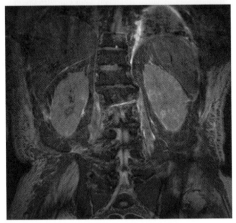

An MRI of thoraco-lumbar spine and MRI pelvis are undertaken.

a. What organism was grown from the blood culture bottles?
b. What antibiotics, if any, would you give?
c. Describe the MRI abnormalities

Best of five questions

Question 1

A 68 year old lady is transferred to the general ward following a six-week stay in the intensive care unit of a tertiary hospital following a perforated duodenal ulcer repair. She developed a severe ventilator associated pneumonia and gram-negative septicaemia. She required several courses of antibiotics and subsequently grew a fungal line infection. The physiotherapist who was attempting to mobilise the patient commented that her vision was very poor and the patient also reported some visual loss in her right eye which she attributed to losing her glasses. She is referred for urgent ophthalmological assessment. What is the most likely cause of this lady's visual symptoms?

a. Retinal detachment
b. Glaucoma
c. Candida endophthalmitis
d. Cataract
e. Anterior uveitis

Question 2

An 81 year old gentleman who resides in a nursing home has had 6 admissions with recurrent aspiration pneumonia following a stroke. He is admitted to hospital with drowsiness, fever and hypotension. He is diagnosed with urosepsis and responds well to initial treatment with ciprofloxacin. He develops foul smelling diarrhoea 6 days later. What is the most appropriate next step in your management?

a. Continue a ten-day course of ciprofloxacin and give intravenous vancomycin
b. Isolate the patient, discontinue the ciprofloxacin, send stool for Clostridium difficile toxin and commence oral metronidazole
c. Isolate the patient, discontinue ciprofloxacin and change to co-amoxiclav
d. Commence a fourteen-day course of oral vancomycin
e. Treat with oral metronidazole until the diarrhoea stops

Question 3

A 69 year old gentleman is brought to hospital by ambulance following a seizure. He has a pyrexia of 38.3°C with no rash, neck stiffness or photophobia. He is found to have a mild right hemiparesis and a transient expressive dysphasia. A non-contrast CT brain shows no evidence of intracranial bleeding, infarction or a space occupying lesion.

An MRI of brain shows abnormal signalling in both temporal lobes without any mass effect. A lumbar puncture is performed showing a normal opening pressure. Cerebrospinal fluid analysis demonstrates a white cell count of 12×10^9/l with 100% lymphocytes and glucose and protein within the normal range. What is the most probable underlying diagnosis?

a. Multifocal leukoencephalopathy
b. Herpes zoster encephalitis
c. Tuberculous meningitis
d. Multi-infarct disease
e. Herpes simplex encephalitis

Question 4

A 75 year old previously fit lady returns from an organised tour to Southeast Asia. Two days later she presents with bloody diarrhoea that resolves within forty-eight hours. What is the most likely cause?

a. Clostridium difficile
b. Norovirus
c. Amoebiasis
d. Diverticulitis
e. Campylobacter

Answers on page 311

Driving

D O'Neill

Driving: a 'basic' instrumental activity of daily living

Functional assessment is a core element of geriatric medicine. With the development of the specialty, an initial emphasis on assessment of basic activities of daily living has matured into increasing recognition of the importance of instrumental activities of daily living. This is particularly true of driving and other mobility issues: access to transportation is increasingly recognised as an important component of social inclusion and successful ageing: this increasingly means access to the private car. Maintaining social contacts, getting to appointments, access to health care and shopping are among the primary functions of driving in older age groups: 77% of drivers over the age of 55 perceive driving as essential or very important.

Lack of access to transportation is associated with reduced utilisation of health care, and driving cessation is associated with lifestyle losses, including lower life satisfaction, reduced role engagement, depression, restricted activity patterns as well as an increased risk of nursing home entry. Public transport has figured in some guides to geriatric care and is often mooted as a solution to the transportation needs of older people. However, older people do not consider that public transport is adequate or efficient, and it poses problems of security and convenience, as well as a higher risk of injury due to falls and instability; use of public transport by older people has been steadily declining in both Europe and the US, and the first longitudinal study on ageing (HESSOP-2) showed a decline in public transport use in rural areas of Ireland.

Older drivers: a growing population

Although we do not have Irish data, the proportion of older drivers is growing in the developed world. In the US in 2003, about 1 in 7 licensed drivers were 65 or older: by 2029, when the last of the baby-boomers turn 65, the proportion will be close to 1 in 4. One of the key questions about the ageing of the driving population is whether they add significantly to hazard on the roads.

Not only do older drivers have one of the best safety records of any group of drivers in society, but there is also evidence that newer and larger cohorts of older drivers have even better safety records. Sometimes a U-shaped curve is displayed showing that older drivers have a higher crash risk per mile than younger drivers do. This is spurious for several reasons. Not

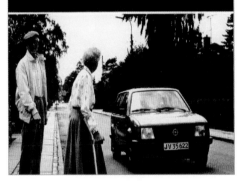

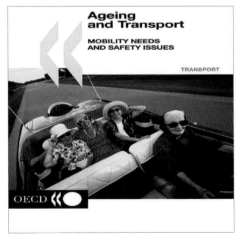

Figure 1: A pictorial representation of how attitudes have changed on older people and driving, with frail older people and safety issues predominating in 1985 and vibrant, energetic older people and a predominant emphasis on mobility in 2001. From OECD reports on older people and mobility

TABLE I
SAMPLE DISEASES FOR WHICH APPROPRIATE ASSESSMENT AND REMEDIATION MAY BE OF BENEFIT
Neuropsychiatric
Stroke
Parkinson's disease
Delirium
Depression
Mild Dementia
Cardiovascular
Syncope
Respiratory
Sleep apnoea
Vision
Cataract
Metabolic
Diabetes
Musculo-skeletal
All arthritides
Iatrogenic
Polypharmacy

only do they drive considerably less miles than their younger peers, but at least two studies have shown that this finding is an artefact of low mileage – if low mileage is controlled for in comparisons with younger drivers, the difference in crash rate disappears. Also, older people tend to drive on roads which are inherently more dangerous - rural and suburban highways are more dangerous than motorways. Finally, old people are more fragile and are more likely to suffer death or serious injury for a given severity of crash than young people are.

Unfortunately, however, the emphasis of many European governments, including Ireland, is to stigmatise older drivers. Older drivers are forced to undergo regular medical checks in most countries of the European Union, despite evidence that this practice is harmful or ineffective. This ageist legislation is not based on any factual evidence and reflects the weakness of organised advocacy for older people in Europe. Geriatricians need to explore and counteract such negative perceptions of older drivers.

Medical aspects: enabling strategies

The role of health in driving cessation demands that emphasis on negative rather than enabling aspects of medical fitness to drive needs to be challenged. Many illnesses present opportunities for interventions which directly or indirectly will improve driving safety and comfort (Table 1). A typical illness with potential for enabling is arthritis. Not only do patients experience many difficulties in driving, but there is also evidence to show that appropriate intervention may improve driving ability and comfort. Many patients do not return to driving after stroke, and rehabilitation and specialised driving re-education may return some of these to independence. Lack of an enabling strategy may negatively influence the relationship between physician and patient.

Skills and resources needed for assessment of fitness to drive

Many professionals working in geriatric medicine initially feel at a loss when confronted with older people who both have age-related illness and drive a car. They often do not realise that their many skills used in clinical decision-making also form the basis of making decisions on driving and mobility. These skills are founded in multidisciplinary assessment, an enabling philosophy and advocacy for older people in the face of nihilism and ageism. In practice the same skills are seen in the integration of clinical assessment and input from the multidisciplinary team in the calculation of risk in other areas of clinical practice such as deciding on discharge to home. Elements of the decision-making process include careful multidisciplinary evaluation, discussion with carers and perhaps a trial visit home.

The elements of this process are very similar to the assessment of fitness to drive. Not only may relatives place security before independence but also a psychometric model is not likely to be helpful. This often surprises clinicians: while psychometric support is important in backing up our diagnostic abilities, it is rarely of help when making decisions about function. For example, the decision that the patient is no longer fit to remain at home and requires placement in a nursing home is much more likely to be taken on the basis of measures of function and behaviour than on psychometric measures.

The premise that the expertise of those who practice geriatric medicine with older people already contains some of the elements necessary for mobility assessments is not a charter for dilettantism. Rather, it is a challenge to us to develop the extra resources required to ensure that we have adequate support when making decisions about enhancing the safe mobility of older people. This has many parallels

TABLE 2		
HIERARCHICAL SCHEME OF DRIVING ASSESSMENT		
LEVEL OF TASK PERFORMANCE		**LEVEL OF RISK**
Strategic		Accepting risk
Tactical		Taking risk
Operational		Dealing with acute danger

with the task of assessing safety at home or capacity to manage financial affairs: in these cases, it is good practice to liaise with an occupational therapist or a neuropsychologist.

At a minimum, the assessment of the impact of illness on mobility in later life requires a careful medical assessment, a collateral history and access to occupational therapy and/or neuropsychology as well as access to a specialist driver assessment. The latter is a *sine qua non* – this is the 'gold standard' of assessment and a number of agencies will assess drivers in Ireland. There may be a case for developing services at a regional level, particularly for those cases where decision-making is not clear after the first assessment. The geriatrician will also need to know the Irish regulations on fitness to drive (very minimalist at the moment, but under review), and be aware of the obligation of the patient to disclose relevant illness to their insurance company.

Models of driving behaviour

While the geriatrician is aided in the assessment and rehabilitation of problems with balance and gait by an understanding of the underlying mechanisms, driving is a complex task, and although there has been progress in developing comprehensive models of driving behaviour, they remain complex and in journals not often frequented by geriatricians. The most useful model for clinicians is a practical scheme with an emphasis on a hierarchy of strategic, tactical and operational factors (Table 2). Strategic performance includes the planning of choice of route, time of day (avoiding rush hour), or even the decision not to drive and to take public transport. Tactical decisions are those aspects of the driving style which are characteristic of the driver and are consciously or unconsciously adopted for a great range of reasons, eg.,decisions on whether or not to overtake, go through amber lights or signalling in good time before turning. Operational performance is the response to specific traffic situations, such as speed control, braking and

signalling. Driving a car requires organisation of action at and between all three levels.

Clinical assessment up to now has tended to dwell on deficiencies on the operational level, i.e. whether an illness affects the subject's appreciation of distracting stimuli or the reaction time to a hazardous situation. This emphasis is misguided: reaction time (a measure which is an integral part of operational tasks) is shortest in the 15 - 25 year age-group, the group with the highest accident rate. It is very likely that decisions at a strategic and a tactical level are much more important in causing accidents. Older drivers are known to use strategic and tactical measures widely to avoid delay, stress and risk by driving less at night and during bad weather, avoiding rush hours and unfamiliar routes, etc.

The application of these three levels of function can be of practical help in decision-making. This is illustrated by studies of drivers with acquired brain damage, particularly stroke. Evidence for impairment at all levels may be collected by discussion with patients and relatives as well as by clinical observation. At a strategic level we would look for evidence of inappropriate planning of trips or lack of selective use of cars. Poor planning, poor judgment, lack of insight and impulsivity affect both strategic and tactical levels. Impulsivity is attributed to disinhibition and/or cognitive impairment. Factors which interfere with the operational level include inadequate visual scanning of the environment, poor visual tracking, slowness in acting and confusion when more complex acts have to be carried out. Right hemisphere lesions seem to produce a more adverse effect on driving skills, possibly relating to visuo-spatial deficits and inattention.

Assessment

The uncertainties underlying models of driver behaviour also affect the art/science of risk assessment. It is better to live with uncertainty and a considered

TABLE 3	
SCHEDULE FOR DRIVING ASSESSMENT IN OLDER PEOPLE	
1	Take a driving/mobility history in all patients
2	Assess the primary impairment
3	Quantify comorbidities which could further reduce driving ability
4	Assess drug and alcohol use which could further reduce driving ability
5	Overall evaluation of potential for maximising driving performance
6	Rehabilitation strategies
7	Overall evaluation of hazard
	• Strategic
	• Tactical
	• Operational
8	If driving too hazardous, consider alternative mobility strategies

TABLE 4
CORE FEATURES OF OLDER DRIVER ASSESSMENT
History
Patient, family/informant
Driving history
Examination
Functional status
Medical illnesses and drugs
Vision
Mental status testing
In-depth cognitive/perceptual testing
On-road Assessment

individualised clinical approach rather than to prematurely adopt guidelines with apparent face validity. Risk assessment in older drivers is affected not only by our understanding of models of driving behaviour as well as by empirical studies of disease and crash risk but also by clinical attributes common to the assessment of function in older patients. A schedule for the assessment of older patients who drive is outlined in Table 3.

Inter-individual variability is extremely important and implies a case by case approach. Factors relating to age-related diseases include not only a different spectrum of illness to younger people, but also the presence of multiple illnesses. In any one patient, is it the arthritis, the dementia, the visual acuity or even the multiple medications which is affecting driving? Within the rubric of one illness there may be multiple influences on driving skills. For example, there is an increased risk of crashes with Parkinson's disease. The illness may involve problems of motor function, depression and impaired cognitive function. Rather than stating that Parkinson's disease is dangerous for driving, it is vital to take a phenomenological approach. The depression and the motor function must be treated, psychoactive medications minimized and cognitive function assessed and managed before any decisions are made about fitness to drive.

Interdisciplinary approach
An interdisciplinary approach is probably useful with emphasis on the physician, occupational therapist,

and if possible a specialised driving assessor. A social worker may be very helpful if driving is no longer permitted. However, while it is fair to say that no one (or indeed any) member of the team may be able to accurately predict driving safety, a team approach has been shown to improve general health, functional status and even driving status. A cascade of assessments is appropriate: many drivers can be classed as fit to drive, unfit to drive or appropriate for driver rehabilitation at a clinical assessment: on-road driving assessments should be reserved for when a patient does not clearly fall into one of these patterns.

Most reviews on driver assessment published since 1992 include a common core (Table 4). One of the most important final common pathways of concern in driving is cortical function, when disrupted by syncope, cognitive function, inattention, neglect or personality change. Perception is probably more important than vision. The relative ease of screening for cognitive dysfunction may conceal the difficulties of interpreting mild to moderate degrees of deficit: functional measures may be more important as a predictor of diminished driving skills. This has the useful effect of diverting attention from cognitive measures - easily measured but of uncertain value - to either functional or behavioural measures as surrogates for driving ability.

Clinicians must make an immediate decision on whether the patient is fit to continue driving whilst further assessment is arranged. All decisions and actions should be documented clearly in the patient's notes. For all progressive diseases, re-evaluation should occur regularly: for dementia, it is our practice to recommend a 6 monthly review. It is also important to advise patients and their families of the predicted decline in driving ability on an individual basis, although three years from when the disease becomes clinically obvious may be a reasonable group average. This allows patients to plan for the eventual cessation of driving and to develop alternative transport options. This process has been termed a *'modified Ulysses contract'*. Just as Ulysses bade his crew to tie him to the mast so that he would not succumb to the charms of the sirens, this contract begins the process of planning with the patient an eventual withdrawal from driving.

Risk assessment in dementia

Retrospective studies of dementia and driving from specialist dementia clinics tend to show a high risk, whereas those which are prospective and which look at the early stages of dementia show a less pronounced pattern of risk. In the first two years of dementia the risk approximates that of the general population. A recent systematic review shows that drivers with dementia are poorer drivers than cognitively normal drivers, but studies have not consistently demonstrated higher crash rates. Likely causes for this counter-intuitive finding include a lower annual mileage and restriction of driving by the patient, family and physicians.

These findings are important because many lay people (and some doctors!) assume that dementia is an absolute contra-indication to driving. Apart from the difficulties of diagnosis in the early stages of dementia, it is a heterogeneous condition and its effects on the driving task are complex. For example, deterioration in driving skills was a phenomenon of the early stages of dementia in 10% of the patients in one study. The decision therefore is a clinical one, preferably aided by a full history (including a collateral driving history), interdisciplinary assessment and possibly by an appropriate on-road test. An added factor which is helpful both in assessment and advice is the finding that drivers with dementia who drive accompanied have less crashes than those who drive alone.

Drugs and driving

The potential and actual effect of drugs on driving may be an important factor in the safe mobility of older people: somewhat surprisingly, there is almost no literature on the positive effects of medications! It is likely that medications modifying the impact of the arthritides, Parkinsonism or depression almost certainly increase driving ease and safety. On the negative side, the effect of alcohol is well

established although alcohol dependency is probably less common in older people. One difficulty with psychoactive medications is deciding on the relative contributions of a) the underlying disease severity, b) the medication and c) the altered pharmacokinetics and pharmacodynamics of ageing, to the increased risk of crashes associated with them. Another is agreeing on which drugs are in this classification. Ray et al quote a prevalence rate of 20 - 21% of psychoactive drug use among older drivers and non-drivers, but includes opioids, antihistamines and hypoglycaemics. In this study older tricyclic antidepressants and benzodiazepines were associated with a relative risk of 2.2 and 1.5 respectively for crash risk in older drivers, and there was no increased risk with opioids and antihistamines. These findings support avoidance of these agents where possible, but it is too early to say yet whether a switch from tricyclics to selective serotonin reuptake-inhibitors would be helpful in reducing medication associated morbidity. Any introduction or change in psychoactive medication should be accompanied by a warning not to drive until the patient has habituated to the effects of the medication.

When driving is no longer possible

The actual process of stopping driving, voluntarily or involuntarily, is not well documented. Healthcare professionals need to develop a better understanding of the dynamics of losing this critical capability as well as difficulties that they may experience in trying to alter mobility status. In the absence of cognitive impairment, one quarter of those who give up take account of advice from a physician (usually an ophthalmologist). Physicians are involved in the process of cessation in less than half of those who stop driving due to dementia.

With dementing illness, the decision to stop driving has been seen as an area of difficulty between patient and physician. To a certain extent, the way we deal with driving reflects how we help the patient to deal with the reality of the deficits caused by dementia. A more positive approach has been suggested whereby the issue of driving is treated as a part of a therapeutic programme. The feelings and fears of patients about giving up driving should be explored. The intervention is designed with the patient as collaborator rather than patient and by dealing with the events at an emotional rather than at an intellectual level. The patient must be able to grieve about the disease and in particular about the loss of his car. This in turn enables him to redirect his attention to other meaningful activities that did not involve driving. Although this approach may be hampered by the deficits of dementia, it reflects a more widespread trend towards sharing the diagnosis of dementia with the patient, and I invariably discuss the dementia diagnosis with those who drive.

The overall interdisciplinary assessment should attempt to provide solutions to both maintaining activities and exploring transport needs. The on-road test may be helpful as it may demonstrate deficits to a patient or carer who is ambiguous about the patient stopping driving. At a therapeutic level, members of the team may be able to help the patients come to terms with the losses associated with stopping driving. The occupational therapist may be able to maximize activities and function and help focus on preserved areas of achievement, while the social worker can advise on alternative methods of transport.

The provision of a system of alternative transport which meets the needs of older people who no longer drive is a challenge to society: conventional mass transit public transport is limited in its utility to this group. Tailored transport (paratransit) is expensive, but may have benefits in reducing institutionalization and in improving quality of life. Geriatricians have an advocacy role to ensure that public policy on transportation is developed to take account of the deficiencies of transit and paratransit systems. The Rural Transportation Scheme in Ireland has been a helpful development in this regard.

Future strategies for safe mobility
There is some evidence of a cohort effect reducing relative involvement of older drivers in crashes, as more experienced drivers reach their older years. Other areas of active research include:
• Developing technology to facilitate the driving task. These include alerting systems for somnolence, route guidance systems and speed and braking control systems for collision avoidance
• Improvement of highway systems, lighting and signs
• Training/retraining of older drivers. California has developed the Mature Driver Improvement Programme but analysis does not as yet support a significant effect

It will be important to nourish growing awareness of the importance of equitable access to transport for older people, a group whose mobility needs may increase rather than decrease with age and whose health and well-being will be diminished if that access is not granted.

Suggested further reading
• Drivers Medical Group. At a glance: Current medical standards of fitness to drive. www.dvla.gov.uk/media/pdf/medical/aagv1.pdf.
• Canadian Medical Association. Determining medical fitness to operate motor vehicles. www.cma.ca/index.cfm/ci_id/18223/la_id/1.htm.
• American Medical Association. Physician's Guide to Assessing and Counseling Older Drivers. American Medical Association, Chicago, 2004. Available on www.ama-assn.org/ama/pub/category/10791.html.
• Older people and transportation. Transportation Research Board. Transportation in an Aging Society: A Decade of Experience. Transportation Research Board, Washington DC, 2004. www.gulliver.trb.org/publications/conf/reports/cp_27.pdf.
• Organisation for Economic Co-operation and Development (OECD) Working Group ERS4. Ageing and Transport: Mobility Needs and Safety Issues. OECD, Paris 2001.
• Charlton JL, Koppel S, O'Hare M, Andrea D, Smith G, Khodr B, et al. Influence of chronic illness on crash involvement of motor vehicle drivers. Monash University Accident Research Centre Report No 213, April 2004. www.monash.edu/muarc/reports/muarc213.html.
• Hine J. Travel Demand Management and Social Exclusion. Mobilities 2007;2(1): 109 - 120.
• Oxley J, Whelan M. It cannot be all about safety: the benefits of prolonged mobility. Traffic Inj Prev 2008;9(4): 367-78.

📁 **Case Study 1**

A 69 year old man presents with Parkinson's disease, with significant bradykinesia and tremor, and reports slowing of thinking, although scoring 28/30 on the MMSE. He is on Sinemet 62.5mg BD. He also reports low mood, scoring 11/30 on the GDS. His wife reports a more cautious driving style, but no crashes or traffic violations.

Any clinical encounter involving assessment of driving should have an enabling focus, and not make a decision on fitness to drive until the patient is maximally treated. Not only is this patient reported to drive safely, but clearly has room for more intensive dopaminergic therapy. His driving skills are likely to be improved by increased pharmacological and non-pharmacological therapy. Depression is more challenging for driving safety than antidepressants, but caution is required not to exacerbate his Parkinsonism with an SSRI. The collateral from his wife is likely to be a good reflection of his driving abilities, but some caution is needed to ensure that she is not constrained by fear of transport problems if she is a non-driver. The MMSE, although crudely correlated with driving skills, is an insufficiently specific guide to cognitive fitness to drive in an individual patient, and does not reflect models of driving behaviour.

Case Study 2

Mr. Jones, 74 years old, has had Alzheimer's disease for 4 years, and is beginning to have difficulty managing the central heating and remote controls at home. His son reports more erratic driving, getting lost, and with more scrapes on his car. You suspect that he has not informed his insurance company or the licencing authority of his illness, despite repeated advice to do so.

In the first instance, all discussion on assessment and disclosure should be with the patient and family (and recorded in writing), and this will be facilitated by an early discussion about, and disclosure of, the diagnosis. Breaking of confidentiality should occur if a) there is concern that his driving represents a risk to other road users, and b) the patient and family cannot effect a cessation. In the Irish setting, a conversation with a senior police officer in the patient's local Garda station is probably the most effective option, and disclosure to the licencing authorities is recommended, but probably ineffective.

Case Study 3

A 65 year old driver presents to the outpatient clinic describing a thirty minute history of left upper and lower limb weakness with paraesthesiae which fully resolves. He also remembers hitting into things on the left hand side during the event. Clinical examination is normal. TIA workup is instigated.

The current advice for TIA is not to drive for a month. An ophthalmology assessment is not required if there are no residual symptoms. While all patients with stroke and TIA should be advised (and a written note kept of this advice) to inform their insurance company (otherwise their insurance may be void), the role of the RSA is not clear at this time. With full resolution of symptoms, no on-road assessment is needed.

Case Study 4

Mrs Smith is referred by her family doctor with a hemiparesis due to previous stroke. She had been driving an adapted vehicle quite safely, and with a clean accident record. Her presenting complaint is that of recurrent syncope over the previous three months, usually while standing up. You note that her medications include a long-acting benzodiazepine for several years, and a beta-blocker, and clinical examination reveals slow atrial fibrillation, an MMSE of 28 and a hemiparesis but little else of note.

Syncope is clearly a cause of concern for safe driving, and patients should be advised to stop driving until there has been a full assessment, treatment of aetiological factors and the patient's symptoms settled: there is no specific time frame for this, unlike some other conditions such as TIA. If she stops driving, she can await the final formulation and clearance from you before informing the insurance company, and then resuming driving. An on-road test is not required, as there is no clinical indication for one in terms of reduced driving skills when not suffering syncope. Long-acting benzodiazepines are the only medications consistently associated with a (modestly) increased crash risk in older people, but we do not know whether it is the underlying symptoms, the benzodiazepine dependency profile, or the medications which are at fault, and we do not know that stopping the medication improves the safety profile. However, it is a good point to discuss the benzodiazepine dependency with the patient, clarify whether or not other psychopathology is present (particularly anxiety/depression), and offer a detoxification regime and further assessment/treatment as required.

Data Interpretation

Question 1

A man suffers a stroke with mild left sided weakness. Three days later he has recovered all power in his limbs but he is bumping into objects on his left side especially in confined spaces.

a. What is the likely reason for his current symptoms and how would this be assessed?
b. How would the problem be formally assessed?
c. What are the implications for the man with regard to driving?

Question 2

A 70 year old woman has probable Alzheimer's disease but is functioning well with minimal assistance required from her husband. However when she drives to visit her sister one night she gets lost on the way home. She has had no other problems with driving. You are asked to assess her re continuation of driving.

a. How should she be assessed?
b.. What would be the advice given?

Question 3

An 80 year old fiercely independent lady has severe rheumatoid arthritis and has been discharged from hospital 3 weeks earlier following a right hemiparesis. She has marked deformity of her hands and an impaired grip in both hands but particularly affecting her right hand. She is adamant that she will continue to drive.

a. What is the appropriate initial advice?
b. What assessment is required before a definitive decision on driving?

Best of five questions

Question 1

A man with Parkinson's disease on low dose Levodopa and known depression is having difficulty driving. There have been no reported accidents. How should he be advised?

a. The severity of his Parkinson's disease and depression are such that he should not drive
b. His driving skills may be improved by modifying anti-Parkinsonian medications
c. Treatment of his depression may improve his driving skills
d. The report from his wife is not a reliable guide to his driving abilities
e. All of the above

Question 2

An older woman is losing items at home, has trouble with cooking and her driving has become hazardous and unpredictable. What is the correct advice for this lady?

a. Ask her relative to inform her insurance company
b. Try to modify treatment to improve her cognitive state
c. Discuss possible cessation with the lady and her son
d. Have an open discussion with the patient and family regarding her diagnosis
e. All of the above

Question 3

A man with a history of recent TIA enquires when he can drive again. What do you advise him to do?

a. To refrain from driving for six months
b. To undergo a formal ophthalmology review prior to return to driving
c. To inform his insurance company of the above and stop driving for one month
d. Reporting to the Road Safety Authority is required
e. An on road driving assessment is needed prior to returning to driving

Question 4

A patient with a history of recurrent blackouts attends the OPD. What advice should be given re driving?

a. Tell her to stop driving for one month
b. Inform her insurance company of her syncopes
c. Stop her benzodiazepine
d. Arrange for an on-road test
e. Tell her to stop driving until her diagnosis is clarified and dealt with

Answers on page 311

Oncology

MSN Mohd Sharial, B Bystricky, S O'Reilly

Introduction

The most significant risk factor for the development of cancer is increasing age. Over 50% of cancers are diagnosed in people over the age of 65 years and cancer represents a major cause of mortality in this population. By the year 2020, 60% of all malignancies will affect this age group. Unfortunately, there is a sobering under-representation of older patients in clinical trials and very few trials recruit patients over 85 years. As a consequence, there is a paucity of knowledge regarding how to best approach and treat older patients with cancer, a state of affairs that inadvertently leads to under-treatment. This problem is being slowly rectified by the International Society of Geriatric Oncology and the National Comprehensive Cancer Network who publish and update practice guidelines annually for senior adult oncology. In 2007, publishers of the Journal of Clinical Oncology and the European Journal of Cancer recognized this gap in oncology for older people and dedicated a special edition of each journal to highlighting significant advances made in the evaluation and treatment of older patients and the work that still needs to be done.

Comprehensive geriatric assessment in oncology

One of the main challenges in oncology for older people is the appropriate selection of patients who may benefit from specific therapeutic approaches. Comprehensive geriatric assessment (CGA) is an evaluation tool for frail older patients performed by multidisciplinary teams with the goal of forming a coordinated management plan. To benefit from a CGA, patients should be neither too fit nor terminally ill. A pilot study using CGA in older patients with breast cancer revealed, on average, 1.5 new medical problems per patient. As many as 10% of patients with good performance status (measured by the Eastern Cooperative Oncology Group scale) had limitations in activities of daily living and one third in instrumental activities of daily living. Over 10% of patients had more than two co-morbidities. CGA allows many previously unrecognised health

problems to be uncovered, including depressive symptoms, malnutrition and polypharmacy.

Results of several studies have highlighted the impact of instrumental activities of daily living and depressive symptoms on survival in cancer patients. Evaluation with CGA may, therefore, help to predict cancer related morbidity and mortality but this hypothesis needs to be addressed in a prospective fashion before definitive conclusions can be drawn. In addition, these data should prompt cooperative groups in oncology to integrate CGA into studies that include a high proportion of older patients and to test the impact of CGA-based interventions on outcome measures.

Multidisciplinary collaboration between geriatricians and oncologists represents the best method of assessing an older patient's health status and tumor burden and of devising an individualized treatment plan to address all problems that have been identified. A geriatric oncology task force has proposed that screening patients for vulnerability and frailty prior to CGA will best identify those most likely to benefit from the process. Several indices of vulnerability and frailty have been devised for screening in this clinical setting, but the Vulnerable Elders Survey-13 (VES-13) has been chosen for inclusion in the National Comprehensive Cancer Network guidelines.

The VES-13 consists of one question for age and 12 items assessing self-reported health, functional capacity and physical status. This self-administered survey stratifies older patients into three groups, namely non-frail, pre-frail and frail. Pre-frailty is diagnosed if one to two criteria are present and frailty if more then three criteria are present. The tool helps to identify fit older patients and prevent under-treatment in this group. In addition, the scale identifies frail patients who should then receive CGA with subsequent intervention and tailoring of cancer treatment based on the presence of geriatric syndromes (Figure 1).

All patients over the age of 70 years should have baseline cognitive screening as cognitive impairment

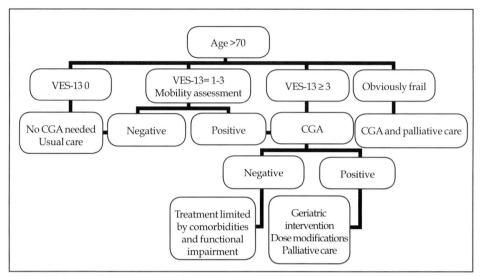

Figure 1: Algorithm for the assessment of older cancer patients using the Vulnerable Elders Survey-13 (adapted from Rodin et al)

increases mortality risk and can be exacerbated by chemotherapy. Comorbidity, polypharmacy, weight loss, body mass index, and reports of fatigue, weakness and exhaustion should be documented, as well as reports about falls or near falls. Dependence for activities of daily living is associated with poor survival rates and dependence for instrumental activities of daily living with poor chemotherapy tolerance. Effective communication with older patients is often complicated by problems such as deafness, reduced visual acuity and cognitive impairment. Older cancer patients also tend to ask less questions, show less proactive behaviour in discussing their cancer diagnosis and physicians tend to spend less time communicating with them.

Quality of life

Health-related quality of life measures assess physical and psychological health as well as social interactions and personal beliefs. Quality of life assessment is an important area of concern in the treatment of older patients, especially those undergoing palliative chemotherapy or radiotherapy. Older cancer patients regard the maintenance and improvement of quality of life as significant goals of cancer treatment.

A number of different questionnaires exist to assess quality of life in cancer patients, but the European Organization for Research and Treatment of Cancer questionnaire (EORTC-QLQ-C30) is the tool most

often used in European clinical trials (www.eortc.be). The validity of this questionnaire is high and has been translated into 81 languages. There are five functional scales, nine symptom scales, one scale to measure global health status and fifteen scales to cover other quality of life issues. Quality of life measurements have been shown to have prognostic significance. In a study of older patients with non-small cell lung cancer, quality of life was a predictor of survival, performance status, the number of metastatic sites and ability to perform instrumental activities of daily living. Another study in patients with colon cancer demonstrated that quality of life, as well as white blood cell count, alkaline phosphatase and metastatic sites, predicted survival.

Health related quality of life may be a primary or secondary end-point in clinical trials to assess the benefits and side effects of experimental drugs. A study of pain control in patients with hormone-refractory prostate cancer, for example, showed significant improvements in pain scores and quality of life in patients taking a combination of mitoxantrone and prednisone versus prednisone alone.

Lung cancer

Lung cancer is the most common cancer in the world and the leading cause of cancer related deaths in western countries. Non-small cell lung cancer constitutes between 80 and 85% of all lung cancer, with small cell lung cancer accounting for the remainder. At the time of diagnosis, the majority of patients already have metastatic disease and systematic palliative treatment is the primary therapeutic option. Over half of non-small cell lung cancers are diagnosed in patients older than 65 years of age with the median age at diagnosis being 70 years. Medical and physiological challenges in older patients and their exclusion from clinical trials render choice of the optimum treatment regime difficult. As a consequence, they are often under treated.

Non-small cell lung cancer

Patients with non-small cell lung cancer can be divided into three groups, namely those for whom potentially curative surgical resection is possible, those with locally advanced disease and those with advanced metastatic disease. Older patients who fulfil the common criteria of operability should be offered surgery (lobectomy or pneumonectomy) with curative intent. Recent trials have suggested that, following potentially curative resection, adjuvant chemotherapy should be offered to patients with stage 2 and 3A disease. Older patients were, however, poorly represented in these studies and the feasibility of cisplatin based chemotherapy in this group can be quite difficult. For patients with small, potentially curable tumours who are not candidates for surgery novel techniques such as stereotactic radiotherapy or radiofrequency ablation focused on the tumour have been used with durable long-term success.

In recent years there has been interest in the use of chemotherapy before surgery to reduce tumour bulk and facilitate potentially curative surgery. Such a strategy is attractive in an older population because pre-operative chemotherapy is generally safer than post-operative chemotherapy and may be more suited to this group. For patients with inoperable locally advanced non-small cell lung cancer that can be encompassed within a radiation field, several studies have shown an advantage in combining chemotherapy with radiation. Evidence from phase 3 studies suggests that fit older patients benefit from concurrent chemotherapy and daily radiation treatment. While such combined modality studies have demonstrated a survival advantage, careful patient selection is required as haematological and non-haematological toxicity are greater.

Unfortunately the majority of patients with non-small cell lung cancer will present with metastatic

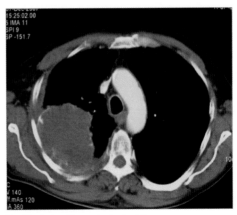

Figure 2: Locally advanced lung cancer invading adjacent rib

involvement. These patients represent a very heterogeneous group with varying comorbidities and disease-related symptoms due to metastatic involvement of the brain, adrenal glands, liver, lung and bone. The treatment needs of this patient group are highly individualised and may consist of palliative chemotherapy, palliative radiation treatment to painful bony sites or best supportive care. Care provision should be multidisciplinary with input from medical and radiation oncology and palliative and primary care. Patients with adequate performance status should be considered for combination platinum based chemotherapy. For frailer patients, single agent chemotherapy has demonstrated a survival advantage compared with no treatment in randomised trials. Novel agents which target genetic alterations in the cancer cell such as erlotinib, an epidermal growth receptor inhibitor, may be used as an alternative to cytotoxic chemotherapy or after first and second line treatment failure. This agent has been found to be well tolerated and has resulted in disease stabilisation in 40% of older patients with previously untreated non-small cell lung cancer.

For patients with metastatic or locally advanced disease, it is important to emphasise the beneficial palliative role of interventional pain management, thoracocentesis and pleurodesis and stent placement for patients with endobronchial tumours.

Small cell lung cancer

Small cell lung cancer accounts for approximately 15 to 20% of lung carcinomas, with chemotherapy forming the cornerstone of treatment. Limited stage disease (that is encompassable within a radiation port) is associated with a median survival time of about 12 to 16 months with a 4 to 5% long-term survival. In extensive stage disease, however, the median survival time is 7 to 11 months.

Small cell lung cancer has a high propensity for early dissemination to bone marrow, brain, liver and lung. The standard therapy for limited stage disease is a combination of chemotherapy and radiation, followed by radiotherapy to the brain as a prophylactic measure for patients with chemotherapy responsive disease. This combined modality approach is associated with increased toxicity but a greater survival benefit. In older populations, however, the addition of radiotherapy to chemotherapy must be carefully evaluated due to the potential for increased toxicity which may abrogate any survival advantage.

For patients with extensive stage small cell lung cancer, platinum based polychemotherapy alone is considered the standard of care. However, patients with responsive extensive stage disease should also be considered for prophylactic cranial radiation as approximately 80% will develop brain involvement. The use of chemotherapy must be tempered by concerns regarding treatment-related toxicity and the impact of comorbidities on tolerance. As in patients with non-small cell lung cancer, management should be multidisciplinary in nature.

Superior vena cava syndrome

Superior vena cava syndrome results from the obstruction of blood flow through the superior vena cava. Lung cancer, especially of small cell type, is the underlying process in approximately 70% of patients with the syndrome, but other known causes include syphilis, tuberculosis, lymphomas and intravascular devices. Dyspnoea is the most common symptom observed, but patients may also present with facial swelling, head fullness, cough, arm swelling, chest pain, dysphagia, orthopnoea, distorted vision, hoarseness, stridor, headache, nasal stuffiness, nausea, and light-headedness.

Physical examination often reveals venous distension of the neck and chest wall, facial and upper extremity oedema, mental changes, plethora, cyanosis, papilloedema, stupor, and even coma. Pemberton's sign is frequently positive. Superior vena cava syndrome may be diagnosed clinically, but chest radiography, CT and MRI are of value in more subtle presentations.

Management of the syndrome includes the relief of symptoms and identification of the underlying cause if it is not yet established. Simple measures such as elevation of the head of the bed and supplemental oxygen can provide significant improvements in symptoms. Corticosteroids and diuretic therapy are often used in complicated cases. Radiotherapy may be effective in superior vena cava syndrome due to malignancy and surgical bypass and superior vena cava stenting may be useful palliative measures in carefully selected patients. When the syndrome is due to thrombus around a central venous catheter, patients may be treated with fibrinolytic or anticoagulant therapy and removal of the catheter. The prognosis of patients with superior vena cava syndrome is dependent upon the course of the underlying illness.

Breast cancer

Although breast cancer is extremely common in older women, there is significant evidence that they are less likely to receive standard care for their disease. Patients presenting with breast cancer can be divided into those with early stage disease, those with locally advanced breast cancer and those with metastatic breast cancer.

For patients with early stage disease, prompt multidisciplinary appraisal in a dedicated breast unit is the gold standard of care. Evaluation should involve surgical assessment, mammography (supplemented if necessary by ultrasound) and tissue diagnosis using a core biopsy. Assessment is followed by appropriate breast conserving surgery or mastectomy with axillary node biopsy and/or axillary clearance. Non-randomised studies published in the early 1980's suggested that hormone therapy with tamoxifen was as effective as surgery for the primary treatment of operable breast cancer in older patients and that tamoxifen could be employed instead of surgery for most patients. Subsequent studies, however, have demonstrated that survival times and progression rates are worse in women treated with tamoxifen alone and a retrospective review of the Geneva Cancer Registry on the prognostic impact of refusing surgery has shown a greater than two-fold increased risk of dying from breast cancer in women who refuse surgery compared to those who consent.

For patients who have breast conserving surgery, or those who are at high risk of local recurrence following mastectomy, radiotherapy will reduce recurrence rates. Ongoing randomised studies are evaluating whether radiotherapy is needed in all patients and whether there may be a subgroup of patients with low risk disease who may be cured with surgery alone. Following curative surgery, adjuvant therapy should be considered for all patients. The relative benefits of adjuvant hormone therapy and chemotherapy in this setting can be calculated using an online web calculator www.adjuvantonline.com. This instrument incorporates patient age, grade and size of tumour, nodal involvement, hormone responsiveness and medical comorbidities to estimate the benefit of adjuvant treatment in this setting. The majority of older patients will have potentially endocrine responsive disease and a minority will have tumours that are hormone insensitive but which may benefit from adjuvant chemotherapy.

For patients with inoperable locally advanced tumours that remain localised to the breast area, a variety of strategies can be pursued once histological confirmation of malignancy has been confirmed and hormone studies have been performed. Consideration may be given to hormone therapy alone, radiation treatment or neoadjuvant chemotherapy with tumour down-staging followed by surgery and subsequent radiotherapy. The management of such patients can be clinically challenging due to problems such as skin ulceration and arm lymphoedema.

Patients who have metastatic disease at presentation, or develop metastatic disease as a consequence of a previously diagnosed early stage lesion, should be offered a multidisciplinary management plan incorporating palliative care and medical, radiation and surgical oncology. Palliative radiotherapy may be administered to painful bony sites and bisphosphonate therapy initiated to reduce the risk of skeletal events and prevent hypercalcaemia. Careful attention should be paid to weight-bearing bones and joints and the potential benefit of orthopaedic evaluation and intervention should be considered. Patients with hormone-sensitive disease may benefit from sequential hormonal therapy followed ultimately by chemotherapy. Intermittent courses of single agent chemotherapy are used for patients with hormone insensitive tumours.

Lymphoma
One half of patients newly diagnosed with lymphoma are over 65 years of age and a significant number are older than 80 years. Non-Hodgkin's lymphoma is more common in older patients than Hodgkin's lymphoma, as 80-90% of patients with Hodgkin's lymphoma are younger than 60 years old.

Non –Hodgkin's lymphoma (NHL)
Although very few differences have been described for morphological and clinical presentations between young and older patients with NHL, the outcome is worse in older patients. This may be at least partly explained by physiological declines in immune function, renal clearance, hepatic metabolism and functional reserves which impact on the choice of optimal lymphoma therapy. Until recently, older patients were considered too frail to receive standard treatment and were treated with low-dose regimens. Recent studies however have concluded that older patients treated with an optimal chemotherapy regimens have improved survival rates. There are nearly 40 subtypes of NHL. The diffuse large B-cell lymphoma subtype is of particular relevance to older people, however, as cure is possible if appropriate first-line therapy can be administered.

The evaluation of patients with lymphoma should include clinical examination, CT scan of the body, full blood counts, bone marrow biopsy, lactate dehydrogenase and β2-microglobulin levels. The Ann Arbor staging classification for NHL has proved to be inappropriate for older patients and prognosis is better described by the International Prognostic Index than stage. This index uses age (younger or older than 60 years), performance status, disease stage, lactate dehydrogenase level and the number of extranodal sites to define four risk categories ranging from low risk to high risk. As the International Prognostic Index is of more relevance for aggressive lymphoma, a separate index, the Follicular Lymphoma International Prognostic Index, has been described for patients with follicular lymphoma.

The presence of comorbidities that will impact on treatment-related mortality and toxicity should be properly evaluated. Older patients often have alterations in the absorption, activation, distribution, metabolism and clearance of drugs which increase the risks of haematological toxicity and febrile neutropaenia in those treated with curative intent. The currently accepted standard of care for diffuse large B-cell lymphoma is a combination of cyclophosphamide, doxorubicin, vincristine, prednisolone and rituximab (CHOP-R) administered every 21 days for six to eight cycles. A dilemma exists, however, as to which lymphoma

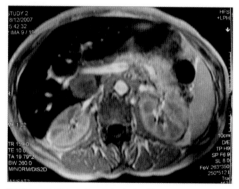

Figure 3: Iron oxide MRI showing liver metastases in colorectal cancer

subdiaphragmatic localization, mixed cellularity histology and Epstein-Barr virus infection, all of which are associated with poor outcome.

Survival rates have been disappointing in older patients in an otherwise highly curable disease. The German Hodgkin's Study Group study evaluated standard dose bleomycin, etoposide, doxorubicin, cyclophosphamide, vincristine, procarbazine and prednisolone in patients older than 60 years, demonstrating increased toxicity without any improvement in outcome over cyclophosphamide, vincristine, procarbazine and prednisolone or doxorubicin, bleomycin, vinblastine, and dacarbazine.

subtypes in older patients should be considered for these potentially curable regimes and which subtypes should be treated with less toxic, though ultimately less effective, options. In making this decision, consideration should be given to age-related factors including frailty, comorbidity and diminished organ function which may compromise ability to tolerate therapy.

The American Society of Clinical Oncology and the European Organisation for Research and Treatment of Cancer have developed guidelines for using granulocyte colony-stimulating factor (G-CSF) to prevent infectious complications in cancer patients. Both societies and the National Comprehensive Cancer Network consider age to be a risk factor for infectious complications and recommend the use of G-CSF in older patients treated with curative intent where the risk of febrile neutropaenia is more than 20%. In making assessments for therapy, comprehensive geriatric assessment tools or the Karnoffsky/Eastern Cooperative Oncology Group performance status can be useful, though more sensitive and user-friendly tools are needed.

Hodgkin's lymphoma (HL)

Despite being typically a disease of younger patients, 10-20% of patients with HL are older than 60 years. In HL, age older than 60 years doubles the risk of relapse and death. Although the International Prognostic Index is used to categorize risk, adverse risk factors are not balanced and increase proportionally in patients older than 60 years in comparison to NHL. Older patients with HL often present with aggressive disease, characterised by symptomatic and advanced-stage disease,

Colorectal cancer

Colorectal cancer is the third most common malignancy (excluding non-melanoma skin cancer) with 2184 new cases diagnosed in 2005 in Ireland alone. The median age at diagnosis is 72 years, emphasizing the importance of providing optimal care for older patients with the disease. A full comprehensive history and physical examination, coupled with necessary laboratory and radiological investigations are important for correct staging and determining suitability for treatment. Carcinoembryonic antigen (CEA) measurement is useful to monitor disease activity after surgery or during treatment. Particular details should be taken to assess end-organ function and comorbidities which may increase the risk of toxicity and decrease the tolerance of chemotherapy.

Surgical resection of the primary tumour, whenever possible, is the only possibility for cure. Neoadjuvant chemoradiotherapy followed by curative resection for rectal cancer has been shown to reduce local recurrence without increasing postoperative complications such as pneumonia and cardiac problems. Adjuvant chemotherapy is now routinely offered to patients with stage III colon cancer and stage II or III rectal cancers as multiagent therapy after removal of the primary tumour improves the overall 3-year survival from approximately 50% to 73%. Active cytotoxic agents include fluorouracil, leucovorin, and oxaliplatin which are used in combination.

Comprehensive geriatric assessment is of critical importance in order to optimize the risk-benefit ratio of treatments for older patients. In metastatic disease, the benefit of chemotherapy is also compelling because colorectal cancer survival without treatment is only 6 months but exceeds 24 months with optimal therapy. The use of approved biologic agents such as bevacizumab, cetuximab and panitumumab should be used with caution, even in fit older patients. There is an increased risk of arterial thromboembolism associated with bevacizumab in patients older than 65 years with a prior history of myocardial infarction or stroke. More data are needed to quantify the activity and toxicity of these agents.

Prostate cancer

Approximately 70% of newly diagnosed prostate cancer patients are over 65 years of age. Due to its prevalence in older people and often indolent nature, the importance of adequately assessing comorbidities and performing comprehensive geriatric assessment before radical treatment cannot be overemphasized. The efficacy of any treatment for patients with limited life expectancy is often difficult to assess because many are likely to die from causes unrelated to prostate cancer.

Early prostate cancer

Epidemiologic data from the United States indicate that 15-37% of PSA-detected prostate cancer might have never presented clinically within the patient's life-time. It has generally been considered that definitive treatments such as radical prostatectomy or radiotherapy should only be offered to patients who are expected to live a minimum of 10 years. Large observational studies, also from the United States, suggest a 30% survival benefit during 12 years after diagnosis for men with early-stage prostate cancer who undergo radical prostatectomy or radiotherapy when compared with no active treatment. In addition, there is no significant difference in 10-year survival after curative radiotherapy in older (70-75 years) versus younger patients. This benefit is not affected by lower performance status in the elderly.

New radiotherapy methods, such as intensity modulated radiotherapy, spare healthy tissues while delivering effective treatment and minimising the acute and late effects of radiotherapy. Treatment with radiation and surgery, however, can still be associated with urinary and bowel symptoms and sexual dysfunction. On the other hand, patients who undergo so called 'watchful waiting' can develop obstructive urinary symptoms or develop metastatic disease with local symptomatology. Primary

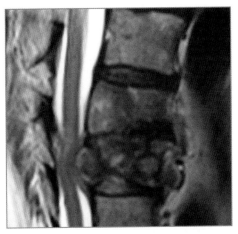

Figure 4: Spinal cord compression from bone metastases complicating prostate cancer

androgen deprivation therapy (with LHRH analogs) is not a definitive treatment, and is not associated with improved survival among the majority of elderly men with localized prostate cancer when compared with conservative management.

Advanced prostate cancer

Japanese research results indicate that the presence of advanced prostate cancer negatively influences the survival of older patients, suggesting that patients with advanced-stage prostate cancer need treatment regardless of age. These studies, however, did not include performance status, a potentially important prognostic indicator, in the multivariate analysis. Androgen deprivation reduces symptoms in 70-80% of patients with advanced prostate cancer, but most tumours progress within 2 years to an incurable androgen-independent state. Docetaxel chemotherapy (usually given in combination with prednisolone) has become the established standard of care for patients with hormone-refractory disease.

Prostate cancer can present initially with bony pain or with neurological symptoms from spinal cord compression. This represents an oncological emergency and must be managed without delay to prevent irreversible loss of neurological function. MRI is considered the gold standard imaging modality for assessing spinal metastatic disease. For patients who are not on hormonal treatment, bicalutamide should be initiated for a few days prior to adding LHRH analog therapy to prevent tumour flare and deterioration of spinal cord compression.

Dexamethasone is the mainstay of pharmacologic therapy for pain associated with vertebral metastases with tapering of doses during radiotherapy treatment. Bisphosphonates may reduce the risk of pathologic fracture and relieve local pain secondary to bony lesions. Radiotherapy is central to the palliative treatment of spinal metastases, assisting in pain management and helping to prevent vertebral collapse and further progression of neurological dysfunction. It is usually administered over a 10-14 day period, but single fractions have also been used with good effect. Radiotherapy is the treatment of choice in diffuse multilevel spinal involvement. Surgical decompression with vertebral stabilisation remains a valid therapeutic approach, especially when rapid neurological deterioration or spinal instability is present.

Conclusion

The high and rising incidence and prevalence of cancer in older people present significant challenges. Non-Hodgkin's lymphoma and ovarian cancer are associated with a poor prognosis in this group, whereas lung and breast cancer usually run a more indolent course. The challenge of managing older patients with cancer is to balance the benefits of treatments such as chemotherapy, radiotherapy and surgery with the risks of treatment-related toxicity in a vulnerable host. For cancer medicine, the development of more effective treatments must be matched by a focus on reducing treatment-related toxicity, improving the evidence base on which decisions are based and preventing ageism from causing suboptimal treatment of those who may gain significantly from anticancer therapy.

Suggested further reading

- Lichtman et al. Geriatric Oncology: A Field Coming of Age. J Clin Oncol. 2007;25: 1821-1823.
- Repetto L et al. Comprehensive Geriatric Assessment adds information to Eastern Cooperative Oncology Group performance status in elderly cancer patients: an Italian Group for Geriatric Oncology Study. J Clin Oncol 2002; 20: 494–502.
- Mass et al. Comprehensive Geriatric Assessment and its clinical impact in oncology. Eur J Cancer 2007; 43: 2161-2169.
- NCCN Clinical Practice Guidelines in Oncology: Senior Adult Oncology. V2.2007, 02/06/2007.
- Rodin M et al. A Practical Approach to Geriatric Assessment in Oncology. J Clin Oncol 2007; 25: 1936-1944.
- Wedding et al. Quality-of-life in elderly patients with cancer: A short review. Eur J Cancer 2007; 43: 2203-2210.
- Tannock et al. Chemotherapy with mitoxantrone plus prednisone or prednisone alone for symptomatic hormone-resistant prostate cancer: a Canadian randomized trial with palliative end points. J Clin Oncol. 1996 Jun;14(6): 1756-64.
- Gridelli C et al. Lung Cancer in the Elderly. J Clin Oncol 2007.25: 1898-1907.
- Crivellari D et al. Breast Cancer in the Elderly. J Clin Oncol 2007. 25: 1882-1890.
- The Non-Hodgkin's Lymphoma Classification Project: Effect of age on the characteristics and clinical behaviour of non-Hodgkin's lymphoma patients. Ann Oncol. 1997;8: 973-978.
- Coiffier B. What treatment for elderly patients with aggressive lymphoma? Ann Oncol. 1994;5: 873-875.
- The International Non-Hodgkin's Lymphoma Prognostic Factors Project: A predictive model for aggressive non-Hodgkin's lymphoma. N Engl J Med. 1993; 329: 987-994.
- Solal-Celigny P, Roy P, Colombat P, et al. Follicular lymphoma international prognostic index. Blood. 2004; 104: 1258-1265.
- Aapro MS, Cameron DA, Pettengell R, et al. EORTC guidelines for the use of granulocyte-colony stimulating factor to reduce the incidence of chemotherapy-induced febrile neutropaenia in adult patients with lymphomas and solid tumours. Eur J Cancer. 2006; 42: 2433-2453.
- Engert A, Ballova V, Haverkamp H, et al. Hodgkin's lymphoma in elderly patients: A comprehensive retrospective analysis from the German Hodgkin's Study Group. J Clin Oncol. 2005; 23: 5052-5060.
- National Cancer Registry Ireland. Cancer in Ireland 1994-2005 a summary.
- Sanoff HK, Bleiberg H, Goldberg RM. Managing older patients with colorectal cancer. J Clin Oncol. 2007; 25: 1891-1897.
- Horiot J-C. Radiation Therapy and the Geriatric Oncology Patient. J Clin Oncol 25; 1930-1935, 2007.
- Lu-Yao GL et al. Survival following primary androgen deprivation therapy among men with localized prostate cancer. JAMA 300; 173-81, 2008.
- Wong Y-N et al. Survival Associated With Treatment vs Observation of Localized Prostate Cancer in Elderly Men. JAMA 2006: 296; 2683-2693.

Case Study 1

A 71 year old female with a history of Barrett's oesophagus is referred by her general practitioner with a two month history of worsening dysphagia, heartburn and weight loss. Her last oesophago-gastroscopy was 5 years ago. Her medications include omeprazole and diclofenac, the latter having been started recently following a road traffic accident.

Although it sounds like diclofenac might be responsible for this lady's symptoms, one has to be alarmed about the presence of weight loss. The history of Barrett's oesophagus which is a pre-cancerous condition should also be taken seriously. These patients should be followed up with regular endoscopies, depending on whether there is dysplasia present or not and this patient was either lost to follow up or has defaulted. Initial investigation in this lady should include a full blood count with haematinics which will highlight any anaemia. Endoscopy is the gold-standard investigation of choice. If there is proven malignancy after biopsy, further investigation should be done including endoscopic luminal ultrasonography, staging computed tomography and staging laparoscopy if warranted. The treatment options are either surgery, neoadjuvant chemotherapy followed by surgery or definitive chemoradiotherapy. The management plan will depend on the extent of the disease and the decision should ideally be made at a multidisciplinary meeting. If malignancy is not detected, stopping diclofenac is warranted with high dose proton pump inhibitor treatment and regular follow up endoscopy (6 months to 1 year depending on whether dysplasia is present).

Case Study 2

A 76 year old man presented to the Accident and Emergency department with a 1 day history of urinary retention. This was preceded by urinary incontinence over the previous 5 days. On further questioning, he also had faecal incontinence. His medication included bicalutamide, leuprorelin acetate injection which is given by his general practitioner every 3 months, diclofenac for back pain and lansoprazole.

The clue to this man's diagnosis lies in his medication. These include bicalutamide and leuprorelin acetate injection for the treatment of prostate cancer. Another clue is that he is also taking diclofenac for back pain. The combination of urinary retention, urinary incontinence, faecal incontinence and back pain in a patient with prostate cancer strongly suggests acute spinal cord compression. This patient should undergo a full neurological examination including a rectal examination to assess for anal tone. Cauda equina syndrome is a manifestation of spinal cord compression below the conus medullaris and often presents with back pain, incontinence of urine or stool, or occasionally saddle paraesthesiae. The investigation of choice is Magnetic Resonance Imaging (MRI) of the spine. If spinal cord compression is suspected, high dose dexamethasone should be started empirically as neurological deficits are irreversible. The treatment of choice is either surgery or external beam radiotherapy, depending on location and whether there are multiple or single levels of compression.

Case Study 3

A 69 year old man was brought to the Accident and Emergency department by his daughter with acute confusion. He recently completed palliative chemotherapy for metastatic lung carcinoma. According to his daughter, he was complaining of chest pain over the previous 3 days and had been taking more than the usual number of painkillers. On arrival, his Glasgow Coma Scale was 12/15. He had pinpoint pupils and also appeared to have occasional myoclonic jerks.

This patient is probably opioid toxic. Other considerations are metastatic disease involving the brain, but the presence of pinpoint pupils and myoclonic jerks with a history of overconsumption of analgesia would point towards the former diagnosis. Chest wall pain from direct extension of lung cancer is quite common and often difficult to manage, and requires a multidisciplinary approach with input from a palliative care team, pain team and an attending oncologist. A combination of opioids, neuropathic agents, paracetamol and non-steroidal anti-inflammatory drugs is often used but there is a delicate balance between optimal pain control and side effects. In the above case, for example, even though the patient is opioid toxic, stopping opioids abruptly or reversing the effects with naloxone will cause rebound pain and withdrawal symptoms which can be distressing. His opioid requirement needs to be adjusted slowly and the simplest way is to convert his oral opioid to a subcutaneous infusion given over 24 hours. This will give the treating physician full control of his opioid requirement which can be adjusted easily.

Opioids are mainly renally excreted and renal function should be checked because impaired renal function will reduce systemic opioid clearance. An alternative would be hydromorphone which is predominantly hepatically eliminated. In certain cases, where a balance between optimal pain control and side effects is difficult to achieve, interventional pain management or palliative radiotherapy may prove invaluable.

Data Interpretation

Question 1

A 68 year old woman with newly diagnosed breast cancer presents to an Accident and Emergency department with pyrexia and confusion. On arrival, her GCS is 13/15. Her temperature is 38.5°C. Her blood pressure is 98/52 mmHg. A collateral history from her daughter reveals that she is attending an oncologist in the hospital. Her initial blood tests demonstrate the following;

WCC	2.1×10^9/l
Na$^+$	136 mmol/l
Hb	10.9 g/dl
K$^+$	4.8 mmol/l
Plt	155×10^9/l
Urea	15.8 mmol/l
Neutrophils	0.3×10^9/l
Creatinine	193 μmol/l
Eosinophils	0.5×10^9/l
Lymphocytes	1.3×10^9/l

a.   Describe the abnormalities
b.   What is the differential diagnosis?
c.   What three immediate management steps would you take?

Question 2

A 76 year old man presents to an Accident and Emergency department with confusion, nausea, vomiting and abdominal pain. His GCS on arrival is 12/15. His blood pressure is 109/65mmHg, his pulse is 98 beats per minute and he is apyrexial. A plain film of abdomen shows faecal loading. A collateral history from his daughter reveals that he recently developed urinary retention and is waiting to see a urologist. His blood tests are as follows:

WCC	9.8×10^9/l
Na$^+$	128 mmol/l

Hb	11.1 g/dl
K$^+$	4.5 mmol/l
Plt	149×10^9/l
Urea	10.1 mmol/l
PSA	11.7 μg/l
Creatinine	131 μmol/l
Albumin	24 g/l
Calcium	2.61 mmol/l
AST	32 u/l
Alkaline Phos	301 U/l

a.   Describe the abnormalities
b.   What is the most likely cause of this man's symptoms?
c.   What is the immediate management?

Best of five questions

Question 1

A 70 year old man who is a heavy smoker presents with a 5 day history of a swollen right arm and increasing dyspnoea on exertion. On examination, there is non-pitting oedema of his right arm and prominent veins bilaterally on his neck. Auscultation of his lungs reveals reduced air entry on the right side with stony dull percussion. Heart auscultation reveals a prominent P2. What is the least likely cause of this man's increasing dyspnoea?

a.   Superior vena cava obstruction
b.   Pulmonary hypertension
c.   Anterior myocardial infarction
d.   Pleural effusion
e.   Pulmonary embolism

Question 2

An 81 year old man with a history of prostate cancer and hypertension presents with a 3-day history of back pain. His general practitioner has prescribed him tramadol with minimal relief. Neurological assessment reveals reduced power graded at 4/5 in his right lower limb with absent knee and ankle reflexes and extensor plantar responses bilaterally. What is the next most appropriate investigation to establish the diagnosis?

a.   Computed tomography of brain
b.   Isotope bone scan
c.   Plain radiograph of lumbosacral spine
d.   Magnetic resonance imaging of spine
e.   Nerve conduction studies

Question 3

A 66 year old woman presents to an Accident and Emergency department with a 1 day history of cough, pyrexia and shortness of breath on exertion. She completed her chemotherapy for Non-Hodgkin's Lymphoma one month previously. Her oxygen saturations are 91% on room air and her pulse is 95 beats per minute. Chest radiograph showed perihilar, fine, reticular interstitial opacification. What is the most likely pathogen responsible for her presumed respiratory tract infection?

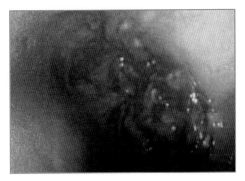

Figure 5: Oesophageal carcinoma

a. Candida albicans
b. Mycobacterium tuberculosis
c. Pneumocystis jirovecii
d. Streptococcus pneumonia
e. Klebsiella pneumonia

Question 4

A 65 year old man presents to his General Practitioner with a 1 day history of frank haematuria. He is referred to the urology service where he undergoes flexible cystoscopy. He is an otherwise healthy man apart from being treated with chemotherapy and radiotherapy for a non-seminomatous germ cell tumour 20 years previously. What is the most likely diagnosis?

a. Renal cell carcinoma
b. Secondary radiation induced transitional cell carcinoma
c. Recurrence testicular carcinoma
d. Benign prostatic hyperplasia
e. Penile carcinoma

Question 5

An 82 year old woman presents to an oncology out-patient department complaining of a one-week history of post-prandial vomiting. Of note, she has recently completed definitive chemoradiotherapy for locally advanced oesophageal carcinoma. Oesophago-gastro-duodenoscopy shows no evidence of disease recurrence. A barium swallow shows reduced motility at the distal oesophagus. Which of the following medications would be least likely to help?

a. Calcium channel blocker
b. Nitrate
c. Tricyclic anti-depressant
d. Botulinum toxin
e. Anti-cholinergic

Answers are on page 311

Skin problems

S Field, S Dennehy, M Murphy

Introduction

Skin disease is a frequent consequence of ageing and many cutaneous disorders become more prevalent with age. Inflammatory dermatoses such as eczema and psoriasis are the most common skin disorders in older people and can have varying clinical presentations. Although they have distinct aetiologies they can be difficult to distinguish.

Eczema/dermatitis

Asteatotic eczema

Asteatotic eczema is a common skin condition of older people that presents with a characteristic cracked or crazy-paving pattern, particularly on the lower limbs. The condition is usually pruritic and often uncomfortable and presents more commonly in winter months and in patients who are hospitalised.

Patients should be encouraged to avoid soaps and other de-greasing agents. Emollients are the mainstay of treatment and bathing in warm water containing dispersible oil and applying a bland emollient is usually sufficient. If necessary, a mild topical steroid, preferably in an ointment vehicle, can be added and applied under the emollient.

Varicose eczema

Varicose eczema occurs on the legs of those with venous hypertension. It is frequently accompanied by ankle oedema, haemosiderin deposition and ulceration. In some patients, varicose eczema disseminates to involve the thighs, upper limbs, trunk and face (id reaction). Patients with varicose eczema appear to have a higher incidence of contact allergic eczema and those responding poorly to treatment should be patch tested.

The affected areas should be soaked in warm water and a dispersible bath emollient. A bland emollient should be used copiously and a moderately potent or potent topical corticosteroid ointment can be applied to inflamed areas if required. Treatment of the underlying venous hypertension may be indicated. Due to the risk of developing contact allergic dermatitis, topical preparations containing antibiotics should be used with caution and corticosteroid preparations should be in an ointment rather than a cream vehicle.

Discoid eczema

Discoid, or nummular, eczema is a common pattern of eczema in older adults. Erythematous, scaly, circular patches develop predominantly on the legs but the trunk and upper limbs can also be involved. Differential diagnoses of discoid eczema include psoriasis, where trunk and scalp involvement predominate, and tinea (ringworm), where the periphery of the lesion tends to be raised. Most patients with discoid eczema grow Staphylococcus aureus from the lesions and an oral antibiotic should be prescribed in conjunction with emollients and topical corticosteroids.

Contact allergic dermatitis

Contact allergic dermatitis is an eczematous reaction that occurs as result of contact with an agent to which the individual has developed a specific acquired delayed hypersensitivity. Contact dermatitis should be considered in those with facial dermatitis (especially the eyelids), hand dermatitis and varicose eczema in particular. A detailed history should be taken and the patient referred for patch testing. Avoidance of the allergen is the mainstay of treatment but emollients and topical corticosteroids may also be required.

Seborrhoeic eczema

Seborrhoeic dermatitis occurs commonly in patients with Parkinson's disease and those infected with HIV and typically involves the scalp, medial eyebrows and nasolabial folds. Eyelid margins, intertriginous areas and the central trunk may also be involved. Overgrowth of the yeast commensal Pityrasporum ovale has been implicated in its aetiology.

Shampoos containing ingredients active against Pityrasporum ovale such as ketoconazole can be applied to the scalp and trunk and, in a more dilute form, to the face. Keratolytics such as tar and salicylic acid can help control scaling of the scalp.

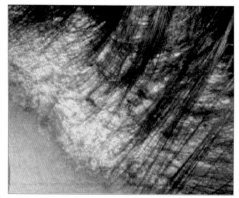

Figure 1: Scalp psoriasis

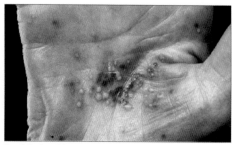

Figure 2: Pustular psoriasis

A 1% hydrocortisone cream or topical tacrolimus ointment can be used on the face for the inflammatory component if necessary.

Atopic eczema

Atopic eczema is a pruritic inflammatory condition with a predilection for the flexures. It is more common in those with a history of atopy and usually begins in childhood. Although up to ten per cent of cases seen in hospital settings start in adults, it is a relatively uncommon condition in older people. Emollients and topical corticosteroids are the mainstay of treatment and, although antihistamines may be useful for pruritus, sedative side effects limit their usefulness in older people. Due to difficulties applying topical treatments, older patients with severe atopic dermatitis often require systemic agents. Azathioprine and mycophenelate mofetil tend to be well tolerated and effective with cyclosporin reserved for more severe cases.

Psoriasis

Psoriasis is one of the most common skin disorders, affecting up to 2% of the population. It commonly presents in early adulthood but can present at any age. Late onset psoriasis tends to run a less severe course than that which presents earlier and patients are less likely to have a family history of the disease. A number of patterns of presentation have been well described.

Plaque-type psoriasis

In this form of psoriasis, well-demarcated erythematous scaly plaques frequently involve sites such as the extensor aspects of knees and elbows, the sacral area and scalp.

Flexural psoriasis

This pattern occurs more frequently in older people and can be a particular problem in those with obesity. Plaques occur in the groin, axillae, umbilicus and inframammary creases. Flexural psoriasis tends to be less scaly than plaques elsewhere and frequently has a moist, glazed appearance. As a result of maceration, secondary bacterial and fungal infections are common.

Erythrodermic psoriasis

Patients with severe plaque-type psoriasis may develop erythrodermic psoriasis. Acute generalised pustular psoriasis is a particularly severe form with sudden florid erythema and crops of small superficial pustules. Cutaneous signs are often accompanied by malaise, pyrexia and arthralgia. It is important to recognise these potentially life threatening forms early, particularly in older people. Patients are at risk of dehydration, high output cardiac failure and electrolyte disturbances and inpatient treatment is usually required. Precipitating factors may be identified which include the withdrawal of systemic corticosteroids, infections and drugs.

Psoriatic arthritis

Psoriatic arthritis affects up to 8% of patients with psoriasis and its prevalence appears to increase with age. Victims with more severe psoriasis, and in particular those with nail involvement, are more at risk with the distal interphalangeal joints most likely to be affected.

Treatments

Topical preparations

Topical preparations form the corner stone of treatment for psoriasis. Emollients can remove scale and improve underlying xerosis and, in some elderly

TABLE 1 SYSTEMIC TREATMENTS FOR PSORIASIS
• Methotrexate
• Acetretin
• Cyclosporin
• Fumaric acid esters
• Biologic treatments (entanercept, infliximab, efalizumab, adalimumab)

TABLE 2 CAUSES OF BULLAE ON LOWER LIMBS
• Bullous pemphigoid
• Porphyria cutanea tarda
• Bullous insect bite reaction
• Cellulitis with bullae
• Bullous erythema ab igne
• Drug eruption
• Dermatitis Herpetiformis
• Phytophotodermatoses
• Bullae secondary to oedema
• Friction bullae

patients with a limited amount of psoriasis, may be all that is required. Useful emollients include traditional preparations such as Silcock's base and Halden's base. For flexural psoriasis, a weak topical corticosteroid is often indicated and this can be combined with an anti-fungal preparation. A weak corticosteroid is the usual first-line treatment for facial psoriasis. Topical tacrolimus is useful for more recalcitrant facial psoriasis but does not appear to be effective for thicker plaques.

The use of potent topical corticosteroids in psoriasis is controversial. They are easy to apply and have good patient acceptability. However, in addition to their well documented local cutaneous adverse effects and risks of systemic effects, they can also cause rebound phenomena and tachyphylaxis in psoriasis and are thought to be associated with the development of pustular psoriasis. As a result, they tend to be used intermittently and in conjunction with other topical preparations such as tar or calcipotriol.

Topical coal tar preparations are useful for limited plaques. Patients and relatives need to be warned of their smell and potential for staining clothing. Dithranol can be effective but its use is now often limited to short-contact applications administered in dermatology departments or as an in-patient regime. Vitamin D3 analogues tend to be better tolerated and more cosmetically acceptable.

Second line treatments
Phototherapy with narrowband UVB (311nm) is an effective treatment for many patients with psoriasis, though remission periods vary widely. The combination of psoralen and UVA (PUVA) is now mainly used for patients for whom narrowband UVB has failed as it is thought to be more carcinogenic. Factors that may limit the number of older people suitable for phototherapy include: ability to stand for 15 minutes in an enclosed unit; availability of transport for two or three sessions per week for 6 to 8 weeks; previous or current cutaneous malignancies; and an ability to tolerate photosensitising drugs.

Systemic treatments for psoriasis (table 1) are reserved for patients with extensive disease or diminished quality of life due to their condition and when other treatments are ineffective or impractical. They are of particular relevance for those with reduced mobility in whom the application of topical treatments may pose difficulties. Methotrexate tends to be particularly well tolerated in older people and the once weekly dosage can be given orally or intramuscularly. Potential side effects include bone marrow suppression and hepatotoxicity and regular monitoring of the full blood count and liver function tests is mandatory. Long-term use of cyclosporin tends to be poorly tolerated in older people but short-term use (2 - 3 months) can be useful for the treatment of disease flares. Newer 'biologic' treatments interfere with key steps in the pathogenesis of psoriasis and offer further treatment options for patients with moderate to severe disease.

Blistering disorders
Bullae can occur in a wide variety of skin conditions that may be particularly disabling in older people. The differential diagnoses of bullae on the lower limb are listed in table 2, but the more common conditions where bullae or vesicles predominate are discussed in more detail.

Herpes zoster
Primary infection with the varicella zoster virus causes chicken pox and is largely a disease of children and young adults. Following primary infection, the virus lays dormant in the dorsal root ganglia and may manifest itself many years later as herpes zoster.

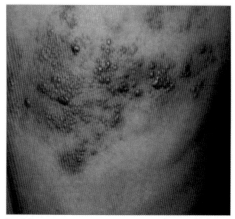
Figure 3: Herpes zoster

TABLE 3
ANTIVIRAL TREATMENT FOR HERPES ZOSTER

ACICLOVIR
- 10mg/Kg intravenously every 8 hours for 7-10 days
- 800mg orally five times daily for 7-10 days

FAMCICLOVIR
- 500mg orally three times daily for 7 days

VALCICLOVIR
- 1000mg orally three times daily for 7 days

Lesions are usually vesicular (less than 0.5cm) and present on an erythematous background. They occur classically in a dermatomal distribution, though multiple dermatomes may be involved in older people and those who are immunosuppressed. The rash is often extremely painful and progresses from vesicles to crusted pustules, usually lasting between two and three weeks.

Where appropriate, patients should be isolated as, although one cannot contract herpes zoster, it is possible to contract chicken pox (varicella) from a patient with herpes zoster if one has not previously been exposed. Nursing and medical staff should be aware of their varicella immunity status. Adequate analgesia is important. Topical saline soaks applied frequently may aid in the removal of crust and topical bactroban or fucidin ointments can be used for secondary bacterial infection. Aciclovir and the newer antiviral agents have been shown to be effective in diminishing the severity and duration of both the rash and acute pain of herpes zoster if given within 72 hours of the appearance of the rash. Perhaps more importantly, they have been shown to decrease the incidence and duration of post herpetic neuralgia (table 3). It is important to maintain adequate hydration while on antiviral therapy and dose reduction should be considered for those with diminished renal function. The role of corticosteroids is controversial and they have not been shown to reduce the severity of post herpetic neuralgia. Ophthalmology opinion must be sought if ophthalmic nerve involvement is suspected i.e. vesicles distributed from the eye up to the forehead. Vesicles present on the tip of nose signify involvement of the nasocilary nerve and the necessity for ophthalmogical examination.

Bullous pemphigoid

Bullous pemphigoid is an acquired autoimmune blistering disease that occurs almost exclusively in older people. Its precise cause is unknown and studies have failed to show a link with underlying malignancy. Tense bullae may erupt on normal looking skin or on an erythematous background, most commonly on the flexor surfaces of the arms and legs. Blisters often develop abruptly but a prodromal phase of pruritus without bullae has been described. Lesions may be clear or haemorrhagic and are frequently quite large and usually pruritic. The mucosa may become involved in 20% of patients.

Skin biopsies demonstrate the pathological hallmark of a subepidermal blister and direct immunofluoresence will show linear deposits of both IgG and C3 at the epidermal basement membrane in most patients.

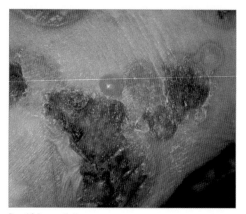
Figure 4: Bullous pemphigoid

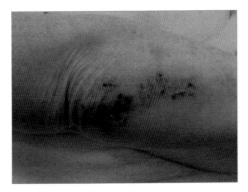

Figure 5: Dermatitis Herpetiformis

Treatment depends on the extent of disease. Localised disease can be treated with a super potent topical steroid (such as 0.05% clobetasol propionate) but more extensive disease usually requires the administration of systemic steroids, at a starting dose of 0.5 mg/kg of prednisolone daily. Once the disease is under control (usually after 2 to 4 weeks) the dose can be initially tapered in 10mg decrements on a weekly or fortnightly basis. Once the dose is less then 20 mgs of prednisolone daily, the decrements should be lowered to 5mgs and the slow taper continued. Relapses are common and require an increase in steroid dose again. Up to 75% of patients will achieve prolonged remission without further therapy after the initial course of oral steroids. Immunosuppressive therapy with azathioprine or mycophenelate mofetil is occasionally required for more recalcitrant disease. Minocycline and nicotinamide have been used as steroid sparing agents.

Pemphigus vulgaris

Pemphigus vulgaris is a rare but potentially lethal immunobullous disorder. It most commonly presents in the sixth decade and is a characterised by oral erosions and flaccid blisters. Due to the fragility of intraepidermal bullae, patients may present with eroded areas only. Oral erosions may precede cutaneous manifestations. Treatment consists of a combination of high dose systemic corticosteroids and immunosuppressive agents. Morbidity from both the disease and its therapy can be significant.

Dermatitis herpetiformis

This is an intensely pruritic, chronic vesicular skin disorder that is usually associated with gluten-sensitive enteropathy. Blisters are symmetrically grouped and most commonly occur on the elbows, knees and buttocks. Due to the intense pruritus vesicles are often excoriated. The diagnosis of dermatitis herpetiformis is usually confirmed by skin biopsy and direct immunofluoresence. Immunofluoresence from clinically normal skin shows IgA deposits at the dermoepidermal junction. All patients with confirmed disease should be commenced on a gluten free diet even if they do not have gastrointestinal symptoms as it is thought to reduce the risk of lymphoma and helps control cutaneous disease. Oral dapsone is a very effective treatment and usually suppresses the very distressing itch of the disease within a few days.

Porphyria cutanea tarda

Porphyria cutanea tarda is the most common form of porphyria and results from a deficiency of uroporphyrinogen decarboxylase. There is frequently a history of alcohol excess and there is an association with hepatitis A, B and particularly C infection. Bullae form in skin exposed to sunshine or trauma. The backs of the hands are most commonly involved but sun-exposed areas such as the forearms, ears and face can also be affected. Bullae are fragile and rupture easily and lesions heal slowly with scarring. Milia, hyperpigmentation and hypertrichosis may also be present.

Skin biopsies of fresh blisters show subepidermal bullae with minimal dermal inflammatory infiltrates but may not be unequivocally diagnostic. The diagnosis may be supported by a full porphyria screen of serum, urine and faeces. Investigations should also include a hepatitis screen, ferritin levels and assessment for haemochromatosis and hepatocellular carcinoma. Treatment includes photoprotection, avoidance of precipitating factors such as alcohol and oestrogens, and phlebotomy to reduce iron overload.

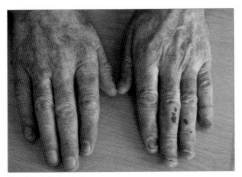

Figure 6: Porphyria cutanea tarda

TABLE 4
INVESTIGATIONS FOR PRURITIS IN OLDER PEOPLE

• Full blood count	• C-reactive protein, ESR
• Liver function tests	• HIV status (if risk factors present)
• Renal function tests	• Faeces for parasites
• Ferritin	• Chest X-ray
• Thyroid function tests	• Skin biopsy (including immunofluoresence)
• Immunoglobulins	

Senile pruritus

Itch associated with xerosis (dry skin) is common in older people and gets worse in winter. It is thought that 'senile pruritus' may be related to loss of neurons in ageing skin resulting in reduced neural inhibition. In the absence of a rash, systemic causes of pruritus should be excluded with relevant investigations (table 4). Morphine and other opioids can cause itch in the absence of a rash and a trial of discontinuing opiate therapy should be considered if this is implicated. It is not unusual for depression to present with pruritus. Treatment options for 'senile pruritus' are outlined in table 5.

Pressure ulcers

A pressure ulcer is an area of localised skin damage, which can extend to underlying tissue such as muscle or bone, caused by pressure, shear, friction, moisture or a combination of these factors. Pressure ulcers can develop in any area of the body but more commonly occur over bony prominences such as the sacrum, coccyx and heels. They are a significant cause of morbidity and it is estimated that between 12 and 20% of adult hospitalised patients may suffer from a pressure ulcer.

Risks for developing pressure ulcers are manifold and include patient related factors (poor mobility, reduced awareness, age, incontinence, both high and low body mass index, malnutrition) and external factors such as the intensity and duration of pressure and the friction or shearing forces between the skin and underlying surfaces. Although many risk assessment tools exist to help predict the development of pressure ulcers, little evidence exists that using a risk tool or scale is better than clinical judgment alone. All patients should be assessed for the risk of pressure ulcer development on admission to hospital or a long-term care facility and this assessment should be repeated at regular intervals, particularly if there are any changes in risk factors.

The prevention and minimisation of pressure ulcers requires a multifaceted approach. A repositioning care plan should be devised and implemented for patients with existing lesions and those identified as being at-risk. The frequency of positional change should reflect the needs of each individual, as should the choice of pressure redistributing mattress. Mattresses made from polyurethane foam act by moulding around the patient and redistributing pressure over a greater surface area while more dynamic systems episodically remove pressure from different areas of the body. Skin should be kept cleansed and lubricated and an emollient should be applied to any dry or cracked areas. Finally, it is essential that the nutritional status of patients should be optimised.

TABLE 5
TREATMENTS FOR SENILE PRURITIS

• Avoidance of harsh cleansers	• Doxepin 10-100mgs daily
• Daily emollient e.g Silcock's base	• Gabapentin
• Topical antipruritic agents eg 1% menthol	• Paroxetine
• Capsaicin (localised area only)	• Thalidomide
• Mild topical steroids	• Oral steroids
• Phototherapy	• Cyclosporin
• Sedating anti-histamine	

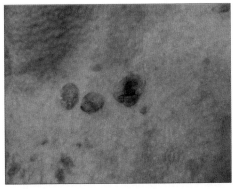

Figure 7: Seborrhoeic keratoses

A grading system for pressure ulcers is described in table 6. The treatment of pressure ulcers involves a combination of pressure relief (in the form of support surfaces), positioning and repositioning, and specific wound care including wound dressings, chemical and surgical debridement, oral antibiotics and antiseptic agents where appropriate.

Lesions associated with ageing

Seborrhoeic keratosis
Seborrhoeic keratoses are extremely common, benign, persistent, sharply demarcated oval lesions that originate in keratinocytes. They range in colour from skin colour to black and often have a 'stuck-on' appearance. Their surface may be smooth, verrucous or cerebriform. Treatment is usually unnecessary but, if occurring in an area of friction, cryotherapy or curettage can easily remove the lesion.

Sebaceous gland hyperplasia
Benign hyperplasia of the sebaceous gland usually occurs on the face and consists of soft pale yellow papules, some of which may have central umbilication. They are common and can mimic basal cell carcinomas. Sebaceous hyperplasia is very common in patients on cyclosporin. Treatment is not required.

Campbell de Morgan spots (Senile angiomas)
These are the most common vascular abnormality, consisting of red ruby papules most commonly on the trunk. Early flat lesions can be mistaken for purpuric lesions. No treatment is required but small lesions respond well to vascular lasers.

Venous lakes
Venous lakes are dark blue to purple blebs that empty when compressed. They are usually located on the lips, ears, face or forearms and are manifestations of chronic sun damage. No treatment is necessary but if bleeding or causing cosmetic distress they can be treated with electrocautery, laser ablation or cryotherapy.

Poikiloderma of Civatte
Poikiloderma of Civatte is a red-brown, mottled pigmentation with telangiectasia and slight atrophy that is seen at the sides, front and V of the neck with sparing of the submental area. It occurs most commonly in women and fair skinned individuals and is a result of photo ageing. Lesions are usually asymptomatic and of cosmetic concern only.

Premalignant and malignant nonmelanoma skin cancers
Solar keratosis (actinic keratosis), squamous cell carcinoma-in-situ (Bowen's disease) and squamous cell carcinomas exist on a spectrum that ranges from early dysplasia to in-situ disease to invasive carcinoma. Invasion occurs when dysplastic cells breech the dermoepidermal junction.

TABLE 6
GRADING OF PRESSURE ULCERS

GRADE 1:
- Non-blanching erythema of intact skin
- Discolouration, warmth, oedema, induration or hardness may also be used as indicators, particularly for individuals with darker skin

GRADE 2:
- Partial thickness skin loss involving epidermis, dermis, or both
- The ulcer is superficial and presents clinically as an abrasion or blister

GRADE 3:
- Skin loss involving damage or necrosis of the subcutaneous tissue that may extend down to, but not through, the underlying fascia

GRADE 4:
- Extensive destruction, tissue necrosis, or damage to muscle, bone or supporting structures with or without full thickness skin loss

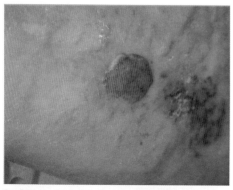

Figure 8: Squamous cell carcinoma

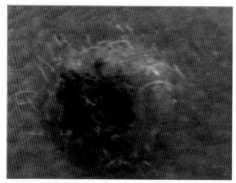

Figure 9: Nodular basal cell carcinoma

Figure 10: Superficial basal cell carcinoma

Solar keratosis

Solar keratoses are found on chronically sun exposed skin and are usually multiple. Lesions are often discrete (commonly more easily felt than seen) and may be keratotic, flat or slightly raised. They vary in colour from flesh-coloured to red with adherent scale or yellow crust. Lesions also vary in size from 1mm

to diffuse involvement of the face and scalp. Other features of chronic photodamage are usually present. The natural history of solar keratoses is controversial and the rate of transformation to squamous cell carcinoma varies widely between studies. Since at least some solar keratoses can progress to squamous cell carcinoma, treatment is indicated. Cryotherapy treats localized lesions effectively but other effective therapeutic options include topical diclofenac sodium, 5-fluorouracil, imiquimod 5% and photodynamic therapy. Treatment should always include advice about photoprotection.

Bowen's disease (squamous cell carcinoma in situ)

Bowen's disease is an intraepidermal squamous cell carcinoma arising from keratinocytes which may become invasive. It frequently occurs on the legs of older females. Lesions consist of well-defined, erythematous patches or plaques with surface scale or crust and are slowly progressive. The development of thickened papular islands, ulceration or fungating areas should raise the suspicion of invasion. A punch biopsy to confirm the diagnosis and exclude invasive disease is advisable. Treatment options are similar to those available for solar keratoses, but the risk of lower limb ulceration with cryotherapy should be considered in older people. Surgical options include curettage or simple excision under local anaesthetic.

Squamous cell carcinoma

Squamous cell carcinoma is the second most common form of skin cancer. Most tumours occur on the head and neck as the greatest risk factor is cumulative chronic exposure to ultraviolet light. Carcinomas present as dull red or skin coloured papules or nodules. Lesions may have a thick keratin crust or surface ulceration and may be friable or bleed easily. Incisional biopsy is advisable for diagnosis. The treatment of choice is surgical excision with 4mm margins. In older patients with multiple lesions, curettage is a reasonable option but the risk of recurrence is higher. In immunosuppressed patients (e.g. renal transplant recipients) with multiple nonmelanoma skin cancers, oral retinoids may reduce the frequency of lesions.

Keratoacanthoma

Keratoacanthomas are solitary lesions that grow rapidly, usually over 2 to 6 weeks. The history is usually of growth of a firm nodule with a crater-like area in the centre. Classical keratoacanthomas have an initial proliferative phase, a mature phase and then involute spontaneously leaving a pitted scar. They are

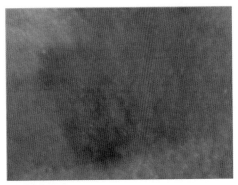

Figure 11: Lentigo maligna

often regarded as abortive squamous cell carcinomas but should be treated in an identical manner with excision.

Basal cell carcinoma

Basal cell carcinomas, the most common form of skin cancer, usually run a chronic course, are destructive and may erode into local structures. Metastases, however, virtually never occur. Most lesions occur on the head and neck and the majority are nodular in morphology, presenting as pearly white or translucent, often domed papules with overlying branched telengiectasia. Central ulceration or crusting is common and lesions frequently bleed on slight injury. Other basal cell carcinoma morphologies include superficial, cystic, pigmented and morphoeic.

Treatment is based on size, site (proximity to other structures such as the eye), morphology, age and the overall health of the patient. Superficial basal cell carcinomas can be treated with cryotherapy, topically with 5-fluorouracil or photodynamic therapy. Nodular

lesions in non-critical sites can be curetted or excised. Morphoeic or basal cell carcinomas in high-risk sites should be excised with clear surgical margins to reduce the risk of recurrence. Radiotherapy can be considered for patients who refuse surgery or are poor surgical candidates due to medical co-morbidities.

Malignant melanoma

Melanoma of the skin is a malignant tumour arising in cutaneous melanocytes and is predominantly a cancer of white-skinned people. The risk of melanoma increases with age and exposure to ultraviolet light is the main modifiable risk factor. Although more females than males develop melanoma, the mortality in males is higher. More recently, the greatest rate of increase in melanoma has been seen in males over the age of sixty years. There are four clinical subtypes of melanoma: superficial spreading melanoma, nodular melanoma, lentigo maligna melanoma and acral lentiginous melanoma. Any naevus which has changed in symmetry size, shape or outline or has become itchy or inflamed should be assessed urgently.

The treatment of melanoma is surgical excision with an appropriate margin. The best prognostic indicator is Breslow thickness (the depth of malignant melanocytes from the granular layer of the epidermis).

Suggested further reading

- *Skin disease in old age, 2nd edition. R Marks 1999*
- *Smith D, Leggat PA. Prevalence of skin disease among elderly in different clinical environments. Australasian Journal on Ageing, 2005; 24: 71-76.*
- *Smith DM. Pressure ulcers in the nursing home. Annals of Internal Medicine 1995;123: 433-442.*
- *Yosipovitch G, Tang MVY. Practical management of psoriasis in the elderly. Drugs Aging 2002; 19(11): 847-863.*

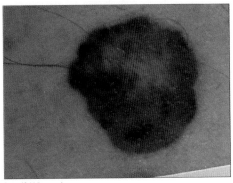

Figure 12: Malignant melanoma

Case Study 1

A 75 year old male has a six month history of an intensely itchy rash over his elbows and buttocks. It waxes and wanes but never clears completely. On examination, he appears malnourished. Skin examination reveals non-specific excoriated papules over the elbows, buttocks and back of his neck.

The blistering nature and intense pruritis associated with this rash is quite suggestive of dermatitis herpetiformis. This diagnosis is supported by the patient's poor nutritional status, suggesting coexisting coeliac disease. The diagnosis can be confirmed by skin biopsy and direct immunofluoresence which shows IgA deposits at the dermoepidermal junction. A positive serum antiendomysial antibody test also supports the diagnosis. The patient should be started on a gluten free diet and oral dapsone can be considered for those who respond poorly to dietary measures.

Case Study 2

An 80 year female with chronic lymphoedema has been admitted via the accident and emergency department complaining of increased swelling of both lower limbs over the previous four weeks. She developed three tense water blisters on her right leg in the previous 24 hours. Clinically there is acute on chronic lymphoedema with pitting to the thighs and oozing of serous fluid. There are three intact tense blisters above the ankle with no surrounding erythema.

These blisters are almost certainly due to oedema. Medical management of the lymphoedema involves elevation of the legs and the use of diuretic therapy. The blisters should be burst with a sterile needle, releasing fluid. Dressing is not always necessary but, if needed, a bland emollient can be used with nonadherent dressings. If new lesions continue to form in spite of an improvement in the lymphoedema, a diagnosis of bullous pemphigoid should be considered.

Case Study 3

A 68 year old male presents for the first time for assessment at a day hospital. He is incidentally noted to have multiple rough erythematous scaling patches on the scalp forehead, cheeks and dorsum of hands. He has male pattern baldness and diffuse photodamage on his arms, head and neck. The patches have been present for a year but have recently become more numerous and scaly. He is fair (skin type 1) and is a semi-retired farmer.

The most likely diagnosis is diffuse photodamage with focal actinic keratosis. Untreated actinic keratoses are often very keratotic and before treatment, scale should be softened with vaseline and lifted. Cryotherapy can be used for focal lesions, but if the area is too extensive (as is probable in this case) topical diclofenac sodium can be used twice daily for 3 months. An alternative is 5-fluorouracil 3 times weekly for 6 weeks or as tolerated. Reaction and crusting can be very florid with 5-fluorouracil, but the more florid the reaction often the better the response. Small areas can be treated in a step wise fashion.

Data Interpretation

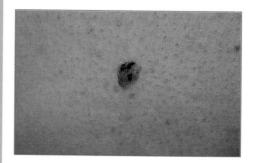

Question 1

A 67 year old female presents with a 2 year history of 20 lesions gradually appearing on her back, chest and inframammary area. The lesions appear as raised, waxy stuck-on skin coloured lesions. They gradually increased in size and became more warty, with some becoming very dark and occasionally itchy. One lesion bled following trauma by her necklace. The above is a representative lesion.

a. What are the lesions?
b. What treatment would you advise?

Question 2

A 70 year old retired outdoor council worker presents with the lesion pictured below on the left side of his neck which has been present for 3 years. It initially started as a small

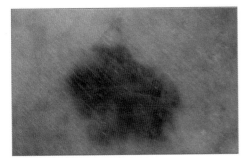

a. Squamous cell carcinoma

b. Basal cell carcinoma

c. Merkel cell carcinoma

d. Keratoacanthoma

e. Seborrhoeic keratosis

Question 2

A 70 year old male was diagnosed with bullous pemphigoid 3 months ago. He has been in remission (no new blisters) for 4 weeks. He is taking prednisolone 40mgs daily and tolerating it well. What would you do next?

a. Stop prednisolone and use 0.05% clobetasol propionate if blisters develop

b. Reduce prednisolone to 10mgs daily

c. Continue present dose of prednisolone and start nicotinamde and minocycline

d. Reduce prednisolone to 30mgs daily today and reduce to 20mgs in 2 weeks if he remains clear

e. Reduce prednisolone to 30mgs and commence mycophenolate mofetil

brown spot but has gradually increased in size over the last 12 months.

a. What is the likely diagnosis?

b. What is the next step in management?

Question 3

An 85 year old female has developed the blisters pictured below on her inner thighs during the last two weeks. New blisters develop every day and have appeared on her abdomen and arms in the past 5 days. For 3 weeks before the blisters developed she had an intensely itchy area on the inner thighs that looked like a 'nettle rash' with wheals. She is systemically well. She started no new medications in the past 6 months and has no oral symptoms.

Question 3

A 70 year male has chronic plaque psoriasis affecting 15% of his body surface area, mainly on his back, buttocks and legs. He lives alone. The plaques itch and he is anxious for treatment. What are the treatment options?

a. Phototherapy PUVA twice weekly

b. Phototherapy narrow band ultraviolet B (TLO1) three times a week

c. Topical coal tar preparation (eg. 5% liquor piscis carbonis in a 0.025% betamethasone ointment) at night to plaques and emollient baths

d. Systemic methotrexate therapy

e. All of the above

Answers are on page 311

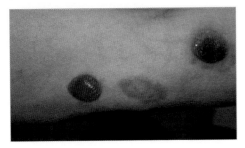

a. What is the likely diagnosis?

b. What investigations would you perform?

c. What treatment would you commence?

Best of five questions

Question 1

An 80 year female presents with a 3 week history of a rapidly growing lesion on her left dorsum of hand. Clinically there is a 1cm nodule which is firm and appears crater like in the centre. What is the likely diagnosis?

Sensory problems

B Ni Bhuachalla, F Kinsella, P Gormley, EC Mulkerrin

The eye

The eye and ageing

As one gets older, anatomical and physiological changes occur in the eye that result in deteriorating function. Most middle aged patients complain that their first sign of 'ageing' is when loss of reading ability (presbyopia) occurs as print is pushed further and further away. In some older patients the 'second vision of old age' develops whereby reading ability is restored due to myopic changes which occur as part of early cataract formation in the crystalline lens. As the cataract density increases, both near and distance vision become reduced. Other changes are independent of the diseases that cause visual decline in older people. In particular, limitations in the ability to accommodate and reductions in pupil size contribute to worsening vision. In addition, the pupil has less capacity to dilate, causing less light to reach the retina. Retinal photoreceptors are less effective in regenerating rhodopsin resulting in delayed dark adaptation. It is not uncommon for older people to specifically complain of difficulty with night vision. Ageing also affects colour vision and contrast sensitivity. Overall, it is thought that perception is negatively affected. Other problems include experiencing glare, which is due to scattering of light by the ageing lens and cornea. Interestingly, there are several visual functions that exhibit little alteration with ageing, for example, how we align two lines with one another (vernier acuity).

Visual assessment

Vision is assessed using the Snellen chart. The patient stands six metres from the chart and the visual acuity in each eye is checked separately. Normal vision is present if the patient can read down to the 6/6 line, whereas visual acuity is merely 6/60 if only the top line can be read. Should the patient be unable to see the top line, he is brought closer to the chart until he can see the top line (eg. if he is able to see the top line at three metres from the chart, his vision is 3/60). A vision of 1/60 equates to counting fingers. Should the patient be unable to count fingers, the ability to detect hand movements is assessed. Should he be unable to assess hand movements, perception of light is checked. It is then important in a patient whose vision is perceptive of light to determine whether projection in all four quadrants is retained or not (as many conditions can result in loss of projection in certain quadrants).

Near vision is assessed using a reading test with the patient's reading glasses on. The vision in each eye is checked separately. In patients with macular problems, Logmar vision is used. The patient reads letters from a distance of 2-3 metres, the advantage being that this is a much more sensitive indicator of visual function than Snellen vision and is particularly important when monitoring patients with maculopathy. Visual fields are assessed by sitting directly in front of the patient with the examiner's eye at the same level as the patient's, and checking the four field quadrants in each eye separately.

Glaucoma

Glaucoma is defined as an optic neuropathy involving a characteristic atrophy of the optic nerve head, often accompanied by typical visual field defects. It is classified in several ways. Firstly it can be congenital or acquired. Glaucoma may also be termed open or closed angle, according to how the aqueous outflow is impaired. Finally, as in all clinical conditions, there may be primary or secondary types depending on the presence or absence of underlying contributory factors.

Glaucoma is often, but not always associated with elevated intraocular pressure. Normal intraocular pressure is 8-21mmHg. Examination of a glaucomatous optic nerve reveals 'cupping', which looks like a 'hollowing out' of the optic nerve. Cupping is associated with the loss of ganglion cell axons.

Primary angle closure

In this type of glaucoma, patients have an anatomically narrow angle. There is no identifiable secondary cause but there may be predisposing risk factors such as family history, female gender and hyperopia. Once the optic nerve shows damage from the high intraocular pressure, the disease is called primary angle closure glaucoma.

Secondary angle closure

Several secondary processes can cause narrowing or closure of the anterior chamber angle including masses, neo-vascularisation and scarring.

Acute angle closure glaucoma

If a patient has a narrow anterior chamber angle (either primary or secondary) they are at risk of the angle acutely closing, with a subsequent acute rise in intraocular pressure and the development of acute angle closure glaucoma. Case 1 illustrates the symptoms and signs of this condition, which requires emergency treatment by an ophthalmologist as blindness can occur in hours to days. Patients who are hypermetropic (long sighted) are at risk of this condition and can be identified as their glasses are magnifiers (similar to readers) but used instead for distance vision.

In acute glaucoma, multi-coloured halos may occur due to the prismatic effect of fluid in the cornea rather than mono-coloured halos which usually occur due to mucus in the corneal tear film (typically due to dry eye disease).

Chronic angle closure glaucoma

Chronic angle closure results if only a portion of the angle is blocked at a time and develops scarring. Over time, the angle may become progressively more closed. In this variant of the disease, the intraocular pressure may be normal or only slightly elevated, in which case symptoms are unlikely to occur. Patients with chronic angle closure glaucoma may have more damage to the optic nerve and peripheral vision when the diagnosis is established compared to patients with symptomatic acute glaucoma, due to the absence of symptoms and delayed presentation. Chronic simple glaucoma (figure 1) is similar in this respect.

Chronic simple glaucoma (primary open angle glaucoma)

Five percent of patients over 70 years of age suffer from chronic simple glaucoma (also called primary open-angle glaucoma). In many cases it remains undetected. Fifty percent of primary open angle glaucoma patients have normal intraocular pressure, referred to as normal or low tension glaucoma. The first sign of glaucomatous damage is identified by nerve fibre layer analysis (showing defects seven years prior to visual field defects), followed by changes in the optic nerve head (cupping) and lastly visual field defects. In advanced cases there is evidence of optic disc cupping (figure 1) and visual field (especially nasal) loss. Progressive peripheral visual field loss is generally followed by central field loss. There are no anatomical factors that identify eyes that are at risk.

Earlier cases of chronic simple glaucoma are generally diagnosed when an elevated intraocular pressure is detected by an optician. As visual field loss that has occurred cannot be recovered, patients should be encouraged to have an intraocular pressure check by their optician every two years.

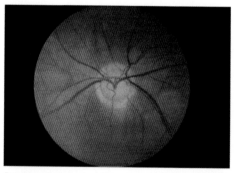

Figure 1: Excavated optic disc and nasal displacement of vessels typical of disc cupping in chronic simple glaucoma

Cataract

Cataract is due to opacification of the crystalline lens (figure 2) and the best method of gauging cataract severity is by observing the amount of red reflex obscuration through the undilated pupil (mimicking what the patient experiences). Nowadays, surgery is offered to patients once they have considerable symptoms with either their distance or near vision. It is no longer necessary to wait until the cataract is mature and the patient blind.

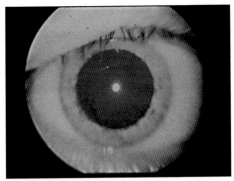

Figure 2: Obscuration of the red reflex due to cataract formation

Macular degeneration

Age related macular degeneration (ARMD) is a progressive degenerative disorder of the retinal pigment layer. In its early stages it does not cause significant visual loss. There are two types, namely 'wet' and 'dry'. Clinical findings of 'dry' ARMD include pigment abnormalities and drusen in the fundus. Patients with 'wet' ARMD have choroidal neovascularisation when examined by fluorscein angiography. Leaky vessels exuding blood and fluid can cause acute deterioration in vision.

A promising therapy for 'wet' type age related macular degeneration has been developed in recent years. It involves a series of injections of a vascular endothelial growth factor (VEGF) inhibitor (pegaptanib/ranibizumab/bevacizumab) directly into the vitreous under local anaesthesia. Treatment stabilises vision in over 90% of patients and improves vision in one-third of cases but it is expensive and time consuming. In addition, complications such as endophthalmitis, cataract formation and detached retina can occur.

Patients with sub-foveal lesions are primarily treated with anti-VEGF treatment and if not responsive to this, have photodynamic therapy whereby the verteporphyrin is infused intravenously and activated by an infra red laser resulting in coagulation of the choroidal neovascularisation. This treatment stabilises vision in 50% of cases but generally does not improve visual acuity. Patients with significant 'dry' ARMD (large soft drusen, geographic atrophy, hyperpigmentation) benefit from Lutein which replaces the macular pigments which thin as patients age. It slows dry ARMD progression, and lessens the risk of wet ARMD.

The National Institute for Health and Clinical Excellence published an appraisal document in 2007 recommending that those with neovascular ARMD and best corrected vision greater than 6/60 should be treated with ranibizumab. However in practice, patients with vision worse than this are often treated with a VEGF inhibitor. Thermal laser photocoagulation, another treatment used to treat exudative ARMD, is only used where the lesion is extra foveal. Antioxidants such as vitamins C and E and β-carotene may help to prevent progression to neovascular ARMD, though evidence from clinical trials is limited.

Floaters & flashing lights

Many patients have small floaters that have been present for many years and these are generally of no significance. The sudden appearance of large floaters where ophthalmoscopy reveals no abnormality is generally due to acute vitreous separation which can result in retinal tear formation and retinal detachment (figure 3) and warrants prompt ophthalmological referral. The other major cause of sudden floaters is vitreous haemorrhage. This is diagnosed by getting the patient to move the eye in various directions and finally to look directly at the ophthalmoscope. Moving opacities against the red reflex are diagnostic (figure 4). The usual underlying causes of vitreous haemorrhage are retinal detachment or proliferative retinopathy (either diabetic or due to previous branch venous obstruction).

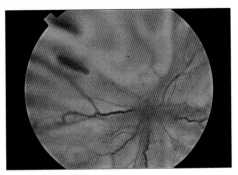

Figure 3: Retinal tears and retinal detachment

Flashing lights can represent retinal tear formation and warrants urgent ophthalmological referral to prevent retinal detachment. Unlike the flashing lights of migraine (which are typically zig-zag in shape, dance up and down in front of the patient and move from one part of the visual field to another within a few

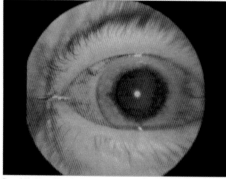

Figure 4: Moving opacities against the red reflex, diagnostic of vitreous haemorrhage

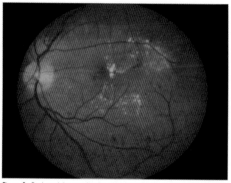

Figure 5: Focal exudative maculopathy with rings of hard exudation due to leaking microaneurysms

minutes), flashing lights due to retinal tears typically occur in elderly patients and are generally located in the temporal field of vision, continue for several days, and appear like tiny momentary streaks of lightning.

Another type of flashing light generally confined to older people is that due to occipital lobe ischaemia. In this condition there are constant multiple flashes in front of both eyes persisting for months or even years and not uncommonly associated with frightening visual hallucinations (which are rarely mentioned unless specifically questioned about). The realisation that there is an organic basis to their symptoms is a great comfort to these patients who are frequently under the misapprehension that they are having psychiatric symptoms.

Diabetic retinopathy

The two types of diabetic retinopathy that result in visual loss are maculopathy and proliferative retinopathy. All diabetic patients must have an annual dilated fundal examination to detect these treatable conditions. Of the three forms of maculopathy (focal exudative, diffuse oedema and ischaemic), only the commonest - focal exudative (figure 5) - can be readily diagnosed by the non-ophthalmologist, and only then with pupillary dilatation to allow adequate macular inspection. Diffuse oedema, recognised by the stereoscopic methods of examination employed by ophthalmologists, and ischaemic maculopathy (diagnosed only by fluorescein angiographic demonstration of capillary non-perfusion) should be suspected where there is an unexplained drop in vision in patients with a relatively 'normal-looking' macula.

The key to diagnosing proliferative diabetic retinopathy (figure 6) is adequate pupillary dilatation

which allows proper ophthalmoscopic inspection of the optic disc and the major vessel arcades (nasal and temporal). Once the disc and arcades have been inspected, move the ophthalmoscope slightly away from the patient, without changing the ophthalmoscopic focus, and this frequently brings previously unseen new blood vessels into view. This is because these vessels grow forward into the vitreous cavity and can be missed if one simply focuses on the optic disc and arcades.

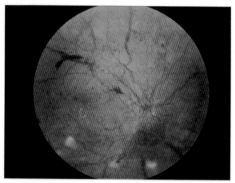

Figure 6: Proliferative diabetic retinopathy with optic disc new blood vessels

Neurological causes of poor vision
Stroke

Many patients with hemiparesis also suffer from a loss of visual field on the same side as the weak limbs (homonymous hemianopia). Older patients can also develop occipital lobe strokes whereby there is no limb weakness but simply contralateral visual field loss. Patients with bilateral occipital lobe infarctions can be left with no peripheral vision, but instead retain a small tunnel of central vision in both eyes.

Consideration of the side of hemianopia should be given when positioning the patient's bed - if a patient's bed is beside a wall, it is important that his hemianopic side faces the wall and his seeing side faces the room in the early stages.

Pituitary lesions

Patients with pituitary lesions, most commonly tumours, initially develop bitemporal visual field loss followed by severe central visual loss as chiasma compression increases. The visual fields and central vision can improve remarkably well following pituitary surgery. The prognosis for visual recovery depends on the amount of optic nerve damage and duration of compression. In patients without advanced optic atrophy, the prognosis for visual recovery is good and duration is short.

Multiple sclerosis

This condition more usually affects younger patients but can sometimes be seen in older subjects. The commonest manifestation is retrobulbar neuritis, typically resulting in loss of vision in one eye associated with pain on eye movement due to stretching of the inflamed ocular nerve. Residual pallor of the optic disc is the typical physical finding noted. Other manifestations include brainstem nystagmus and diplopia.

Diplopia

Uniocular diplopia (present with one eye closed) is due to ocular pathology splitting the visual axis and is most commonly caused by early cataract formation. The more usual diplopia is that which is present with both eyes open and examination will reveal a paralytic squint (dissociation of eye movements). The most important of these are the sixth and third nerve palsies.

In sixth nerve palsy, the patient complains of horizontal diplopia and examination reveals failure of abduction. It is usually due to an acute vascular event and tends to recover in six weeks. Apart from a general vascular work-up, the only investigations warranted at presentation are a blood glucose and ESR, as lateral rectus palsy can be a manifestation of giant cell arteritis. The false localising sign of sixth nerve palsy frequently gives rise to confusion and unnecessary CT scan requests. This false localising sign occurs only in the context of papilloedema and, consequently, a CT scan to exclude raised intracranial pressure is not needed when there is no disc swelling. A CT scan is however warranted if there is no recovery of a sixth nerve palsy after six weeks so as to exclude cavernous sinus pathology such as an infraclinoid aneurysm or metastatic deposit.

In third nerve palsy, there is complete ptosis and the eye is 'down and out' (figure 7). From the diagnostic viewpoint, there are two broad categories of third nerve palsy, namely 'medical' and 'surgical'. The 'medical' palsies are associated with 'pupil sparing' (non-dilatation of the pupil), are generally painless and causes include brainstem vascular lesions, diabetes and Herpes zoster. The initial investigation of these cases is similar to patients with a sixth nerve palsy. By contrast, the 'surgical' palsies are characterised by a dilated pupil and are painful. An expanding posterior communicating artery aneurysm must be excluded as a matter of extreme urgency to prevent subarachnoid haemorrhage.

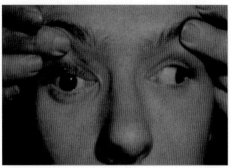

Figure 7: Complete ptosis and 'down and out' eye of right third nerve palsy (lids elevated to show eye position)

Ear, nose and throat (ENT)

History taking is the key to diagnosis in most ENT conditions and time spent in allowing the patient to explain their symptoms is always time well spent.

Examination of the ears

Always begin by looking at the pinna and behind the ear. Conditions such as basal cell carcinoma (figure 8), squamous cell carcinoma (figure 9) and Herpes zoster (figure 10) are obvious. Use the auriscope with the largest speculum that will fit. All parts of the tympanic membrane should be seen and wax removal may be required (figure 11). The Formby Wax Hook is a wonderful tool. Rinne and Weber tests will distinguish between conductive and neural deafness. Many practitioners have the 'AUDIOSCOPE' to perform limited audiometry at the bedside. Audiometry in a sound proofed room is required for accurate assessment of hearing levels. White patches on the tympanic membrane (tympanosclerosis) may indicate scarring and conductive deafness. A perforation may be seen. Cholesteatoma causes chronic discharge, deafness and may cause tinnitus and vertigo - a perforation with dirty grey ragged edges or granulation tissue is a dangerous sign and requires specialist referral.

Presbycusis is diagnosed with the symptom of deafness, often described as 'hard of hearing', which is worsened in the presence of background noise. Definitive audiometry in presbycusis shows deafness increasing at higher frequencies, with both ears

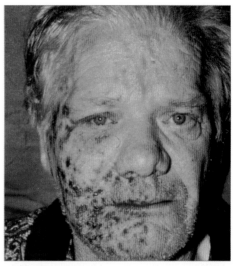
Figure 10: Herpes zoster of trigeminal nerve

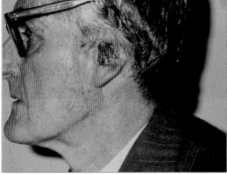
Figure 8: Basal cell carcinoma of ear pinna

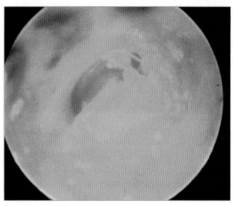
Figure 11: Wax in ear canal

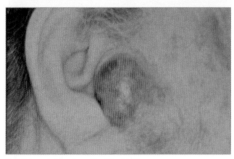
Figure 9: Squamous cell carcinoma of parotid (metastatic)

equally affected. Hearing-aids are helpful but, like a walking stick in arthritis, are an aid, not a cure. In cases of vertigo, look for ear pathology, particularly cholesteatoma, otorrhoea, facial paralysis, nystagmus, and carotid bruits. Also examine the cranial nerves and cerebellar functions.

Examination of the nose

Begin at the outside and look for symmetry,

excoriation or redness of the nasal vestibules or evidence of nasal obstruction such as nasal polypi (figure 12). The nasal septum, turbinates and nasal cavity may be easily assessed with an otoscope and large speculum. Simple nasal polypi are bilateral, pale, fleshy, glistening, relatively avascular, grey, insensitive to touch and are very mobile when touched. They may cause severe nasal blockage, widening of the nasal bones and even destruction of some turbinate bones. Large inferior turbinates are often mistaken for polypi, but hurt when prodded!

Unilateral polypi which are painful or bleed, or

polypi with localized tenderness, are more sinister and may be malignant. Involvement of cheek skin is always a suspicious feature and any unilateral nasal pathology should be regarded with suspicion. Orbital cellulitis may complicate nasal or sinus tumours (figure 13).

Maxillary sinusitis may affect many people. The patient presents with facial tenderness, (but not swelling), purulent nasal discharge, headache, dental pain and malaise. X-rays of sinuses are diagnostic (figure 14). If it becomes chronic, sinusitis usually requires surgical treatment.

Obstruction of the nose may also occur in the nasopharynx as in this case of antro-choanal polyp (figure 15).

Examination of the throat

Remember to look at the lips, cheeks, gums and the floor of the mouth under the tongue, before going on to inspect the tongue, palate, tonsils and oropharynx. The lips may be affected by leukoplakia (figure 16) or squamous carcinoma, especially in pipe-smokers. Surgical excision or radiotherapy are very successful. White patches on the cheeks or gums may be due to lichen planus, leukoplakia (pre-malignant) or candidiasis. If the white patch does not rub off, send for specialist help. Laser treatment is very easy and effective.

Tongue cancer presents with ulceration, induration and mild pain. Early treatment is important as lymphatic spread occurs at a very early stage in this disease. Delay in treatment can be disastrous. Involvement of neck nodes is a very poor prognostic sign. Aggressive therapy with surgery and radiotherapy may improve survival rates to 50%.

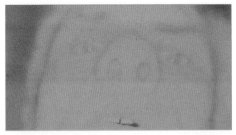

Figure 12: Bilateral simple nasal polypi

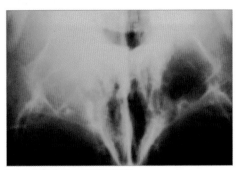

Figure 13: Orbital cellulitis secondary to tumour in sinuses

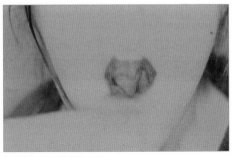

Figure 15: Antro-choanal polyp in nasopharynx

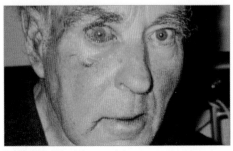

Figure 14: Maxillary sinusitis showing unilateral opacity

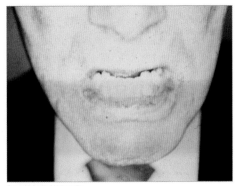

Figure 16: Leukoplakia lower lip

The tongue and palate are supplied by the vagus and hypoglossal cranial nerves and are good indications of disease in the brainstem or skull base. The fasiculating tongue of motor neurone disease or immobile tongue of bulbar palsy are diagnostic. Unilateral hypoglossal paralysis may be due to cancer in the nasopharynx (figure 17). The tongue is part of the digestive system and may be shiny and beefy in iron deficiency or thin and cracked in vitamin deficiency states.

Hoarseness is a serious symptom if it lasts for more than 3 weeks - especially in older smokers. Other warning symptoms are otalgia and haemoptysis. Cancer of the larynx is now becoming more common in women. If diagnosed early, laryngeal cancer has excellent survival prospects as the vocal cords have no lymphatic supply and metastases occur late (figure 18). Neck nodes are again a poor prognostic sign in patients presenting with hoarseness or dysphagia (figure 19).

In globus pharynges, cricopharyngeal muscles go into a state of spasm and give a feeling of a lump in the throat and the need to 'double swallow' to get food down. A barium swallow will help in the diagnosis. Note that flexible oesophagoscopy may easily miss tumours in the lower pharynx or upper oesophagus. Foreign bodies in the oesophagus are easily spotted and removed (figure 20).

Clinical findings of common ENT pathologies in older people

Ramsay Hunt Syndrome

Ramsay Hunt Syndrome is typically associated with reactivation of latent Varicella zoster residing within the geniculate ganglion. Herpes simplex type 2

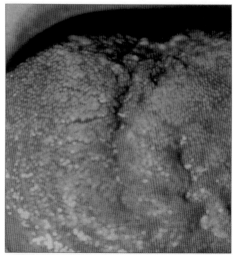
Figure 18: Carcinoma of vocal cord

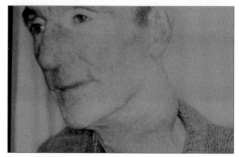
Figure 19: Cervical lymphadenopathy

can also be a precipitant of the syndrome. Auditory and vestibular symptoms are due to inflammation of the eighth cranial nerve, but the fifth, ninth and tenth cranial nerves may also be involved. The facial paralysis seen in Ramsay Hunt syndrome is usually associated with a lower probability of recovery in comparison to Bell's palsy, a similar condition in which Herpes simplex is postulated to be the cause.

Meniere's disease

Meniere's disease is caused by increased pressure within the endolymphatic gland spaces of the inner ear. The aetiology is unknown and the symptoms may quickly disappear or become progressively worse. The diagnosis can only be made where there is the triad of vertigo, tinnitus and hearing loss.

When assessing these patients, a detailed history

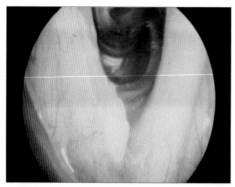
Figure 17: Unilateral paralysis of the tongue

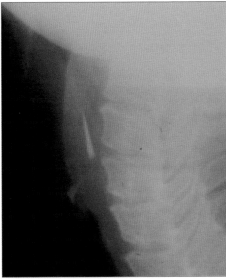
Figure 20: Bony foreign body in upper oesophagus

and neurological examination must be undertaken to exclude more sinister disease processes. During attacks, Romberg's test will be positive. The Dix-Hallpike manoeuvre will help to exclude a diagnosis of benign paroxysmal positional vertigo. Audiology is essential and will show low frequency, unilateral sensorineural hearing loss. The hearing loss worsens during attacks and incompletely recovers between attacks, so that hearing will progressively deteriorate in a step-wise fashion.

Management of Meniere's disease during the acute phase involves control of the distressing symptoms of vertigo and nausea. Prochlorperazine, cyclizine and benzodiazepines control symptoms due to their anticholinergic, antiemetic and sedative properties. Long-term prophylaxis includes salt restriction, diuretics, cessation of smoking and stress reduction. Severe cases can be controlled by labyrinthine destructive treatments by either medical (gentamicin) or surgical means.

Benign paroxysmal positional vertigo
Several particle repositioning manoeuvres have been devised and have been found to be effective in treating benign paroxysmal positional vertigo. These include the Brandt-Daroff exercises, the Epley and modified Epley manoeuvres and the Semont and modified Semont manoeuvres. They are also helpful in diagnosing

benign paroxysmal positional vertigo if nystagmus is not evident – resolution of symptoms following the manoeuvre is diagnostic. Medications are not usually helpful for the short attacks of vertigo experienced by the patient with this condition.

Suggested further reading
- *Jacobs D S. Primary Open Angle Glaucoma. Up-To-Date 2008.*
- *Weizer J S. Angle Closure Glaucoma. Up-To-Date 2008*
- *Jacob D S. Cataract in Adults. Up-To-Date 2008.*
- *Arroyo J G. Age-related Macular Degeneration: Epidemiology, etiology and diagnosis. Up-To-Date 2008.*
- *Arroyo J G. Age-related Macular Degeneration: Treatment and Prevention. Up-To-Date 2008.*
- *Fraser C E, D'Amico D J. Classification and Clinical Features of Diabetic Retinopathy. Up-To-Date 2008.*
- *Bienfang D C. Overview of Diplopia. Up-To-Date 2008.*
- *Arroyo J G. Retinal Tear and Detachment. Up-To-Date 2008.*
- *Avery RL. New Treatments for Age-Related Macular Degeneration. Lancet. 2007 Oct 27;370(9597): 1479-80.*
- *Brown DM, Regillo CD. Anti-VEGF agents in the treatment of neovascular age-related macular degeneration: applying clinical trial results to the treatment of everyday patients. Am J Ophthalmol. 2007 Oct;144(4):627-37.*
- *Evans JR. Antioxidant vitamin and mineral supplements for slowing the progression of age-related macular degeneration. Cochrane Database of Systematic Reviews 2006, Issue 2. Art. No.: CD000254. DOI: 10.1002/14651858.CD000254.pub2.*
- *Hatt S, Wormald R, Burr J. Screening for prevention of optic nerve damage due to chronic open angle glaucoma. Cochrane Database of Systematic Reviews 2006, Issue 4. Art. No.: CD006129. DOI: 10.1002/14651858. CD006129.pub2.*
- *Mayor S. Targeted screening may be a cost effective way to detect glaucoma. BMJ. 2007 Dec 1;335(7630): 1114.*
- *Van Overdam KA, Bettink-Remeijer MW, Klaver CC, Mulder PG, Moll AC, van Meurs JC. Symptoms and findings predictive for the development of new retinal breaks. Arch Ophthalmol. 2005 Apr;123(4): 479-84.*
- *Gordon-Bennett P, Ung T, Stephenson C, Hingorani M. Misdiagnosis of angle closure glaucoma. BMJ. 2006 Dec 2;333(7579): 1157-8.*
- *Hilton M, Pinder D. The Epley (canalith repositioning) manoeuvre for benign paroxysmal positional vertigo. Cochrane Database of Systematic Reviews 2004, Issue 2. Art. No.: CD003162. DOI: 10.1002/14651858. CD003162.pub2.*

Case Study 1

A 78 year old woman presented to her GP with severe left sided headache and vomiting. She had associated severe pain in her left eye with reduced vision. She was also experiencing light halos. Further questioning confirmed that the halos were multi-coloured. She had been unwell for several days with coryzal and flu like symptoms and took an 'over the counter' nasal decongestant the previous day. Past medical history included hypertension, type 2 diabetes mellitus and urge incontinence. Her medications were as follows: amlodipine, ramipril, metformin, atorvastatin and oxybutynin.

On examination she had no features of meningism and no lateralizing neurology. However her left eye was red with a poorly reactive mid dilated pupil (4-6mm). The cornea appeared cloudy. Her GP was concerned regarding her symptoms and signs and referred her for urgent ophthalmology review.

Gonioscopy confirmed a shallow anterior chamber in the left eye. Her intraocular pressure was 60mmHg. Pupillary dilatation was performed. The diagnosis was acute angle closure glaucoma precipitated by medication which was subsequently discontinued. A topical ophthalmic beta blocker and alpha agonist were used to reduce both intraocular pressure and inflammatory response, in addition to intravenous and oral acetazolamide. Analgesia and antiemetics are important therapeutically as they also assist in lowering intraocular pressure. She subsequently proceeded to a laser peripheral iridotomy, which is the definitive treatment.

Case Study 2

An 80 year old man presented to his GP having been told by his optician that his discs appeared 'cupped' and that further ophthalmology review was advised. He denied any history of trauma or any episodes of red or painful eyes. Past medical history included hypertension, hypercholesterolaemia, osteoporosis and osteoarthritis. Medications included bisoprolol, atorvastatin, paracetomol, calcium and vitamin D. On fundoscopy the optic disc did appear cupped.

He was referred for ophthalmology review and had a more extensive examination. This confirmed that he had peripheral field changes (both nasal defect and arcuate scotoma). Gonioscopy, a technique which involves use of a special lens for the slit lamp, allowed visualization of both anterior chamber angles. These were open and normal in both eyes. Of note, intraocular pressure was also normal. He was diagnosed as having primary open angle glaucoma and was commenced on a topical beta-blocker twice daily. He was unable to tolerate this therapy however, as he became increasingly dyspnoeic. A topical prostaglandin was commenced instead, which apart from having little systemic effects had the added advantage of once daily dosing. Of interest, his visual acuity was normal on formal assessment.

Case Study 3

An 80 year old gentleman complained to his GP of a progressive decline in his vision. He had attended his optician several times in recent years as he had become increasingly short-sighted. Despite spectacle correction the deterioration had continued. Both eyes were affected although his right was worse than his left. He had particular difficulty driving at night and reading road signs. He commented that his near vision was relatively good. He gave no history of redness or pain in either eye. There was no history of trauma. Past medical history included hypertension, COPD and Type 2 diabetes. He had a 30 pack year history of smoking. Medications included aspirin, ramipril, bisoprolol, atorvastatin, metformin, tiotropium and budesonide nebulisers.

On examination with the direct ophthalmoscope, the GP detected that there was darkening of the red reflex. It was not possible to see the fundus clearly. He correctly diagnosed that this patient had developed cataracts in both eyes. He advised the patient to stop smoking and made a referral for a non-urgent comprehensive ophthalmology review (subjective refraction, establishment of type and extent of lens opacity, dilated fundus examination). He also arranged for the patient to see him at more regular intervals in the interim, with the aim of improving his blood pressure and diabetic control in anticipation of future surgery. His ophthalmologist confirmed a diagnosis of nuclear sclerosis. The patient went on to have surgery under local anesthesia.

Case Study 4

A 76 year old woman presented to her GP with an acute disturbance of her vision, which had occurred over a period of days. She noticed that when she looked at objects that she knew to have straight edges, they appeared distorted. In describing this, she commented that doors and window blinds looked 'curved'. She also felt that the visual acuity in her left eye had significantly deteriorated. Past medical history included hypertension, hypercholesterolemia, myocardial infarction and hypothyroidism. Medications included thyroxine, amlodipine, bisoprolol, atorvastatin, aspirin and clopidogrel. She was a lifelong smoker of twenty cigarettes a day. She also had a high body mass index.

Upon dilated fundoscopy, some oedema in the macular area was noted, suggestive of possible choroidal neovascularisation. Small hemorrhages and exudates were also visible on the retina. The GP was concerned by her symptoms and signs and referred her for urgent ophthalmology review. Her visual acuity was formally assessed and dilated fundus examination was performed using the slit lamp. Neovascularisation was confirmed with fluorescein angiography. A diagnosis of 'wet' age related macular degeneration (ARMD) was made.

Case Study 5

A 68 year old woman became concerned when she suddenly experienced black 'cobweb' like material floating across the field of vision in her left eye. She also noticed as she looked up and down that she experienced bright flashes of light which lasted only seconds. These were not painful. She had no headache and initially no reduction in visual acuity. There was no history of trauma. Suddenly however, a shower of black dots seemed to fall over her field of vision in that eye. It intensified and dramatically she lost vision – only being able to count fingers in that eye when she presented to her GP. Past medical history included hypothyrodism, osteoarthritis and bilateral hip replacements. Medications included thyroxine and regular paracetamol. Of note, she had been severely myopic for many years.

She was referred to eye casualty and diagnosed with a vitreous haemorrhage due to posterior vitreous detachment. Ultrasound confirmed this (it was not possible to see the posterior or peripheral retina due to blood in the vitreous). Thankfully there was no evidence of retinal detachment (retinal elevation on ultrasound heralds impending retinal detachment). She had to be monitored carefully as patients with vitreous haemorrhage have a 40% chance of retinal tear due to posterior vitreous detachment. She was consequently monitored weekly until the blood cleared. Both eyes were examined. Over time her vision improved with no intervention.

Case Study 6

A 78-year-old gentleman presented to his GP. He had been diagnosed as having Type 2 diabetes five years previously and had known retinopathy. He had some difficulty with his diabetic control in the past and had of late been commenced on insulin. His control was now much tighter with his most recent HBA1C being 7.9%. He was disappointed however, as he felt his vision was worse.

Fundoscopy confirmed an increasing number of cotton wool spots. These represented superficial layer retinal infarcts which were precipitated by the lower plasma volume (itself induced by treating hyperglycaemia) in some marginal vessels.

Case Study 7

A patient presented to Accident & Emergency with a left facial droop and reduced power in his left upper and lower limbs. He had a background history of hypertension, hypercholesterolaemia and ischaemic heart disease. Medications included aspirin, atorvastatin, bisoprolol, ramipril and isosorbide mononitrate.

On examination it was noted that he was in fast atrial fibrillation. Cardiovascular examination revealed no murmurs or carotid bruits. Neurological examination confirmed an upper motor neuron lesion of the seventh cranial nerve. He also had a left hemianopia and left visual field neglect. Not unexpectedly, he had also had left sided sensory loss and neglect. Power was 4/5. Despite the deficit in power being relatively mild, his rehabilitation was slow and difficult. This in a significant way was secondary to his visual field deficit and neglect and although he achieved discharge home he required assistance of one with all personal activities of daily living.

Case Study 8

A 72-year-old patient presented to her GP with severe right sided ear pain and a right sided facial droop. She felt her hearing had deteriorated in that ear and was experiencing tinnitus. She had increased lacrimation on the right side. She was also complaining of severe unsteadiness and she described the room as 'spinning'.

On examination, vesicles were visible in the auditory canal and auricle. She had no other focal neurology. Past medical history included infection with Varicella zoster infection and a diagnosis of Ramsay Hunt syndrome was made. She was commenced on oral valcyclovir 1000mg tds for one week. The predominant goal of treatment was to reduce the intensity of the pain and to help prevent the occurrence of post herpetic neuralgia. Evidence from clinical trials, supports the above approach especially if the treatment is initiated within 72 hours of onset of symptoms.

Case Study 9

A 65 year old gentleman was referred by his G.P. for a specialist ENT opinion. He had experienced recurrent episodes of vertigo, preceded by right-sided aural fullness over the previous 5 years. These episodes were becoming more frequent. His tinnitus in the same ear became worse with the episodes of vertigo. Other features elicited on questioning were hearing loss and nausea, which worsened with the episodes of vertigo.

Audiometry showed low frequency sensorineural hearing loss in his right ear. MRI brain and MRI of his internal auditory canals showed no pathology. The diagnosis was Meniere's disease.

Case Study 10

A 70-year-old patient presented to her GP concerned by symptoms of severe unsteadiness occurring episodically over the previous two weeks. This unsteadiness was associated with a severe sense of rotation or the room spinning with some symptoms of nausea during the attacks. These episodes began after a sudden postional change such as lying down or turning in bed. The vertigo began after a delay of a few seconds after moving and lasted no more than thirty seconds. She was very clear about the fact that the episodes were provoked by changes in posture or sudden movement.

Her GP was very thorough, but review of systems revealed no other neurological symptoms. Her hearing was normal bilaterally. Neurological examination was normal. When performing the Dix-Hallpike manoeuvre, the vertigo and nystagmus were worse with her head to the left side and this indicated that the affected ear was on the left side. The diagnosis was clear – benign paroxysmal positional vertigo.

Data Interpretation

Question 1
An 80 year old man with a background history of hypertension and severe COPD presented to his GP with multiple bruises and an increased frequency of 'bumping' into objects. He denied any unsteadiness or focal neurological symptoms. He agreed that his peripheral vision had markedly deteriorated.

a. What would you expect to find on fundoscopy?
b. What is the most likely diagnosis?
c. What agent would you choose to treat this condition, given his past medical history?

Question 2
A 75 year old lady with a history of sleep apnoea and hypertension suffered acute loss of vision. This was preceded by disturbance of her vision whereby lines and edges appeared distorted and curved over the previous few days.

a. What is the main differential diagnosis based on this presentation?
b. How is this condition classified?
c. What treatments exist?

Question 3
A 65-year-old gentleman complained of intermittent episodes of vertigo. These episodes persisted only for a few minutes but sometimes were accompanied by emesis. He felt he was increasingly unsteady between attacks. He denied any hearing loss.

a. What test would you do to clarify the diagnosis?
b. What is the most effective treatment?

Question 4
A 70-year-old patient presented with hearing loss and tinnitus but he did not have vertigo.
a. What is the likely diagnosis?
b. What is the differential diagnosis?
c. What is the prognosis?

Best of five questions

Question 1
A 70 year old gentleman presented to his GP with gradually reducing visual acuity over several years. He had attended his optician frequently to alter the prescription for his glasses. He had particular difficulty driving at night. His medical history included type 2 diabetes and hypertension. He had a 30 pack year history of smoking.

What is the most likely diagnosis?
a. retinitis pigmentosa
b. chronic simple glaucoma
c. cataract
d. central retinal vein occlusion
e. diabetic retinopathy

Question 2
A 65 year old woman presented to her GP for a 6 monthly assessment of her type 2 diabetes. It was noted that her blood pressure was sub-optimally controlled at 150/90mmHg. She mentioned she had been experiencing multiple flashes in front of both eyes for a period of months. On more detailed questioning, she commented that she had been suffering from low mood and felt very anxious. When asked directly she admitted to having experienced visual hallucinations.

What is the likely diagnosis?
a. Proliferative diabetic retinopathy
b. Occipital lobe ischaemia
c. Retinal detachment
d. Migraine
e. Uncontrolled hypertension

Question 3
A 78-year-old lady presented to A&E with sudden onset of left sided facial droop. She had normal visual fields. Peripheral nervous system examination did not reveal any lateralising signs. She was very unsteady however and could not walk unaided. She had severe pain in her right ear.

What is the next most appropriate course of action?
a. MRI brain
b. CT brain
c. Examination of auditory canal
d. Varicella zoster serology
e. Lumbar puncture

Question 4
A 65 year old lady presented to her GP with vertigo, nausea

and vomiting which had been persistent for several hours. There was no obvious provoking factor. She did not have hearing loss. Of note, she did not have any cardiovascular risk factors and was on no medications. She had experienced symptoms like this on two other occasions over the previous month. She was referred to A&E and investigations included a CT brain which was normal.

What is the most likely diagnosis?

a. Brainstem infarct

b Cochlear Meniere's disease

c. Vestibular Meniere's disease

d. Benign Paroxysmal Positional Vertigo

e. Acoustic Neuroma

Answers are on page 311

Palliative care

S O'Hanlon, P Sheahan

Introduction

Palliative care has existed in some form since the 19th century. The medieval hospice was a 'house of rest and entertainment for pilgrims, travellers, strangers, destitutes and the sick'. The modern hospice movement is based on a philosophy of care rather than a place of care. Its founder, Dame Cecily Saunders, who originally trained as a nurse, said: *'I have become more and more aware of the problems of the dying, particularly of the hopeless advanced case of cancer. I do think that they are deserted by the doctors. I want to find ways of alleviating their physical and mental distress'.*

She was advised by the surgeon she was working with to 'go read medicine; it is the doctors who desert the dying'. She trained as a doctor and after qualifying did some clinical research in St. Joseph's Hospice, where she introduced the regular administration of analgesia for pain control. She founded St. Christopher's Hospice in 1967 and, based on her following statement, the modern hospice movement began. *'You matter because you are you, you will matter until the last moment of your life and we will help you not only to die peacefully but to live as fully as possible until the moment you die'.*

In 2005, the World Health Organisation defined palliative care as 'an approach that improves the quality of life of patients and their families facing the problems associated with life threatening illness, through the prevention and relief of suffering by means of early identification, and impeccable assessment and treatment of pain and other problems, physical, psychological or spiritual.'

Palliative care was initially developed for people dying of cancer but now it is increasingly used in other diseases such as heart failure, chronic obstructive pulmonary disease and progressive neurological conditions. This chapter aims to provide an outline of the principles and practice of palliative care with a particular emphasis on the older population.

Principles of palliative care

Specialist palliative care is provided by a multidisciplinary team under the direction of a consultant in palliative medicine. The team consists of the consultant, junior doctors, specialist palliative care nurses and nurses with a skill mix to meet the needs of the patient, a dedicated physiotherapist, occupational therapist, social worker and chaplain. The specialist team should have access to support services including speech and language therapy, pharmacy, complementary therapy, volunteer co-ordinator and dietetics. Access to palliative care should be based on need and offered as needs develop, before they become unmanageable.

Palliative care should be provided wherever the patient is – at home, in hospital or in continuing care. The most common reasons for referral to specialist palliative care services are complex symptom management, rehabilitation, respite and terminal care. Such care, however, should be available to those individuals whose illnesses show clear evidence of progression with increasing symptom severity, increasing complexity of care needs and declining level of function, in whom a specialist could say 'I would not be surprised if this patient died within the next year'.

Previous perceptions of palliative care were that it was only relevant in the last few weeks of life (figure 1). However, many patients and families need palliative support and care alongside other therapies which may prolong life and so a new concept of palliative care has developed (figure 2).

Palliative care in older people

Palliative Medicine and Geriatric Medicine both aim to improve the dignity and autonomy of patients and to improve quality of life by working to make patients as independent as possible within the constraints of illness. Both specialties involve multidisciplinary team-working and provide

TABLE I
SELECTED DRUGS REPORTED TO CAUSE SEIZURES
• Provides relief from pain and other distressing symptoms
• Affirms life and regards dying as a normal process
• Intends neither to hasten nor postpone death
• Integrates the psychological and spiritual aspects of patient care
• Offers a support system to help the patient live as actively as possible until death
• Offers a support system to help the family cope during the patient's illness and in their own bereavement
• Should be applicable early in the course of illness, in conjunction with other therapies that are intended to prolong life, such as chemotherapy or radiotherapy
• Should be available based on needs, not on diagnosis or life expectancy

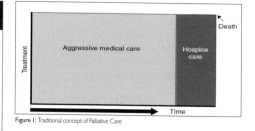

Figure 1: Traditional concept of Palliative Care

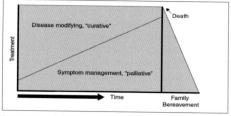

Figure 2: New concept of Palliative Care
These figures are adapted from 'Living Well at the End of Life' by Joanne Lynn and David Adamson, used with permission of the author and RAND corporation

care across all care settings, yet there has been little integration between the two specialties. Should palliative care for older people, therefore, be considered as a separate entity? It is generally believed that palliative care services should be based around need, and that age should not be a factor. However the needs of an older population may be different to those of a younger group. In addition there are separate challenges which affect older patients, and older carers. The 2004 WHO report 'Better Palliative Care for Older People' described it as 'a public health priority' and identified the following special needs of older people:

• Older people are more commonly affected by multiple medical problems of varying severity
• The cumulative effect of these may be much greater than any individual disease, and typically lead to greater impairment and needs for care
• Older people are at greater risk of adverse drug reactions and of iatrogenic illness
• Minor problems may have a greater cumulative psychological impact in older people
• Problems of acute illness may be superimposed on physical or mental impairment, economic hardship and social isolation

Challenges in palliative care for older people

Older patients are more likely to have palliative care needs, but are less likely to be referred and less likely to receive home care and inpatient palliative care than younger patients. Variation in service provision compounds this difficulty with access. The average age of informal carers, most of whom are women, is increasing and younger retired people will have a pivotal role in caring for the oldest old in the future. Patients with older carers have worse access to palliative care and greater problems with social isolation.

Patients should be able to choose the place of their dying and, in most surveys, about 75% of patients would choose their home. Keeping patients at home may be difficult and the majority of older people die in acute and long stay units where facilities are not always appropriate to patients' needs. The availability of single rooms at the time of death is highest in private nursing homes and lowest in acute hospitals. The majority of staff in these areas have not received any formal training in palliative care. In addition, there is also a low level of access to palliative care services in long stay facilities.

Referral of older patients to palliative care is often determined by estimated survival but establishing an accurate prognosis is difficult, especially in the very old or those with non-malignant conditions. A systematic review of models to predict prognosis in non-cancer patients revealed that none could do this successfully. This is a very heterogeneous group and survival times vary widely. There are more data for patients with cancer, but survival still varies.

A key challenge faced when attempting to enhance quality of life for older people at the end of life is the preservation of autonomy and dignity in the face of inevitable paternalism. Laws on decision making at the end of life are based on the principles of autonomy and self-determination. To uphold these principles, patients must be kept informed about their health at all stages of their care. It is not right that families are informed while the patient remains ignorant. Patients must be involved directly in their own care and this requires an improvement in communication between doctors, families and patients.

Caring for patients dying with cancer was the original focus of palliative care, and services usually cope better with patients dying from malignancy than those with non-malignant conditions. However, more people now die of chronic cardiovascular, cerebrovascular and respiratory diseases, representing a disparate range of conditions with clinical courses that are difficult to predict. Specialist palliative care services, therefore, need to work in harmony with lead clinicians from other disciplines.

Non-malignant conditions

Dementia
The median survival for dementia is 4.5 years, with inevitable progressive declines in cognition and function that render the assessment of need and delivery of care very difficult. End-stage, distressing symptoms such as severe confusion, agitation and aggression are particularly difficult to treat. Carers carry a huge burden and may have little support or education about the condition. There is also a lack of specialized institutional care units to manage those with severe end-stage disease. Ethical issues such as parenteral feeding, resuscitation and how aggressively to manage acute illness pose difficult challenges.

Cardiac failure
Mortality rates in patients with heart failure are worse than many cancers. Periods of symptom control may be interspersed with periods of severe disease exacerbations which can be frightening, prolonged and lead to stepwise deterioration. Almost one in three patients will require hospital admission in any one year. Symptoms such as shortness of breath and pain are common and difficult to control and often undertreated by doctors. A study comparing a heart failure clinic with a palliative care clinic found that the patients complained of identical symptoms: pain, loss of independence, difficulty in walking, anxiety, fatigue, breathlessness, constipation, nausea, vomiting and difficulty sleeping.

Disease management is frequently complex, with many patients on multiple medications. Home oxygen may be required and night sedation should be considered for those with nocturnal dyspnoea. The course of the disease is very difficult to predict, ranging from progressive decline to sudden cardiac death, and deciding when these patients should be referred to palliative services can be challenging.

Chronic Obstructive Pulmonary Disease (COPD)
Patients with severe COPD have poor quality of life and studies have shown that their needs may not be addressed as well as those of patients with lung cancer. Their symptom load is particularly heavy in the final year of life as symptoms of breathlessness may be heightened by anxiety and fear of loss of control. The clinical course is one of progressive irreversible deterioration. Patients may reach a point where standard treatments do not improve symptoms and, in such cases, palliative care is necessary and appropriate. Morphine and benzodiazepines can help to treat severe dyspnoea in end-stage disease, but often at the expense of a worsening of carbon dioxide retention. Short-acting benzodiazepines may ease anxiety and concerns regarding accumulation and dependency are not a factor in the terminal phase.

Progressive neurological conditions
Motor neurone disease, multiple sclerosis and Parkinson's disease are just some of the neurological conditions which cause reduced quality of life, increased morbidity and shorter survival.

While there are a wide variety of symptoms associated with the diseases mentioned above, it is important to note that most patients have multiple symptoms. One study of patients referred to a palliative care service noted that the median number of physical symptoms reported was six. Symptoms

- 'Pain is an unpleasant sensory and emotional experience associated with actual or potential tissue damage, or described in terms of such damage'
- 'Pain is a complex sensation, encompassing a whole range of factors including physical, emotional, spiritual and social. All of these intertwine to form what Saunders describes as the total pain experience'
- 'Pain is whatever the experiencing person says it is'

may be due to the underlying disease itself, its treatment, general debility or concurrent illnesses. Each symptom requires careful assessment in order to treat appropriately.

Pain

When people think of cancer, they associate it with pain and suffering. Patients dread the pain of cancer more than anything. It is important to remember that intractable pain is the exception not the rule and, by using the World Health Organisation Analgesic Ladder, up to 90% of pain can be controlled. Pain is not just a physical entity and physical pain does not always imply suffering. Physical pain may be just the tip of the iceberg as pain may also be psychological, social and spiritual.

Pain is experienced by 75% of people with cancer at some point in their illness and more than two-thirds of patients will experience more than one pain. It is under-recognised and under-reported, especially in the older population where patients with cognitive dysfunction pose particular problems. One-third of older people in the community report that pain is an important symptom, while physicians have a tendency to under-treat pain due to both malignant and non-malignant disease. In a study of pain management in older patients with cancer, those over 85 years of age were least likely to receive drugs such as opioids. Another study showed that nearly 30% of older patients in long term care units did not receive analgesia despite daily complaints of pain.

Pain in cancer may be caused by the cancer, its treatment, generalised debility (eg. pressure sores) or may be secondary to other conditions such as arthritis. The important first step in the management of any pain is to identify and treat the cause, if possible, while at the same time prescribing appropriate analgesic medication to control the symptom. When treating pain, it is necessary to know what the patient's interpretation of the pain is and to be aware that perception of pain is greatly influenced by the patient's mood, morale and the meaning of the pain for them eg. 'Does it mean that cancer has returned?'

Pharmacological management of pain

When prescribing in palliative care, it is important to use as few medications as possible, stop any unnecessary medications, monitor for adverse effects and review prescriptions regularly. The World Health Organisation analgesic ladder (figure 3) offers a useful guide for pain management and is based on the following principles:

- Regular medication should be prescribed with the aim of preventing pain from occurring
- Appropriate PRN medication ought to be available for breakthrough pain in doses that reflect the regular prescribed dose
- Medication should be prescribed orally as first choice and the strength of the analgesia should depend on the severity of pain rather than the stage of the disease or the person's prognosis. The response to the analgesia should be assessed
- In cancer pain, one drug is rarely sufficient and appropriate adjuvant analgesia should be prescribed. The most important thing is to use the right drug, at the right dose and at the right time intervals, and to prescribe appropriate adjuvant analgesics

Step 1

Paracetamol or non-steroidal anti-inflammatory drug (NSAID) +/- adjuvant analgesics. If pain not controlled, move to

Step 2

Combination of weak opioid + paracetamol +/- adjuvant analgesics. An example of a weak opioid is Codeine Phosphate. If on the maximum dose of Step 2 and pain is not relieved, there is no point switching from one weak opioid to another, move to

Step 3

A strong opioid + paracetamol + an adjuvant analgesic. The strong opioid of choice is morphine.

Morphine

The starting dose of morphine should be tailored

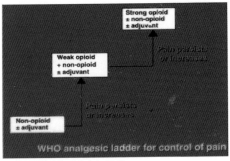

Figure 3: World Health Organisation Analgesic Ladder

to each patient. Opiate naïve patients should receive 5mg of an immediate-release morphine preparation every four hours and as required. If already on a weak opioid, the patient should be switched to 10mg of an immediate-release morphine preparation every four hours and as required. After one day of treatment, the total dose over the previous 24 hours should be calculated and divided by six to give the new four-hourly dose. This dose should also be used as required. Doses should be reviewed every 24-48 hours until adequate pain control is achieved. At this point the formulation may be changed to a sustained release one, containing the same total amount per day, but in one or two doses only.

In contrast to paracetamol and non-steroidal anti-inflammatory drugs, opioids do not have a dose ceiling above which there is no added therapeutic benefit. Older patients may seem to require a lower dose of morphine than younger patients, but side effects such as drowsiness and constipation tend to be more severe. It is also important to be aware of the need to adjust the frequency of dosing from four to six hourly in older patients with impaired renal and liver function.

Side effects of opioids and symptoms of toxicity include:
• Nausea and vomiting, which may be treated with metoclopramide, domperidone or haloperidol
• Constipation, for which regular laxatives should be prescribed, eg. lactulose and senna
• Drowsiness - the patient should be advised that this usually improves after three to five days
• Dry mouth - appropriate mouth care should be prescribed
• Hallucinations, which may respond to haloperidol 1.5mg – 3mg orally
• Respiratory depression, which is only seen at doses above those required for analgesia or if the drug has accumulated due to renal impairment or infection

Alternative strong opioids for cancer pain include oxycodone, hydromorphone, fentanyl and buprenorphine, the latter two preparations being available in patch form.

Non-steroidal anti-inflammatory drugs
Caution should be exercised when using non-steroidal anti-inflammatory drugs in patients with asthma, renal impairment, cardiac failure or a history of peptic ulcer disease. A proton pump inhibitor gives some gastric protection but non-

TABLE 3
APPROXIMATE DOSE EQUIVALENCE TO ORAL MORPHINE

Drug	Potency ratio with morphine	Duration of Action
Tramadol	0.2	4-6 hours
Oxycodone	1.5-2	4-5 hours
Hydromorphone	7.5	4-5 hours
Buprenorphine SL	60	6-8 hours
Methadone	5-10	8-12 hours
Codeine	0.1	3-6 hours
Morphine SC	2	3-4 hours

SL = sublingual   SC = subcutaneous

steroidal anti-inflammatory drugs may precipitate acute pulmonary oedema in older people at quite low doses.

Adjuvant analgesics

The use of adjuvant analgesics should be considered at every stage of the ladder. Suggested adjuvant analgesics are:

1. Steroids, which can be used for pain secondary to raised intracranial pressure, liver pain or neuropathic pain.
2. Amitriptyline, which is started at a dose of 10 mg nocte and titrated upwards according to response. Side effects, which include constipation, dry mouth, hypotension, falls and urinary retention may be particularly bothersome.
3. Anticonvulsants, which can be used for neuropathic pain. Carbamazepine, gabapentin and pregabalin are now commonly prescribed. It is important to remember to start with low doses (for example 25mg bd of pregabalin) and to titrate up every five to seven days according to response.
4. Bisphosphonates, which are used for skeletal metastatic disease. There is evidence from randomized placebo controlled trials that they can reduce pain due to skeletal secondaries from breast, prostate and lung cancer and reduce the rate of bone related complications. They are also used in multiple myeloma. The analgesic effect may take up to two weeks to develop and it is important to monitor renal function and to be aware of the potential to develop hypocalcaemia and osteonecrosis of the jaw.

Non pharmacological adjuvant pain management strategies include:

5. Radiotherapy, which is effective at reducing pain due to local tumour effects of skeletal metastases.
6. Anaesthetic techniques for difficult pain such as that caused by the coeliac plexus in pancreatic cancer.
7. Physiotherapy for management of lymphoedema.
8. Acupuncture and relaxation therapies.
9. Surgery/splints.

Shortness of breath

Breathlessness, like pain, is what the patient says it is. Breathlessness can be extremely frightening and it is essential to manage this fear. This symptom is common in respiratory conditions and in advanced disease with an incidence of 94% in chronic lung disease, 83% in heart failure and up to 70% in cancer. In palliative medicine, shortness of breath may be due to lung cancer, end stage congestive cardiac failure, COPD, motor neurone disease, pulmonary embolism or infection. Indeed, a single patient may have many causes of dyspnoea. For example, a patient with lung cancer may have anaemia, a pleural effusion and background COPD.

Given the wide range of causes, it is important to investigate appropriately, diagnose the cause and treat any reversible contributing factors. Treatment may include:

- Oxygen – if oxygen saturation is < 90%, a trial of O_2 is indicated
- Bronchodilators – if bronchoconstriction is present
- Antibiotics – for respiratory tract infections
- Diuretics, angiotensin converting enzyme inhibitors and nitrates – for heart failure
- Drainage of a pleural effusion
- Anticoagulation for thromboembolism
- Steroids – if known obstructive airways disease or in emergency obstruction
- Superior vena caval stenting
- Benzodiazepines – for anxiety or intractable breathlessness in dying patients
- Morphine – for symptomatic treatment near the end of life

Nausea & vomiting

Nausea and vomiting occur in up to 70% of patients with advanced cancer. It may be multifactorial in aetiology and management requires assessment of the underlying cause or causes which include:

- Medications - opioids, chemotherapy, antibiotics or non-steroidal anti-inflammatory drugs
- Metabolic – uraemia and hypercalcaemia which may be associated with symptoms of constipation, confusion, drowsiness and abdominal pain
- Infection
- Increased intracranial pressure due to cerebral secondaries or meningeal disease (a history of headaches that are worse in the morning is suggestive)
- Gross ascites, constipation, hepatomegaly or faecal impaction
- Bowel obstruction, especially if the patient has intra-abdominal disease
- Radiotherapy
- Peptic ulceration

Any reversible cause should be treated and anxiety that may be exacerbating symptoms should be managed appropriately. Medications should be reviewed and stopped if necessary and the most appropriate anti-emetic (table 4) should be prescribed regularly and on a PRN basis. Use a non-oral route if vomiting prevents drug absorption or nausea prevents compliance. A subcutaneous route allows the use of a syringe driver which facilitates re-evaluation of treatment at regular intervals and optimal dosing. Treatment should be changed if there is no improvement after 24 - 48 hours. Add or substitute a second anti-emetic if there is still no improvement. If nausea and vomiting remain intractable, add a third line anti-emetic. If the patient has been symptom-free for 72 hours, the subcutaneous route should be discontinued and the patient switched to oral equivalents. The final common pathway for prokinetic drugs is cholinergic and antimuscarinic drugs should not, therefore, be concurrently prescribed as the prokinetic action will be blocked.

Constipation

Constipation is a symptom that is often overlooked but may cause severe distress and precipitate delirium or bowel obstruction. It can be caused by disease processes as disparate as intra-abdominal malignancy, Parkinson's disease or diabetes. It may also be triggered by immobility, painful defaecation and medication. If related to opiate treatment, constipation may become more troublesome as the dose increases. Ideally, this side effect should be anticipated in patients on opiate therapy and prophylactic measures should be considered when starting opiate analgesics.

Patients should initially be assessed for faecal impaction by performing a digital rectal examination. If present, impaction may require manual evacuation or rectal suppositories. The mainstay of treatment is a stool softener used in combination with a stimulant laxative. Treatment may be short or long-term, depending on the precipitating factors. Patients should be advised to maintain an adequate intake of fibre and develop a regular bowel habit. Sitting on the toilet after breakfast takes advantage of the gastrocolic reflex. In the case of established severe faecal overload, enemas or suppositories should be used first if impaction is low in the rectum. Subsequently, an osmotic agent such as macrogol (polyethylene glycol) may be added, particularly if impaction is higher in the bowel.

TABLE 4
ANTI-EMETICS COMMONLY USED IN PALLIATIVE CARE

FIRST LINE
- Prokinetic agents (such as metoclopramide and domperidone) – for gastric stasis, gastritis, decreased gut motility or subacute bowel obstruction
- Drugs acting principally in the area postrema / chemoreceptor trigger zone (such as haloperidol 1.5mg od or bd) - for most chemical causes of vomiting e.g., hypercalcaemia, morphine, uraemia, toxins from infection or bowel obstruction
- Drugs acting principally on the vomiting centre (such as cyclizine 50mg tds orally or 150mg by subcutaneous infusion over 24 hours) - for mechanical bowel obstruction, raised intracranial pressure or motion sickness
- Dexamethasone may be useful in cases of raised intracranial pressure

SECOND LINE
- Dexamethasone and levomepromazine are useful options when first line antiemetics fail to relieve nausea and vomiting satisfactorily. Dexamethasone is normally added to the existing regime whereas levomepromazine is normally substituted for the first line anti-emetics
- Lorazepam – for anxiety

THIRD LINE
- 5HT3 receptor antagonists (such as ondansetron and tropisetron) were developed primarily to control chemotherapy-induced nausea and vomiting. They are useful when there is a large release of serotonin from enterochromaffin cells or platelets, for example during chemotherapy or when radiotherapy has damaged the gut mucosa

Terminal care

Terminal care is a continuum of palliative care and describes the care that is offered during the period when death is imminent and life expectancy is limited to hours or days. It is important to recognise when death is imminent, but at times this may be difficult. The terminal phase patient may deteriorate gradually with increasing fatigue and profound weakness. They may sleep more and more, essentially becoming bedbound, and may have difficulty taking tablets or anything more than sips of fluids.

- Pain which may be due to urinary retention, constipation, soreness from lying in the one position or from a pressure sore
- Noisy and moist breathing
- Restlessness and agitation which may be due to a full bladder, incontinence, pain, hypoxia, fear or medication
- Nausea and vomiting - continue anti-emetics by the most appropriate route
- Sweating - keep the patient cool, use a fan, and change the bed linen on a regular basis. Use cotton nightwear
- Jerking/twitching may be myoclonic jerks due to excessive opiates in which case the appropriate response is to reduce the opioid. Alternatively it may be due to uraemia or an altered neurological state, in which case low dose midazolam by continuous infusion would be appropriate
- Confusion may have many causes including drugs, infection or renal failure

Some people with cancer, however, and many patients with respiratory or cardiac disease may experience life-threatening episodes prior to the event. It is important to confirm the person is dying, ensuring there is no reversible cause for the deterioration, for example hypercalcaemia, infections or opioid toxicity. Confirming imminent death allows unnecessary treatments and investigations to be discontinued and the patient, family and others to be informed of what is happening. Exacerbations of pain or nausea are unusual in the terminal phase in patients who have previously had these symptoms well controlled.

Management of the terminal phase

The patient, family and carers should be made aware of what is happening and their needs and worries identified and addressed. Realistic goals should be agreed and the patient, family and carers made aware that these may change as the patient's condition deteriorates. If not already addressed, difficult issues such as hydration, feeding and resuscitation may need to be discussed and explained. Spiritual issues should be addressed and spiritual care offered. Changes in management should be explained to the family giving as much or as little information as they need, always taking into account the express wishes of the patient in this regard. As comfort is the priority, all non-essential investigations and medical and nursing procedures should be discontinued. All non-essential medication should also be stopped, but analgesics, anxiolytics, anti-emetics and anticholinergics remain important pharmacological tools in the terminal phase. Any drugs used should be prescribed by an appropriate route, for example oral, subcutaneous, buccal, rectal or transdermal, but the subcutaneous route is the preferred option. It is important that PRN doses of medication are also prescribed and available.

If patients can no longer take morphine orally, this can be given via a subcutaneous infusion instead at half the 24-hour oral dose due to the greater bioavailability by the subcutaneous route. The PRN subcutaneous morphine dose is one-sixth of the 24-hour dose by subcutaneous infusion. Oral anti-emetics can also be switched to the subcutaneous route and, if nausea and vomiting are not present, they should be prescribed subcutaneously on a PRN basis. If respiratory tract secretions are present, changing position may be of benefit and anticholinergics such as hyoscine hydrobromide may be added to a syringe driver and prescribed PRN, but are only effective in 50 - 66% of patients.

Benzodiazepines such as midazolam can be used for terminal agitation, fear, breathlessness, intractable hiccups or seizures. Once-off subcutaneous doses of 5mg can be used but it can then be added to a syringe driver if necessary. Haloperidol or levomepromazine may be useful for nausea or terminal agitation with or without delirium and can also be added to a syringe driver if required.

Research in palliative care for older people

Comparatively little research has been performed on the palliative care needs of older people. There is a particular paucity of studies in older patients with non-malignant conditions. The resultant lack of an evidence-base in this area renders treatment difficult. It is recognised, however, that palliative care is a difficult area in which to perform research. There is difficulty in recruitment and patients vary widely in their disease stage, symptoms and survival. Many trials have high attrition rates and it can be difficult to obtain consent and ensure that there are no ethical issues. These challenges mean that research methodologies are often limited to observational studies, case reports and questionnaires. There are few randomised controlled trials.

A recent study showed that patients do wish to participate in palliative care research. Their priorities were emergency treatments, pain management and improving doctors' abilities to understand patients. Older patients were most concerned about difficulties getting to their general practitioner's surgery. Finally, they were also increasingly availing of complementary therapies, possibly because of their perceived safety.

Suggested further reading

- *World Health Organisation. Better Palliative Care for Older People. Davies E, Higginson I, eds. Europe: WHO, 2004.*
- *The National Council for Palliative Care. The Palliative Care Needs of Older People. Briefing Bulletin No. 14. http://www.ncpc.org.uk/.*
- *The National Council for Palliative Care. Improving Palliative Care Provision in Older People in Care Homes. http://www.ncpc.org.uk/.*
- *Cartwright A. Dying when you're old. Age and Ageing 1993; 22: 425–30.*
- *Robine JM, Michel JP, Herrmann FR. Who will care for the oldest people in our ageing society? BMJ 2007; 334: 570-571.*
- *Gott M, Seymour J, Bellamy G, Clark D, Ahmedzai S. Older people's views about home as a place of care at the end of life. Palliative Med 2004; 18: 460–7.*
- *Ahmed N, Bestall JC, Ahmedzai SH, Payne SA, Clark D, Noble B. Systematic review of the problems and issues of accessing specialist palliative care by patients, carers and health and social care professionals. Palliat Med 2004; 18: 525–42.*
- *AGS Panel on Persistent Pain in Older Persons. The management of persistent pain in older persons. Journal of the American Geriatrics Society, 2002, 50: S205–S224.*
- *Bernabei R et al. Management of pain in elderly persons with cancer. Journal of the American Medical Association, 1998, 279: 1877–1882. www.cks.library.nhs.uk*
- *Skilbeck J, Mott L, Page H, Smith D, Hjelmeland-Ahmedzai S, Clark D. Palliative care in chronic obstructive airways disease: a needs assessment. Palliative Med 1998; 12: 245-54.*
- *Aminoff BZ, Adunsky A. Their last 6 months: suffering and survival of end-stage dementia patients. Age Ageing (2006) 35: 597–601.*
- *ABC of palliative care. BMJ.*
- *Doyle D, Hanks G, Cherny N, Calman K eds. Oxford Textbook of Palliative Medicine 3rd edition. Oxford: Oxford University Press, 2004.*
- *Burt J, Raine R. The effect of age on referral to and use of specialist palliative care services in adult cancer patients: a systematic review. Age Ageing 2006; 35(5): 469-476.*
- *Grande GE, Farquhar MC, Barclay SIG, Todd C. The influence of patient and carer age in access to palliative care services. Age Ageing 2006; 35(3): 267-273.*
- *Dainty P, Leung D. An evaluation of palliative care in the acute geriatric setting. Age Ageing, March 12, 2008;*
- *Addington-Hall JM, Higginson IJ, eds. Palliative care for non-cancer patients. Oxford, Oxford University Press, 2001.*
- *Coventry P, Grande GE, Richards DA, Todd CJ. Prediction of appropriate timing of palliative care for older adults with non-malignant life-threatening disease: a systematic review. Age Ageing 2005; 34: 218–227.*
- *Kübler-Ross, E. On Death and Dying. 1969, Macmillan: New York.*
- *Advisory Group, Marymount Hospice Cork and Atlantic Philanthropies, 2005.*

Case Study 1

A 76 year old-man presented with worsening back pain of 3 months' duration. He lost his ability to walk in the previous two days and became incontinent of urine. On examination, he had power graded at 2 out of 5 in both lower limbs globally, a sensory level at L1 and lower limb hyperreflexia.

This presentation is highly suggestive of spinal cord compression and an MRI confirmed an infiltrating tumour at the L1 level compressing the spinal cord. His PSA was 4,600ng/ml and a diagnosis of metastatic prostate carcinoma was made. The patient received emergency radiotherapy to his lumbar spine and had good resolution of his pain. His mobility improved and he was able to walk with a stick.

Spinal cord compression is a medical emergency. Typical symptoms are back pain exacerbated by coughing or sneezing and not relieved by bed rest, reduced sensation and power below the level of the lesion, and urinary or faecal incontinence, urinary retention or constipation. The earlier treatment is commenced, the greater the preservation of function. The median survival of metastatic spinal cord compression is 3 months. MRI is the investigation of choice. Dexamethasone 16 mg should be promptly given intravenously to reduce peri-tumour oedema as speed is of the essence to minimize permanent cord damage. Oncology and neurosurgical opinions should be sought immediately. Fewer than 10% of patients with established paraplegia from metastatic disease ever walk again.

Case Study 2

A 77 year old man with Stage 4 non-small cell lung cancer presented with headache for two days which was worse in the morning and associated with dizziness and a feeling of fullness in the head. He also complained of breathlessness which was exacerbated by lying down. On examination, he was tachypnoeic, had non-pulsatile dilated neck veins, dilated veins in the arms and chest, facial oedema and cyanosis. Chest X-ray showed widening of the mediastinum.

This presentation is very suggestive of superior vena cava obstruction which was proven with a CT scan of thorax. The aetiology may be compression or invasion of the superior vena cava by mediastinal nodes or tumour or thrombus within the vein. Sixty percent of patients have an undiagnosed cancer at presentation. Unless the patient has severe symptoms, definitive treatment should be delayed until histological diagnosis is made.

Management consists of sitting the patient up and delivering oxygen if appropriate. Intravenous dexamethasone may be useful and anxiolytics and opioids may be helpful if the patient is breathless. Definitive treatment depends on the underlying cause, severity of symptoms and the expertise available locally. Stenting results in good palliation of symptoms after 48 hours and is the treatment of choice if symptoms are severe, the expertise is available or the obstruction recurs post-radiotherapy. If a venogram confirms the presence of a clot, thrombolysis and anti-coagulation are the treatments of choice. If thrombus has formed around a Hickman Line, removal of the line will usually lead to resolution of the obstruction.

Radiotherapy will not provide immediate relief, and anticipated life expectancy should be weeks for the patient to gain benefit. Chemotherapy should be considered if the cause is a chemotherapy-sensitive tumour, for example, small cell lung cancer, lymphoma or testicular cancer.

Case Study 3

An 82 year old man was admitted with an inferior myocardial infarction and acute renal failure. His echocardiograph showed severely impaired cardiac function and he deteriorated progressively over 2 weeks. His chest pain and shortness of breath were well controlled with morphine but he was noted to have intermittent agitation and discomfort. There was no obvious cause for this.

A referral was sent to the palliative care team who identified that the patient was constipated, faecally impacted and was suffering from overflow. He was distressed by abdominal cramps and each time he suffered incontinence he became agitated and restless. He was given a phosphate enema with good effect and commenced on regular macrogol. His constipation resolved quickly and his distress abated.

Data Interpretation

Question 1

An 83 year old woman with early Alzheimer's disease, hypertension and chronic kidney disease and who completed chemotherapy for small cell lung cancer 3 weeks previously is admitted with a 24-hour history of confusion and drowsiness. Her general practitioner stopped her donepezil tablet 2 days previously and switched her from 10mg bd of sustained release morphine to a Fentanyl '25' patch to get better control of her back pain. The following are her some of her blood results:

Hb 8.9g/dl   Urea 13.9 mmol/l
WCC 3.2 x 10⁹/l   Creat 213 μmol/l
Neutrophils 1.2 x 10⁹/l   Calcium 2.3 mmol/l
Plt 223 x 10⁹/l   Sodium 126mmol/l

a. List the abnormalities detected.
b. What is the most likely cause of her confusion and drowsiness?

Question 2

A 79 year old woman is taking 100mg of tramadol four times daily for dorsal back pain due to skeletal metastases from breast cancer. She finds that this is not controlling her pain and is requesting better analgesia.

a. What alternative analgesia would you recommend according to the World Health Organisation analgesic ladder?
b. What is the approximate daily oral morphine dose equivalent of the current tramadol dose?
c. Name one pharmacological and one non-pharmacological adjuvant analgesic therapy that may be helpful in this case.

Best of five questions

Question 1

An 80 year old lady admitted with inoperable ovarian carcinoma has sudden onset severe shortness of breath. She has no previous lung disease. She was started on ibuprofen on admission 2 days ago for abdominal pain, and is also taking paracetamol and codeine. Her Hb is 12.4g/dl, white cell count 8.5 x 10⁹/l, urea 11 mmol/l, creatinine 120 μmol/l and D-dimers 205ng/ml. What is the most likely cause of her sudden onset dyspnoea?

a. Acute pulmonary embolism
b. Respiratory tract infection
c. Cardiac failure
d. Lung metastases
e. Pleural effusion

Question 2

A 72 year old man is being treated in a nursing home for terminal metastatic prostate carcinoma. He has a background of chronic kidney disease and ischaemic heart disease. He is taking morphine 5mg four hourly for back pain. He begins to experience nausea, drowsiness and hallucinations. What is the most likely problem?

a. Acute on chronic renal failure secondary to morphine
b. Acute urinary retention
c. Cerebral metastases
d. Acute psychotic reaction
e. Morphine toxicity

Question 3

A 91 year old lady who has metastatic colorectal carcinoma presents with severe nausea. Her haemoglobin is 8.2g/dl, white cell count 12 x 10⁹/l, urea 32mmol/l, creatinine 420 μmol/l and corrected calcium 3.4mmol/l. What are the three most appropriate initial management steps?

a. Blood transfusion, dialysis and haloperidol as an antiemetic
b. Blood transfusion, rehydration and metoclopramide as an antiemetic
c. Withdrawal of all unnecessary medications, morphine for comfort and cyclizine as an antiemetic
d. Rehydration with normal saline, an intravenous bisphosphonate and haloperidol as an antiemetic
e. Rehydration with 5% dextrose, an intravenous bisphosphonate and domperidone as an antiemetic

Answers are on page 311

Seizures

J Lynch, N Delanty

Introduction

Many older patients present for clinical assessment following an episode of collapse and this is responsible for a significant burden on healthcare systems. An epileptic seizure is an important consideration in the differential diagnosis of collapse. Old age is the most common time to develop new-onset seizures. Epilepsy, defined as recurrent seizures is a cause of significant morbidity and mortality and this is particularly true in the older population. The scale of the problem is perhaps under-recognised in the U.K. and Ireland and appropriate treatment of epilepsy involves a multidisciplinary approach. The approach to the use of antiepileptic drugs (AEDs) in older patients differs from that used in the younger population because of differences in metabolism and concomitant polypharmacy. The introduction of many newer anticonvulsants to the physician's armamentarium also makes management more complex. The prognosis of epilepsy in older patients, in general, is good if properly managed.

Definitions and classification

The 'International League Against Epilepsy' (ILAE) published a revised 'Classification of the Epilepsies and Epileptic Syndromes' in 1989. An 'epileptic syndrome' is defined as 'an epileptic disorder characterised by a cluster of signs and symptoms customarily occurring together'; this includes type of seizure, aetiology, chronicity, diurnal and circadian cycling and sometimes prognosis. Epilepsy is not a single disease entity but rather infers a liability to clinically manifested seizures and encompasses a wide range of aetiologies. Broadly speaking, 'epilepsy syndromes', which must involve more than seizure type and whose identification is based on a complex of symptoms and signs, may be categorised according to whether they are generalised or partial, idiopathic or symptomatic (Figure 1). An idiopathic epilepsy syndrome refers to a syndrome which is solely epilepsy and for which there is no underlying structural brain lesion. They are presumed to have a large genetic contribution. A symptomatic epilepsy syndrome refers to the occurrence of epileptic seizures secondary to a known (lesional) or inferred (non-lesional) structural brain abnormality and is more likely to begin in the elderly than an idiopathic epilepsy syndrome.

An epileptic seizure is the manifestation of an abnormal and excessive synchronised discharge of a set of cerebral neurons. This manifests suddenly and transiently in a number of ways with motor, sensory and psychic phenomena. The exact nature of the clinical presentation will depend on which area of the brain is involved and on the pattern and rate of spread. In focal epilepsy, a seizure may be simple partial, with no impairment of consciousness or complex partial, associated with impairment of consciousness. Simple partial seizures may have motor manifestations such as isolated limb jerking.

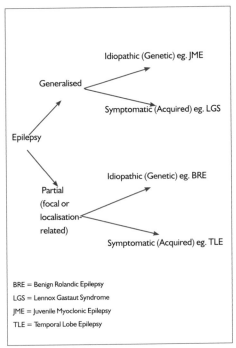

BRE = Benign Rolandic Epilepsy
LGS = Lennox Gastaut Syndrome
JME = Juvenile Myoclonic Epilepsy
TLE = Temporal Lobe Epilepsy

Figure 1: Classification of epilepsies

Sensory symptoms may be described as a tingling, numbness, burning or pain. Other partial seizure expressions include experiential phenomena such as déjà vu, jamais vu, depersonalisation and unreality; affective symptoms such as fear, anger and laughter without mirth (gelastic); illusions of size and shape, or structured hallucinations, eg. visual, auditory, gustatory or olfactory.

Complex partial seizures frequently cause automatisms, defined as involuntary motor actions which occur during or in the immediate aftermath of epileptic seizures, in a state of altered level of consciousness. These can include lip smacking, fiddling or fidgeting movements of the hands, walking, quasi-purposeful movements such as turning a page of a book which is perhaps upside-down and uttering meaningless words (ictal speech). Complex partial seizures arise from the temporal lobe in about 80 – 85% of cases and from the frontal lobe in about 10 -15%. Occipital and parietal seizures are rarer.

Simple partial and complex partial seizures may give rise to secondary generalised convulsions. Seizures may however also be generalised from the outset as occurs in primary generalised epilepsy. Generalised seizures indicate diffuse cortical and subcortical involvement. Motor changes are bilateral and more or less symmetrical. Simultaneous EEG recordings would show bilateral and grossly synchronous activity over both hemispheres. In older patients generalised seizures are usually secondary rather than primary generalised and as such they usually arises from an underlying partial or focal epilepsy, although a focal onset to the seizure may not be clinically apparent. During a tonic-clonic seizure the patient will fall to the ground if standing. There is a brief period of tonic flexion and then a longer phase of rigidity and axial extension, with the eyes rolled up, the jaw clamped shut, the limbs stiff, adducted and extended and the fists often clenched. Respiration ceases which often leads to cyanosis. This tonic period usually lasts approximately 10 - 30 seconds and is followed by the clonic phase which encompasses convulsive movements of all four limbs and facial muscles. It may be associated with urinary or bowel incontinence. There is invariably a post-ictal phase characterised by deep sleep or confusion. The plantar responses are often extensor during this time. A Todd's paralysis (and other focal signs, such as dysphasia) may last hours to sometimes days in the elderly. Generalised seizures may have other forms including typical and atypical absences, myoclonic, clonic, tonic and atonic seizures. However, these generalised seizures usually occur in the symptomatic generalised epilepsies which usually affect a younger population, and are usually associated with learning disability.

Epidemiology and aetiology

There is a bimodal age–dependent incidence pattern for epilepsy, with an initial peak in the first year of life and another rise in late life. In a study of an unselected population of over 2 million people in England and Wales between 1991 and 1995 the prevalence of treated epilepsy was 6.53 per 1,000 in the 70 - 74 years age group and 7.73 in the over 85 age group. The incidence of treated epilepsy in these age groups was 82.8 and 153 per 100,000 respectively.

The single most common risk factor for the development of epilepsy in older patients is cerebrovascular disease. The term 'vascular epilepsy' is sometimes used in this context. Small vessel disease may be clinically silent but can be detected as diffuse small white matter lesions on magnetic resonance imaging (MRI) of the brain. The individual often may not have a clinical history of stroke but rather a number of risk factors for cerebrovascular disease. In acute stroke, a symptomatic seizure may occur within the first few hours and may not need to be treated if isolated and not prolonged. However, seizures occurring weeks or months following (remote symptomatic seizures) a stroke are associated with an increased mortality and imply the development of epilepsy and should be treated. Seizures are associated with large and small vessel disease but are more common in the former. Haemorrhagic strokes, either primary parenchymal or secondary to infarction, are associated with a greater risk of epilepsy. Seizures may also occur during or in the first few hours following a subarachnoid haemorrhage. A number of factors are implicated in seizure activity following stroke including ischaemia, oedema, cytotoxicity and altered neurotransmitter activity. Dementia is associated with epilepsy in 10% of patients. This is particularly so for Alzheimer's disease. The risk is not so clearly defined for Pick's disease or fronto-temporal dementia. Creutzfeldt-Jakob disease is frequently associated with myoclonic seizures.

It is estimated that at least 15% of all cancer patients will have a symptomatic neurologic complication

TABLE I
SELECTED DRUGS REPORTED TO CAUSE SEIZURES
Antibiotics including penicillin
Antihistamines
Antidepressants
Antipsychotics
Baclofen
Chorambucil
Cyclosporine
General anaesthetics
Hypoglycaemics
Isoniazid
Nalidixic acid
Opioid analgesics
Sympathomimetics
Theophyllines
Other, eg. bupropion

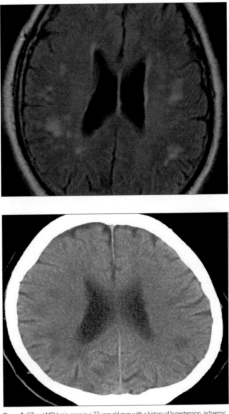

Figure 2. CT and MRI brain scans in a 77 year old man with a history of hypertension, ischaemic heart disease, and previous coronary artery bypass surgery who presented with new-onset complex partial seizures. Both imaging modalities show peri-ventricular and sub-cortical ischaemic white matter disease

during the course of their disease. There are a number of mechanisms by which seizures may occur in cancer. They may occur as a direct consequence of a primary brain tumour or metastases. Brain tumours present as a seizure in approximately 20% of patients with metastases. There is an inverse correlation between tumour grade and seizure frequency in primary brain tumours. Slow-growing, indolent tumours such as low-grade gliomas, gangliogliomas and oligodendrogliomas are often associated with seizures. The epileptic phenomenology associated with tumours is related to their location as in other causes of lesional epilepsy eg. mesial temporal sclerosis.

A Cochrane review of published studies regarding AED prophylaxis in individuals with brain tumours concluded that evidence is inconclusive, neither for nor against prophylaxis. Specific decisions to treat will depend on individual cases. It is therefore reasonable to withhold anti-epileptic medication until the first seizure has occurred. However, melanoma metastases are associated with a 50% incidence of seizures because of the predilection of this tumour to cause haemorrhagic metastases in the grey matter, and thus it may be justifiable in these cases to commence anticonvulsant therapy prophylactically. Cancer is also indirectly associated with seizures i.e. cerebrovascular disorders eg. infarction and haemorrhage; metabolic eg. electrolyte disturbance, organ failure; infections e.g. bacterial, viral, fungal, parasitic; treatment-related eg. chemotherapy,

radiation, supportive medications; paraneoplastic eg. paraneoplastic limbic encephalitis. Idiopathic primary generalised epilepsies with onset in older age have been reported but it is a rare phenomenon.

Trauma is common in older patients and may give rise to a subdural haematoma which can be associated with seizures. Older patients are at risk of subdural haematomas because of underlying brain atrophy, prominent bridging veins and possibly anticoagulation. They often present with chronic rather than acute subdural haematomas and these patients have been shown to benefit from prophylactic anticonvulsants. Seizures are uncommon in the immediate aftermath of head trauma.

Multiple metabolic and infective conditions are associated with the development and exacerbation of seizures in older patients including renal and hepatic impairment, cardiac disease, electrolyte disturbance particularly hyponatraemia which can itself be precipitated by AED use (carbamazepine and oxcarbazepine), hypoglycaemia, hyperglycaemia and hypothyroidism. Seizures are a frequent complication of hypoxic encephalopathy following cardio-respiratory arrest and may be associated with myoclonic status epilepticus.

Numerous drugs have been reported to cause or predispose to seizures, Table 1. The frequent occurrence of polypharmacy in older patients leaves this group of patients at particular risk. The role of drugs in reducing the 'seizure threshold', the physiological concept of an individual's susceptibility to a seizure, can range from definite to circumstantial. It is often only after post-marketing surveillance that the exact risk of seizure associated with a particular drug becomes clear.

A drug may lower the seizure threshold in a number of ways. Theophyllines antagonize the action of the endogenous anticonvulsant adenosine. Penicillin and other antibacterial agents may directly or indirectly antagonise a receptor subtype of the inhibitory neurotransmitter γ-aminobutyric acid (GABA). Isoniazid has an anti-pyridoxine effect.

Other drugs may indirectly lead to seizures. These include insulin and oral hypoglycaemic agents which can cause hypoglycaemia, diuretics and SSRIs which can cause hyponatraemia and immunosuppressive therapy which can contribute to CNS infections. Antipsychotic agents are commonly used in older patients and may predispose to seizures. Phenothiazines are more likely to lower the seizure threshold than butyrophenones and thus haloperidol has been the drug of choice in agitated patients.

The newer antipsychotics are also associated with seizures. Clozapine-related seizures appear to be dose-related and more likely to occur if there is a rapid titration. However, at present, it is thought that risperidone, olanzapine and quetiapine are not associated with a significantly increased risk of seizures. Tricyclic antidepressants can cause seizures in overdose, usually accompanied by a prolonged QRS duration on the electrocardiogram. Withdrawal of anticonvulsants and benzodiazepines can also cause acute symptomatic seizures

Diagnosis of epilepsy and seizures in older patients

The diagnosis of epilepsy can be difficult to make in older patients. It is, above all, a clinical diagnosis. It is often difficult to obtain a complete history of events from the patient and so a collateral history from a witness is of paramount importance and is probably the most important 'investigation' that can be performed. The doctor should firstly enquire about the events preceding the collapse; was there a warning or aura, palpitations, pallor, pre-syncope, staring episodes, impairment of consciousness or focal limb movements? Questions should be asked concerning the circumstances of the collapse, the relationship to posture, the duration of unconsciousness, involuntary movements, incontinence, cuts and bruises and tongue biting. Post-ictal symptoms and signs including confusion, drowsiness, Todd's paresis, headache and rapidity of return to baseline should also be directly enquired about.

The important differential diagnosis of collapse in older patients includes convulsive syncope which may result from neurally-mediated reflex syncope, postural hypotension, cardiac outflow obstruction and cardiac arrhythmias. In convulsive syncope patients may exhibit some seizure-like activity upon losing consciousness; this is not however truly 'epileptic' in origin. Less common mimics include periodic leg movements of sleep, rapid eye movement (REM)-behaviour disorder and psychogenic non-epileptic seizures, which can occur in the elderly.

The routine laboratory investigations which should be sought, include full blood count, urea and electrolytes, serum glucose, thyroid function tests, ECG and CXR. Additional tests such as echocardiography, Holter monitoring, implantable loop monitoring which records cardiac rhythm over a few weeks to months, tilt-table testing and carotid and basilar artery angiography will depend on individual cases. Occasionally, complete or almost complete occlusion of one carotid artery may present as a contralateral tremor, particularly on change of posture, which may be mistaken for a partial seizure ('limb-shaking TIA').

Magnetic resonance imaging (MRI) of the brain provides the most sensitive and specific imaging for most symptomatic seizures including the detection of arteriovenous malformation, tumours and strokes (Figure 2). However, computed tomography (CT)

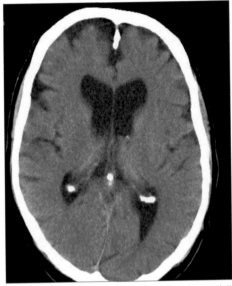

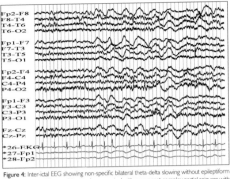

Figure 4: Inter-ictal EEG showing non-specific bilateral theta-delta slowing without epileptiform abnormalities in a 78 year old man who presented with new-onset complex partial seizures with secondary generalisation (same patient as in Figure 3).

Figure 3: CT brain scan showing non-specific atrophy in a 78 year old man who presented with new-onset complex partial seizures with secondary generalised tonic-clonic convulsions.

is more sensitive for brain haemorrhage. It is also cheaper and still more readily available than MRI and therefore is often the only imaging which is performed. In addition, CT imaging alone may be adequate in those with a clear history of cerbrovascular disease or stroke. MRI, particularly using coronal sequences through the temporal lobes is the imaging method of choice for detecting mesial temporal sclerosis, the presence of which may make excisional surgery a possibility for intractable partial epilepsy. However, de novo medically intractable partial epilepsy is not common in older patients.

The role of electroencephalography (EEG) is often unhelpful in the elderly with a history of collapse. It is associated with a significant proportion of false positive and negative results. With advancing age, 10–40% of normal individuals develop non-specific abnormal EEGs, such as theta slowing over the temporal regions (Figure 4). Conversely, many older patients with epilepsy have normal EEGs. Approximately 30% of people with epilepsy will have an abnormal EEG after one recording. This rises to 80% after four EEGs but this volume of EEGs is not justified in most cases and underlines the importance of a good clinical and collateral history. Only 10 – 20% of those with post-stroke seizures have an abnormal record, sometimes revealing periodic lateralising epileptiform discharges (PLEDs)

over the site of the infarct or haemorrhage. Despite the above, an EEG recording is often invaluable when non-convulsive status is suspected in those with an acute confusional state. On occasion, video EEG and ECG monitoring in a specialised setting can give invaluable information in complex diagnostic cases.

Management

The goal of seizure management in older patients is to achieve improved or complete seizure control with minimal or no side effects. It is important that both the patient and the caregivers understand the diagnosis, possible seizure precipitants and rationale for treatment. This ideally requires a multidisciplinary approach between geriatrician, neurologist, general practitioner and epilepsy nurse specialist. The diagnosis of epilepsy is made when a patient has two unprovoked seizures. In the general population, treatment is not usually instituted until the occurrence of a second seizure. The risk of seizure recurrence is increased by concomitant risk factors such as cerebrovascular disease or dementia. Therefore most physicians will commence older patients on AED treatment after a first definite seizure if there is an 'enduring predisposition' to epilepsy. This is further justified because a second convulsion may result in a hip fracture or other significant injury, which may be devastating to older individuals.

There are a number of lifestyle issues that should be discussed between the patient, caregiver and physician or epilepsy nurse specialist. Driving is prohibited by Irish law until a patient with epilepsy is seizure-free for at least one year (regardless of whether on AED treatment or not) or if there is a consistent pattern of nocturnal seizures only for a period of two years or more. Common precipitants of seizures should be discussed including sleep deprivation and alcohol withdrawal. It is recommended that a patient with epilepsy should have as regular a sleep pattern as possible. It is usually not necessary to prohibit alcohol altogether but restriction to 4 units at any one time is advised with the caveat that seizures are more likely to occur in the withdrawal phase, 24 – 48 hours following alcohol ingestion.

The choice of anticonvulsant medication involves both consideration of pharmacokinetics (the factors determining the dose of a drug and time course of its concentration in the plasma) and pharmacodynamics (the relationship between drug concentration and pharmacological response as a function of time). The metabolism of drugs in older patients is different from that in younger individuals and this has an impact both on the choice and amount of drug prescribed. In general, there is altered volume of distribution, lower protein binding, impaired hepatic metabolism, less enzyme induction and slower renal elimination with older age. Idiosyncratic drug reactions are also more common in older patients. There is also a rationale for concurrently prescribing bone protection medication because of the increased risk of osteopenia and osteoporosis secondary to long-term use with enzyme-inducing AEDs, guided by findings from DEXA scanning.

Polypharmacy provides an additional challenge when prescribing AEDs. Many older people are also taking medication for hypertension, cardiac disease, respiratory disease and infection. These medications can affect the pharmacokinetics of AEDs and vice versa. It is important to know the primary mechanism of AED drug clearance and whether or not it is a cytochrome P450 enzyme inducer or inhibitor. Phenytoin, phenobarbitone, primidone and carbamazepine are hepatic enzyme inducers. They may also auto-induce their own metabolism, particularly carbamazepine. Many drugs including cimetidine (ranitidine has no effect), isoniazid, propoxyphene, erythromycin and calcium-channel blockers such as verapamil and diltiazem (nifedipine has no effect), danazol, fluoxetine and valproate inhibit the metabolism of carbamazepine and therefore increase its plasma level, leading to toxicity. Clonazepam, felbamate, phenobarbital, phenytoin and primidone induce hepatic enzyme activity and so decrease the plasma level of carbamazepine.

Some of the newer AEDs such as gabapentin and levetiracetam are excreted by the kidney. Drugs with a high degree of protein binding displace AEDs leading to a decreased total level of AED but a higher free fraction.

Clinical assessment is the best way to assess AED toxicity rather than relying on serum levels which may be inaccurate, dependent on time taken from last dose and do not routinely calculate free fractions. Toxicity may exist for one individual in the setting of a 'normal' serum level, and conversely, another individual may have no adverse consequences despite a 'toxic' level. Common symptoms of toxicity include diplopia, ataxia, falls, fatigue, nausea and vomiting and psychomotor retardation. Signs suggestive of toxicity include ataxia, new onset finger-nose dysmetria and nystagmus. If there is clear evidence of toxicity and the treatment is efficacious it would be prudent to reduce the dose rather than switching to an alternative agent. The AED may need to be changed if there are chronic and intolerable side effects or if a lower dose does not adequately control the epilepsy.

Individual anticonvulsants

Phenytoin
Phenytoin is effective against partial and generalised seizures in all age groups but may paradoxically increase myoclonus and absence seizure frequency in primary generalised epilepsy. It is often prescribed as a continuation of intravenous therapy commenced for status epilepticus and has the advantage of once daily dosing. It is a hepatic enzyme inducer and is about 90% protein-bound. It is, therefore, prone to drug interactions. It also displays unusual pharmacokinetics in that it is initially metabolised in a first order kinetic fashion by the hepatic P450 mixed oxidase system and as such a particular fraction of the drug concentration is eliminated at any one time and so its concentration is predictable. However, when the level of phenytoin saturates the enzyme responsible for its breakdown, it displays zero order kinetics and so its concentration may readily increase and lead to toxicity. Relatively small increases in dose can therefore lead to large increases in serum levels. It is initially metabolised by the CYP2C9 isoenzyme and then by the CYP2C19 isoenzyme at higher concentrations. The CYP2C19 isoenzyme also metabolises topiramate, so phenytoin toxicity may occur more readily when the two drugs are used in combination. The interaction between phenytoin and warfarin is unpredictable,

making close monitoring of the INR mandatory. Frusemide clearance can be increased by as much as 50%. Acute dose-related adverse effects of phenytoin include ataxia, nausea and vomiting, motor slowing and lethargy. Idiosyncratic adverse effects including skin reactions in 5% of patients may occur within the first two months of therapy. Phenytoin has also been associated with lymph node enlargement and exacerbations of myasthenia gravis. Its long-term use is associated with cerebellar degeneration, gum hypertrophy, hirsutism, acne and osteopenia. Although commonly used, these problems make it unsuitable as a first line agent for chronic use in older patients.

Carbamazepine

Carbamazepine is effective against partial and secondary generalised seizures. Like phenytoin, it may worsen myoclonic and absence seizures. It is metabolised by CYP3A4. It induces its own metabolism. It is bound to both albumin and α1-acid glycoprotein (AGG) at 65 - 85% of the total drug. It takes from 4 - 8 hours to reach peak plasma levels. It has excellent bioavailability. In gastrointestinal disease the absorption of carbamazepine may be significantly reduced. It shares many of the same side effects as phenytoin which are more prevalent after the initiation of therapy, although, in general, it is better tolerated and has less long term side-effects. It may cause fatigue and depression. It is also implicated in idiosyncratic reactions including rash, haemopoeitic abnormality and hyponatraemia. Older patients are more susceptible to rash. It is available in long-acting formulation helpful in reducing the risk of peak dose toxicity and facilitating a twice daily scheduling. It is prudent in older adults to start at 100 - 200mg nocte to reduce the risk of adverse reaction and to double this dose every fortnight to a level of 400 - 1200mg daily, depending on response and tolerability. Although equally effective to both lamotrigine and gabapentin in a randomised clinical trial comparing the three agents in 593 elderly patients (mean age 72 years) with newly diagnosed epilepsy, it was less well tolerated.

Phenobarbital

Phenobarbital is also effective against partial and generalised seizures. Many older patients who have suffered epilepsy for much of their life may still be on this drug. There is a lack of evidence regarding its specific metabolism in older patients although it is thought to have a reduced clearance. It is not highly protein bound. It can often be sedating and associated with psychomotor retardation even if a patient has been taking it for many years. Sometimes, this may only be apparent in retrospect, following slow drug withdrawal. It has a propensity for multiple drug interactions. It is not a first-line agent in a patient newly diagnosed with epilepsy. If a patient has been successfully treated with it for years with minimal or no side effects there is little reason to change or stop it. However, one may consider reducing or weaning a patient from it very slowly, if it is poorly tolerated and changing to another AED. It is has a long elimination half-life of 75 - 120 hours. If one allows that it takes five half-lives to reach a steady state, then phenobarbital can often be safely reduced by 15mg every month. There is a risk of worsening seizure control if weaning from an AED and so reduction should be performed slowly to minimise this risk. The safest means of weaning from any AED is to know its half-life and allow five half lives for it to attain its new serum concentration. Therefore, one should request its serum concentration after five half-lives have elapsed if one is using serum concentrations to aid in accurate titration of dosage for individual patients.

Valproate

Sodium valproate is a broad-spectrum anticonvulsant. It is highly protein-bound and has good bioavailability. It takes one to eight hours to reach peak plasma levels. It is a hepatic enzyme inhibitor and so may prolong the action of other AEDs if used in combination. It is available in a slow-release formulation with twice daily scheduling and this is recommended. It can be associated with weight gain (30% of all patients), hair loss, haematological manifestations including thrombocytopenia and rarely, pancreatitis and acute hepatic failure. Ten per cent of patients develop a dose-related tremor, and this is sometimes confused with essential tremor or even the tremor of idiopathic Parkinson's disease in the elderly. It improves with dose reduction, and is usually not severe enough to necessitate withdrawal of the drug. Valproate also has a variety of metabolic effects resulting from disruption of mitochondrial metabolism. It may result in hypocarnitinaemia, hyperglycinaemia, and hyperammonaemia. When hyperammonaemia is severe, stupor, coma or death can result. Patients with coexisting hepatic dysfunction are particularly at risk. The usual starting dose in adults is 200mg at night increasing by 200 mg increments to a maintenance dose of between 600 and 1600mg per day, again depending on individual response and tolerability.

Gabapentin

Gabapentin is generally prescribed as monotherapy in older patients with partial epilepsy. It is not protein-bound and is excreted in an unchanged form via the kidneys. In younger adults it is usually prescribed three times daily because of its relatively short half-life. However, in older adults it is often prescribed as a twice-daily dose because of decline in the creatinine clearance with ageing. An initial target dose of 300 - 400mg bd, achieved over approximately three weeks after commencing at 100 mg bd, may be reasonable. If commenced too rapidly side effects such as drowsiness and dizziness are common. It is otherwise well tolerated and has minimal drug interactions. It may cause somnolence, ataxia and dizziness at higher doses and occasionally may paradoxically worsen seizure frequency, as indeed can all anticonvulsants. Its mode of action is unclear but it increases brain GABA levels and it may bind to a calcium channel receptor in the cerebral neocortex and hippocampus. It is now frequently used for painful diabetic neuropathy, trigeminal neuralgia, and other neuropathic pain syndromes.

Lamotrigine

Lamotrigine is licensed as adjunctive or monotherapy in partial and generalized epilepsy. It is 55% bound to plasma protein and it is metabolised by the liver. It does not induce or inhibit hepatic enzymes. However, its metabolism is induced by phenytoin, carbamazepine, phenobarbital and other enzyme inducing drugs. Its levels are increased by valproate. Lamotrigine is thought to function by blockade of voltage-gated sodium channels. It is prescribed as a twice-daily dose. It must be titrated from 25mg once a day to reduce the risk of allergic rash. If used as monotherapy or with a hepatic enzyme inducer the dose may be increased by 25mg every week to achieve a maintenance dose of 200 - 400mg daily. However, if it is combined with an enzyme inhibitor such as valproate the dose should be increased more cautiously by 25mg every second week and initially prescribed as 25mg on alternate days. Lamotrigine is usually titrated to 100 mg twice daily. The incidence of rash is 5%. The rash is usually mild but it may progress to bullous erythema multiforme and even Stevens-Johnson syndrome, which may be fatal. The most common side effects of lamotrigine are headache, nausea and vomiting, diplopia, dizziness, ataxia and tremor. Lamotrigine, is however, usually well tolerated. Significant cognitive adverse effects are uncommon.

Oxcarbazepine

Oxcarbazepine is used as adjunctive or monotherapy in partial epilepsy. It shares many characteristics with carbamazepine but has a unique molecular structure which gives it a number of advantages. The pharmacological action of oxcarbazepine is mediated primarily through its 10-monohydroxy metabolite (MHD). Oxcarbazepine is about 70% and MHD about 40% protein bound. It is rapidly metabolised in the liver. There is no auto-induction and fewer interactions with other drugs compared to carbamazepine. It does not interact with warfarin, cimetidine, erythromycin, verapamil or dextropropoxyphene. It is often commenced at 150mg twice daily to achieve a target dose of 450 – 600 mg twice daily over a number of weeks. It is associated with rash in 5% of patients as compared to 10% with carbamazepine. Cross-reactivity with rash associated with carbamazepine is only 33%. The most common dose-related side effects are fatigue, headache, dizziness and ataxia. There is a greater risk of hyponatraemia than with carbamazepine but it is usually asymptomatic and mild. The risk of hyponatraemia is increased in older patients and with concomitant diuretic usage. Carbamazepine may be replaced by oxcarbazepine at a carbamazepine:oxcarbazepine ratio of two:three.

Levetiracetam

Levetiracetam may be prescribed as adjunctive or monotherapy in partial or primary generalised epilepsy. It has a novel binding site to SV2A (synaptic vesicle protein 2A) but its exact mechanism of action is poorly understood. Levetiracetam and its metabolites are excreted through the kidneys. Impaired renal function would necessitate prescribing a lower or sometimes, a once-daily dose. It achieves peak plasma concentration within 0.6 to 1.3 hours. No clinically significant drug interactions have been reported with warfarin, digoxin or other anticonvulsants, except occasionally and inconsistently with phenytoin when it approaches saturation levels. Its most common side effects are somnolence, asthenia, dizziness and headache. It is usually well tolerated in the elderly. It should generally be commenced at a dose of 250 mg twice daily and titrated to 500 - 1500 mg twice daily depending on tolerability, efficacy and creatinine clearance. Case series reports suggest that it may be particulary effective for seizures and myoclonus following hypoxic brain damage.

Topiramate

Topiramate is a broad-spectrum drug that can be used

in both partial and generalised epilepsy. It has excellent bioavailability and reaches peak plasma levels in two hours. It has 15% protein binding. It is metabolised by the P450 microsomal enzyme system in the liver. It does not generally affect the concentrations of other anticonvulsants except for phenytoin by the 2CYP19 pathway as described above. However, it is itself affected by hepatic enzyme inhibitors and inducers. Topiramate and its metabolites are eliminated renally. It has several mechanisms of action. It causes blockade of sodium channels, enhancement of GABA-mediated chloride influx and modulatory effects on the GABA receptor, and also has actions at the AMPA receptor. It is a very effective anti-epileptic medication in many cases and is often used in medically refractory seizures. Adverse effects include ataxia, confusion, dizziness, fatigue, paraesthesia in the extremities, somnolence, depression, agitation and slowness of speech. These adverse events are prominent in approximately 15% of patients. It is also associated with weight loss, which is usually dose-related and is more likely to occur in overweight patients. It also carries a risk of renal calculi because of its carbonic anhydrase inhibition.

Zonisamide
Zonisamide is a broad-spectrum drug originally developed in Japan, but now available worldwide, that has a somewhat similar profile to topiramate, although the two drugs have not been formally compared in terms of efficacy and tolerability. Structurally it is a sulphonamide derivative, and it should therefore be avoided in any individual with a remote history of sulphonamide hypersensitivity. It has low protein-binding, is metabolised via CYP 3A4, and is excreted via the urine. It has a long half-life and can be administered once daily, which could be potentially an advantage in an elderly individual who requires directly observed therapy, eg. by a public health nurse or other visting carer. However, there is little in the published literature about the use of this AED in the elderly.

Other AEDs such as felbamate, clobazam, clonazepam, ethosuximide, tiagabine, piracetam, vigabatrin and acetazolamide are rarely prescribed to older adults. Newer AEDs with novel mechanisms of action such as lacosamide and retigabine are shortly to be released as add-on agents in individuals with refractory partial epilepsy.

Rescue medication
In patients with refractory epilepsy or a history of convulsive seizures, it is important that family members and carers be instructed in seizure first aid and the administration of a rescue benzodiazepine preparation. Traditionally this has been with either rectal diazepam or sublingual lorazepam but these are now being superseded by buccal midazolam. This is generally embraced as a convenient and humane addition to care by families and carers and can also be administered intranasally. Buccal midazolam is generally administered in the event of complex partial seizure activity lasting five minutes or longer, for the occurrence of serial seizures or at the beginning of any convulsive seizure. Onset of action is rapid and post-administration drowsiness may occur. 10mg in one ml is the standard dose in adults but the dose could be halved in the frail elderly.

Status epilepticus
Status epilepticus has traditionally been defined as a condition in which epileptic seizures persist for 30 minutes or more; however, it is now being operationally redefined as continued seizure activity for ten minutes or longer or recurrent serial seizures without return to baseline. There are various types of status epilepticus, dependent on the underlying seizure semiology. Status epilepticus of any seizure type can cause neuronal damage, and in some cases the physiological sequelae can cause significant morbidity or death. This section will focus on tonic-clonic status epilepticus and epilepsia partialis continua.

Tonic-clonic status epilepticus
Tonic-clonic status epilepticus is a medical emergency and can be defined as continuous tonic-clonic seizure activity lasting ten minutes or recurrent seizures persisting over 30 minutes. Mortality for all ages for tonic-clonic status is 5 - 10% and depends on aetiology and seizure duration. Frequently, there is a premonitory phase during which seizure frequency may be increased in the preceding hours. Urgent therapy at this point can often lessen or prevent the development of status epilepticus. Tonic-clonic status epilepticus may be considered to have two phases; phase 1 (phase of compensation), and phase 2 (phase of decompensation). During the first phase, there is a marked increase in cerebral metabolism, with increased cerebral blood flow and glucose delivery. There are appropriate systemic physiological changes including catecholamine release with consequent hyperglycaemia and increased cardiac output. This is usually associated with sweating, fever, and

sometimes vomiting. After about 30 – 60 minutes there is the phase of decompensation characterised by loss of cerebral autoregulation and systemic hypotension. This in turn can result in cerebral oedema. Additionally, pulmonary oedema and cardiac arrhythmias, hypoglycaemia and electrolyte disturbances including hypo- and hyperkalaemia, lactic acidosis and hyponatraemia can develop. Further complications include acute tubular necrosis, renal and hepatic failure and disseminated intravascular coagulation. Tonic-clonic status epilepticus can result in permanent neurological damage including greater susceptibility to future seizures, hemiparesis and decline in level of cognitive functioning.

The management of status epilepticus in older patients is not different from the standard approach in younger adults. Treatment of tonic-clonic status epilepticus combines specific anti-convulsant therapy and supportive measures. The first priority is to maintain an adequate airway, with delivery of supplemental oxygenation if necessary and is best done with anaesthetic expertise, with a low threshold for airway intubation if respiratory function is compromised. It is equally important to prevent and treat hypotension. Regular evaluation of vital signs and neurological observations should be performed. Continuous pulse oximetry and ECG monitoring and regular glucose, arterial blood gas and electrolyte recording are recommended. Additionally, blood should be checked for coagulation screen, magnesium, AED levels and a sample saved for possible future analysis.

If hypoglycaemia is suspected or detected it should be treated immediately with 50ml of 50% glucose intravenously (IV). Thiamine (250mg) should be co-administered IV if there is any suspicion of alcoholism or poor nutritional state. There is a caveat to good glucose control; hyperglycaemia in status epilepticus may worsen neurological damage and therefore, glucose should only be administered to those individuals in whom hypoglycaemia is suspected rather than in a general fashion to everyone with status epilepticus. The correction of acidosis, rhabdomyolysis and hyperthermia is best done through control of motor seizure activity in status epilepticus and management of severe metabolic disturbance is best managed in the intensive care unit. Patients should be closely monitored for acute renal and/or hepatic failure which can occur with hypotension, disseminated intravascular coagulation,

and hypersensitivity reactions to AEDs. Cerebral oedema will often require continuous intracranial monitoring and frequently require treatment with dexamethasone or mannitol and occasionally neurosurgical decompression depending on the underlying cause. Investigations should also be directed to identifying the underlying aetiology and this will often include brain imaging and lumbar puncture. When seizure activity is not controlled rapidly then intensive care unit admission will be necessary.

The specific drug treatment of status epilepticus may vary between physicians and institutions because of the lack of good comparative trials but it is very important that each institution has a protocol for its management. Lorazepam is the preferred drug in the premonitory or early stage of status epilepticus. A single injection of two to four milligrams is highly effective in many patients and the drug has a longer initial duration and a smaller risk of cardio-respiratory depression than diazepam. Once status epilepticus is established in a patient who is not already taking phenytoin, a phenytoin infusion IV at 15 - 20 mg/kg at a rate of 50 mg/min can be commenced. Phenytoin loading IV can be associated with cardiac arrhythmias and therefore must be done with continuous ECG monitoring. Fosphenytoin at 15mg/kg of phenytoin equivalents may be given at 100mg/min as an alternative to phenytoin and although more expensive, is associated with a lower risk of thrombophlebitis, especially when there is very poor intravenous access. Phenobarbital may be administered as an intravenous infusion at 10mg/kg at a rate of 100mg/min as an alternative to either phenytoin or fosphenytoin.

Tonic-clonic status epilepticus which is refractory to benzodiazepine and phenytoin/phenobarbital (i.e. seizures continuing for 60 – 90 minutes) may require general anaesthesia with propofol or thiopental and should be administered in the intensive care unit. Propofol may be administered as a 1 - 2mg/kg IV bolus initially, repeated if necessary and then followed by a continuous infusion of 1 - 15 mg/kg per hour titrating the dose with EEG findings (targeting a burst suppression pattern) and aiming to gradually reduce the dose. When seizures have been controlled for 12 hours, the drug dosages should be slowly tapered over 12 hours. Propofol is relatively easy to use but requires ITU monitoring and is fast-acting but there is limited data on its antiepileptic effects.

Thiopentone may be administered as an alternative to propofol, when the patient is intubated and receiving artifical ventilation as a 100-250mg IV bolus given over 20 seconds. Further 50mg boluses may be given every 2 - 3 minutes until seizures are controlled, followed by a continuous IV infusion to maintain a burst suppression pattern on the EEG (usually 3-5mg/kg/h). Thiopentone may be slowly withdrawn 12 hours after the last seizure. Barbiturates such as thiopentone have good antiepileptic properties but can cause marked hypotension and can have a long half-life because of saturable kinetics.

Tonic-clonic status epilepticus will usually respond to the above treatments. However, the common causes of status epilepticus remaining refractory to treatment include inadequate dosage of antiepileptic drug infusion, failure to continue old AED regimen, medical complications of status epilepticus and failure to address the underlying aetiology of status epilepticus.

Epilepsia partialis continua

Epilepsia partialis continua may be defined as spontaneous regular or irregular clonic muscle jerking of cerebral cortical origin, sometimes aggravated by action or sensory stimuli, confined to one part of the body and continuing for hours, days or weeks. The muscle jerking may be widespread or confined to one muscle group. Complex epilepsia partialis continua implies an associated impairment of consciousness which usually manifests as a confusional state which can be continuous or fluctuant both in time and severity. Epilepsia partialis continua can result from any of a number of causes including acute or chronic encephalitis, cerebrovascular disease, brain tumour, brain abscess, brain infarct, brain haemorrhage, metabolic disturbance e.g. non-ketotic hyperglycaemia particularly when associated with hyponatraemia.

Reported scalp EEG abnormalities with epilepsia partialis continua include continuous or frequent spike, with or without slow wave abnormalities. As the duration of epilepsia partialis continua lengthens, the scalp EEG is less likely to detect abnormalities. Therefore, a high index of clinical suspicion is necessary to treat appropriately. When recognised and treated, the prognosis for recovery from epilepsia partialis continua is usually very good with relatively low risk of permanent neurological damage when compared to prolonged tonic-clonic

status epilepticus. However, there is a strong risk of recurrence. When identified early epilepsia partialis continua often responds well to phenytoin, carbamazepine or phenobarbital. Steroids have been reported to be of benefit in some instances. However, epilepsia partialis continua which has been occurring for a prolonged time can be refractory to therapy and antiepileptic treatment is directed at preventing secondary generalisation. The risk of neuronal damage resulting from prolonged complex epilepsia partialis continua is less certain. Treatment should include administration of benzodiazepines with concomitant antiepileptic medication such as carbamazepine, phenytoin or levetiracetam.

Post-ictal phenomena

Epilepsy remains a clinical diagnosis and knowledge of post-ictal phenomena may help in seizure recognition and occasionally aid in localisation or lateralisation. Post-ictal mood disturbance including depression, anxiety or mania may occur following seizures of temporal lobe origin. Post-ictal depression can vary from mild to severe and can last up to two weeks. Post-ictal psychosis can occur particularly with temporal lobe epilepsy. It typically follows a cluster of complex partial seizures, is often preceeded by a post-ictal lucid interval and can last from a few hours to a few weeks. The post-ictal psychosis is characterised variously by delusions, hallucinations, thought disorder or mania. Post-ictal psychosis may require treatment with a short course of benzodiazepines or antipsychotics. Complex motor seizures arising from the frontal lobe of the dominant hemisphere (usually left-sided) can give rise to post-ictal dysphasia. Complex partial seizures arising from the frontal or temporal lobes often give rise to post-ictal confusion lasting a few minutes to hours on occasion.

Frontal (contralateral pre-central gyrus), parietal and occasionally temporal seizures can give rise to post-ictal Todd's paresis (contralateral weakness) which may be very transient or last a few hours. However, it is not generally appreciated that Todd's paralysis can sometimes last several days, especially in older patients. Occipital (and parietal) epilepsy can result in post-ictal blindness (eg. hemianopia). Generalised seizures often result in drowsiness and fatigue. Both complex partial and secondary generalised seizures are associated with post-ictal amnesia for the event.

Prognosis

The use of appropriate treatment with caution

regarding the potential side effects is associated with a good outcome for seizure management in the older population. It is estimated in these circumstances, that control will be achieved in 70% of patients. It is more difficult to achieve control when there is an associated underlying neurodegenerative condition. Regular follow-up is necessary to achieve good results. Epilepsy is associated with significant morbidity in older patients. Patients may suffer falls, lacerations, burns and fractures because of seizures. A patient with epilepsy may suffer loss of confidence and its diagnosis may worsen depression. There is an extensive differential diagnosis for epilepsy and collapse in older patients and the importance of a good collateral history to ensure the correct diagnosis is essential. Treatment must be tailored to suit the individual patient and to encompass the different physiology of older patients and strong possibility of drug-drug interactions. Ideally, the carers should be involved and a multidisciplinary approach employed. Adequacy of control should primarily be judged by the patient, family and carers. Epilepsy in older individuals is an under-recognised clinical entity which brings difficult diagnostic and therapeutic challenges. However, when managed well the prognosis is often very good.

Suggested further reading

- Cohen N, Strauss G, Lew R, Silver D, Rect L. Should prophylactic anticonvulsants be administered to patients with newly-diagnosed cerebral metastases? A retrospective analysis. J Clin Oncol 1988; 6: 1621-24.
- Delanty N (Editor). Seizures. Medical causes and management. Humana Press 2001.
- Delanty N, Vaughan CJ, French JA. Medical causes of seizures. Lancet 1998; 352: 383-90.
- Hauser WA. Seizure disorders: the changes with age. Epilepsia 1992; (Suppl 4): S6-14.
- Lackner TE, Cloyd JC, Thomas LW, Leppik IE. Antiepileptic drug use in nursing home residents: Effect of age, gender, and comedication on patterns of use. Epilepsia 1998; 39: 1083-87.
- McAreavey MJ, Ballinger BR, Fenton GW. Epileptic seizures in elderly patients with dementia. Epilepsia 1992; 33: 657-60.
- McKeon A, Vaughan C, Delanty N. Seizure versus syncope. Lancet Neurol 2006: 171-180.
- Murphy K, Delanty N. Drug induced seizures. General principles in assessment, management and prevention. CNS Drugs 2000; 135-46.
- Ramsey RE, Macias FM, Rowan AJ. Diagnosing epilepsy in the elderly. Int Rev Neurobiol 2007; 81: 129-151.
- Rowan AJ, Ramsey RE, Collins JF, et al. New onset geriatric epilepsy. A randomised study of gabapentin, lamotrigine, and carbamazepine. Neurology 2005; 64: 1868-1873.
- Sabo RA, Hanigan WC, Aldag JC. Chronic subdural haematomas and seizures: the role of prophylactic anticonvulsive medication. Surg Neurol 1995; 43: 579-82.
- Sheorajpanday RV, De Deyn PP. Epileptic fits and epilepsy in the elderly: general reflections, specific issues, and therapeutic implications. Clin Neurol Neurosurg 2007; 109: 727-743.
- Shorvon S. Handbook of epilepsy treatment. Blackwell Science 2000.
- Stephen LJ, Brodie MJ. Epilepsy in elderly people. Lancet 2000; 355: 1441-46.
- Wallace H, Shorvon S, Tallis R. Age-specific incidence and prevalence rates of treated epilepsy in an unselected population of 2,052,922 and age-specific fertility rates of women with epilepsy. Lancet 1998; 352: 1970-3.
- Willmore LJ. Management of epilepsy in the elderly. Epilepsia 1996; (Suppl 6): S23-33.

📂 Case Study 1

A 73 year old left handed man was referred for a second opinion following three generalised tonic-clonic convulsions that had occurred over the preceding 10 months. The patient had no early risk factors for partial epilepsy and had experienced no prior seizures. His first seizure had occurred as he was eating breakfast, beginning with an aura of an 'odd' taste in his mouth and then evolving rapidly into a tonic-clonic seizure that was witnessed and reliably described as such by the patient's wife. He sustained a vertebral fracture during the convulsion and he reported that it took two days for his memory to return to normal.

During his initial hospitalisation, the patient was started on phenytoin. When a generalised rash developed, the drug was discontinued and the patient was then switched to sodium valproate. After leaving the hospital, the patient stopped taking the drug because he felt that the drug was causing a rash; he did not seek medical advice or direction at that time. Four months after his initial seizure and taking no anticonvulsant medication the patient experienced a third convulsion, after which he was started on lorazepam. At the time of referral, he was being treated with lorazepam 0.5mg bd. The patient had a history of asthma since childhood and at the time of referral was using a steroid inhaler regularly and a salbutamol inhaler as required. However, it emerged during the history that he had used a combination proprietary bronchodilator medication shortly before two of his three convulsions. This contained 130mg theophylline, 25mg ephedrine and 10 mg hydroxyzine. He was not using this medication regularly and he was not using it or any other medication at the time of consultation. He neither smoked nor consumed alcohol, and was otherwise well. General physical examination, vital signs, and neurological assessment were unremarkable. An MRI study performed after his first seizure showed a small area of increased signal in the periventricular white matter on T2-weighted images, possibly consistent with small vessel ischaemic cerebrovascular disease. No other abnormalities were identified. A routine EEG performed at the time showed mild generalised slowing of the background without epileptiform abnormalities.

A diagnosis of late onset partial epilepsy, manifesting as partial seizures with rapid secondarily generalised tonic clonic convulsions, was made and it was thought that two of the patient's three seizures had been exacerbated by the proconvulsant ingredients in his asthma medication. The patient was advised to avoid any drug containing theophylline because such drugs could potentially lower his seizure threshold. He was started on gabapentin and given a dose escalation schedule to reach a target dose of 600 mg tid over two weeks; simultaneously, his dosage of lorazepam was tapered until it was discontinued. When seen on follow-up 10 weeks later, the patient was doing well and had experienced no further seizures. He continues to be seizure-free and receives occasional short-term prednisolone therapy as required for asthma exacerbation.

This case illustrates that seizures may be precipitated by the proconvulsant properties of some medications even if they are only taken on an as required basis.

📁 Case Study 2

A 74 year old gentleman was referred to the neurology clinic by his general practitioner following numerous collapses associated with involuntary movements which had not improved with AED treatment. The patient lived alone. He had no early risk factors for partial epilepsy. His first collapse occurred 18 months ago. He had been watching television and had arisen five minutes previously to make lunch. While standing he experienced a premonitory feeling that he was going to collapse. He attempted to sit down but next recalls wakening on the floor with evidence of urinary incontinence. He was unsure for how long he had lost consciousness. This event was unwitnessed. He presented to his GP following a similar unwitnessed event four months later. He did not give any history suggestive of partial seizures. He suffered from chronic obstructive airways disease and was being treated with a twice daily salbutamol inhaler. He had a trans-urethral resection of the prostate performed for benign prostatic hypertrophy four years previously. He was a lifelong smoker of 20 cigarettes a day and drank alcohol occasionally. He was a widower of five years. Routine blood tests, ECG, Holter monitoring and CT brain did not reveal any abnormality. An EEG was not performed initially. He was treated by his GP with carbamazepine which was well tolerated. However, he had a further three events despite carbamazepine levels being within the therapeutic range. His son who described his father as becoming pale and falling to the ground from a standing position witnessed one of these events. He had myoclonic type jerking of his upper limbs with urinary incontinence. There was no tongue biting. The patient required five minutes to recover following the event but was able to proceed normally after that. There was no evidence of postural hypotension. Routine blood tests and ECG were again normal. EEG revealed some generalised non-specific slowing. MRI brain was normal except for very minimal vasculopathic change. Repeat Holter monitor confirmed runs of bradycardia with the heart rate as low as 40 beats per minute. A diagnosis of cardiogenic syncope was made. Carbamazepine was discontinued. A permanent pacemaker was inserted and the patient remained free of convulsive syncopal episodes one year later.

This case underlines the difficulty distinguishing between convulsive syncope and seizures, particularly when the events are relatively infrequent and unwitnessed. It also demonstrates the importance of a good collateral history and the value of questioning for postictal disorientation and fatigue.

📁 Case Study 3

A 72 year old lady was referred to the neurology clinic

with suspected dementia. She had experienced a generalised tonic clonic seizure 12 months previously and had been commenced on phenytoin. In the six months prior to presentation she had episodes of confusion, staring and wandering lasting for a few minutes and often associated with fatigue afterwards. She did not suffer any further convulsions. She had not suffered a stroke previously. However, she had been treated with diuretics for hypertension for a number of years. She had no early risk factors for partial epilepsy. General physical examination was normal. Neurological examination did not identify a dementia. There was no focal neurological deficit. EEG revealed right mid-temporal spikes. MRI showed mild atrophy and isolated peripheral white matter hyperintensities which were reported to be consistent with small vessel ischaemia. A diagnosis of localisation-related or partial epilepsy manifesting as frequent partial seizures was made. A second anticonvulsant was felt to be appropriate. Carbamazepine was not used because of the potential for developing hyponatraemia in light of the fact that she was already being treated with a diuretic. Sodium valproate was added instead.

When she returned to the clinic eight weeks later her husband described that there had been a general deterioration in her level of cognition and mobility. She was now in a wheelchair and had a marked postural tremor of both hands. She had finger-nose dysmetria and could not walk without the assistance of another person. General physical examination was normal. Routine blood testing revealed only a marginally low albumin. EEG displayed generalised slowing. MRI of brain did not show any new findings. Total phenytoin level was 16.7mg/l (ref 10 - 20) and valproate level was 54 mg/l (ref 50 - 100), both of which were within the therapeutic range. However, free phenytoin level was 3.9 mg/l and free valproate was 22mg/l both of which were high. Her dosage of valproate and phenytoin were both reduced and maintained at the lower end of the therapeutic range. Her level of cognition and mobility improved dramatically with modest improvement of her tremor.

This case illustrates the difficulty in prescribing multiple medications to older patients. It demonstrates the importance of considering protein-binding characteristics and how easily a small change in dose may result in a dramatic decline in level of functioning.

Case Study 4

An 83 year old lady was referred to the neurology clinic with focal motor seizures. She had no early risk factors for partial epilepsy. She first noticed left leg jerking episodes three months previously which could last from 10 to 30 minutes. These consisted of involuntary, irregular movements occurring without any impairment of consciousness and had occurred approximately 20 times since onset. She had never had a convulsion. She was attending the nephrology clinic with chronic kidney disease but did not require dialysis. She had also suffered a myocardial infarction six years previously. She was receiving treatment for hypertension and hypercholesterolaemia with amlodipine and pravastatin and was also on aspirin. Routine blood tests were notable for chronic renal impairment only. EEG revealed left temporal and central slowing and MRI of brain showed a large parasagittal meningioma. She was diagnosed with localisation-related lesional partial epilepsy. She was felt to be medically unfit for surgery. Treatment with lamotrigine was commenced. However, she developed an erythematous maculo-papular rash on her trunk with one mouth ulcer. Lamotrigine was discontinued and the patient was commenced on carbamazepine. This was well tolerated and reduced her seizure frequency to once a month. She did not have any further convulsions. She later became dependent on haemodialysis. During dialysis she had a cardio-respiratory arrest, which lasted 5 minutes. She remained comatose for 24 hours but slowly became more alert. However, it was noticed that she began to develop frequent myoclonic movements of all four limbs after one week. Levetiracetam was commenced at the low dose of 125 mg bid in view of her renal failure and this resulted in a modest improvement in her myoclonus. She improved to her pre-cardiac arrest cognitive status. Her partial seizures continued to occur once a month and it was decided to continue her on both AEDs.

This case underlines the importance of knowing both the common side effects of frequently used AEDs and the mechanism of drug excretion in patients with organ failure. It also underscores the fact that each AED is not necessarily effective against every seizure type.

Data Interpretation

Question 1

An 84 year old gentleman with hypertension had two secondary generalised convulsions over a two-year period. CT brain showed extensive small vessel cerbrovascular disease. He was on treatment with a thiazide diuretic and aspirin. Treatment was commenced with carbamazepine retard at 200mg twice daily. Four weeks later he present to A&E with confusion, lethargy and dizziness.

His routine bloods showed the following;

FBC	normal
Na$^+$	120mmol/l
K$^+$	4.2mmol/l
Urea	6.4mmol/l
Creatinine	98μmol/l

a. Describe the abnormality
b. What is the most likely diagnosis?
c. What medication change would you make to improve treatment?

Question 2

A 75 year old gentleman had been treated with phenytoin 300mg once daily for 7 years. He suffered approximately one seizure every 18 months and his phenytoin level was within the therapeutic range. However, after suffering three generalised tonic-clonic seizures within six weeks his phenytoin had been increased to 350mg once daily. Five days after taking the increased dose he presented to A&E with unsteadiness, nausea and vomiting.

His blood test results were as follows;

FBC	normal
Na$^+$	129mmol/l
K$^+$	4.4mmol/l
Urea	5.2mmol/l
Creatinine	104μmol/l
Phenytoin	25.1mg/l (ref 10 - 20mg/l)

a What are the abnormalities?
b. What is likely to be causing his symptoms?
c. What is the mechanism of this phenomenon?

Question 3

A 79 year old woman suffers a large left middle cerebral artery territory stroke. One year later she suffers a first generalized tonic-clonic seizure and later develops intermittent confusion and frequent clonic movements of her distal right upper limb, which has persisted for five days.

A non-sleep-deprived scalp EEG is requested. The EEG is reported as showing:

Delta waves in the left temporal region
Underlying alpha rhythm
Frequent focal spike and wave activity in the left temporal region

a. Which of these findings may be considered 'normal'?
b. What is the cause of the involuntary movements of the right upper limb?
c. What is the first line treatment for this condition?

Best of five questions

Question 1

What is the commonest cause of new onset epilepsy in the elderly?

a. Metastatic brain disease
b. Small vessel cerebrovascular disease
c. Primary brain tumour
d. Electrolyte disturbance
e. Herpes encephalitis

Question 2

Which of these is most likely to represent a post-ictal phenomenon following a seizure of occipital lobe onset?

a. Confusion
b. Dysphasia
c. Todd's paresis
d. Psychosis
e. Hemianopia

Question 3

Which of these medications is most likely to cause a Stevens-Johnson syndrome?

a. Phenytoin
b. Topiramate
c. Lamotrigine
d. Levetiracetam
e. Phenobarbital

Answers are on page 311

Answers

1. ASSESSING OLDER PATIENTS

Data interpretation answers:
Question 1:
Answer: b. Hyponatraemia commonly causes confusion. There is no striking evidence of infection and no hypercalaemia. Hyperkalaemia and mild anaemia do not generally cause confusion
Question 2:
Answer: a. Though the weakness resolved, this patient has a new onset expressive dysphasia persisting more than 24 hours which is an indication of stroke
Question 3:
Answer: c. The aim should be to return this man to his baseline independence and rehabilitation has the potential to do this

Best of five answers:
Question 1: C
Question 2: E
Question 3: B

Best of five answers:
Questions 1:
Answer d. Resuscitation should begin immediately and antibiotics should be given as quickly as possible – aim to give within one hour of presentation to the A&E. The source of infection may not have been determined and in this instance broad spectrum cover should be instituted. Blood cultures are desirable but should not delay administration of antibiotics. Platelets should be given when the count is less than 5 X 109 regardless of bleeding. Serum lactate is a well documented prognostic tool in sepsis. Patients with a level of 4mmol/l or greater in the presence of sepsis should have goal directed treatment instituted

Questions 2:
Answer a. Circulating catecholamines are increased with aging, however receptor response is decreased

Question 3:
Answer e. The mortality rate approaches 50% at one year

2. THE EMERGENCY DEPARTMENT

Data interpretation answers:
Question 1:
Answer: perforated appendicitis. It is not uncommon for elderly patients to present atypically with serious conditions

Questions 2:
Answer:
• injuries at different stages of healing
• frontal facial injuries
• unkempt appearance, missing dentures
• frailty
• predominantly hidden injuries (under clothes)
• prone to agitation
• fear of been 'put in a home'
• hovering caregiver
• 'accident prone' patient

3. MEMORY PROBLEMS

Data interpretation answers:
Question 1:
a. ECG to check QT interval
b. If the QTc interval is greater than 450 msec or shows more than 25 percent increase above baseline, neuroleptics should be avoided until potassium levels are restored and the QTc normalises. A sitter should be used to calm the patient. Low dose lorazepam or trazadone might be considered. If the QTc is normal, intravenous fluids with added potassium should be started and a low dose oral atypical antipsychotic medication can be commenced

Best of five answers:
Question 1: C
Comment: Stroke can certainly cause delirium and may be difficult to recognise if motor signs are absent. However, a CT brain can be traumatic for

patients with acute confusion. Assessment should start with a good history and physical examination and with investigations such as ECG, chest X-ray and basic bloods. Postoperative delirium occurs in up to 40% of patients after elective joint replacement and is even more common after emergency hip repair. A large variety of problems could have precipitated delirium, and a proper assessment of the patient is essential. Anaesthesia of itself is not often the cause of delirium unless there has been significant perioperative hypoxia or hypotension. It is dangerous to prescribe blindly without a full assessment of the patient. Not all patients with delirium require pharmacotherapy. Haloperidol is often the treatment of choice, but one would wish to consider substance withdrawal and to examine for parkinsonism before using neuroleptics. Finally, silent myocardial infarction is a well-recognised cause of delirium

Question 2: C

Comment: Haloperidol is an excellent choice for the majority of patients with significant agitation. Additional 'as needed' doses should be allowed 4 hourly until the optimal daily dose is attained. Bedrails increase the height from which patients will fall from bed and hence the risk of injury and may increase paranoia and agitation in delirious patients. Uncomfortable procedures should be avoided unless absolutely essential. Also, it is not uncommon for delirious patients to remove bladder catheters themselves, with risk of urethral injury. Benzodiazepines can cause disinhibition and respiratory depression. If high doses of haloperidol are required for more than a few days, a small dose of lorazepam could be introduced cautiously. Delirium is a transient disorder in most patients, but resolution of all symptoms may take some time

Question 3: D

Comment: Prominent visual hallucinations and parkinsonism with a low dose of a relatively mild antipsychotic suggest Lewy body dementia. Atypical presentation of Alzheimer's disease is possible but less likely. It would not be unreasonable to perform a CT brain scan here, but a subdural haematoma is unlikely

4. STROKE AND HYPERTENSION

Data interpretation answers:
Question 1:
a. Hypernatraemia, hyperkalaemia, dehydration, severe hypoglycaemia
b. Her hemiparesis and confusion may be due to neuroglycopaenia or may be a Todd's paralysis following a hypoglycaemic seizure. Her hypernatraemic dehydration may indicate prolonged reduced consciousness and also may be contributing to her confusion. The high potassium may reflect some tissue breakdown due to a prolonged lie on the floor
c. She needs immediate 50% dextrose, repeated until normoglycaemic and intravenous fluids preferably 5% or 10% dextrose

Question 2:
a. He has high serum creatinine with mild hyponatraemia and hypokalaemia
b. He has arteriopathy with associated renal disease and so goal BP is < 140/80mmHg. Beta-blockers are contra-indicated in peripheral vascular disease and he has hyponatraemia and hypokalaemia, which would be worsened by a diuretic. Appropriate treatments would include an angiotensin receptor blocker or potassium sparing diuretic. Given his PVD and prior stroke, clopidogrel monotherapy is the anti-platelet agent of choice

Question 3:
a. This woman should have warfarin therapy as she has atrial fibrillation, cardiomegaly and she is over 75 years of age. If she doesn't want to commence warfarin or has a contraindication to warfarin, her aspirin should be increased to a higher dose
b. Digoxin therapy should be commenced with concurrent correction of her hypokalaemia. Betablocker therapy is indicated given her biochemical hyperthyroidism but care must be taken given her probable LVF. Amiodarone should be avoided in thyroid disease
c. As well as rate control, carbimazole should be commenced with consideration of radioactive iodine for definitive treatment

Best of five answers:
Question 1: D
Question 2: C
Question 3: D
Question 4: E

5. BONE AND JOINT DISORDERS

Data interpretation answers:
Question 1:
a. Osteoarthritis
b. Standing radiographs of knees
c. Reassurance, paracetamol and isometric knee exercises

Question 2:
a. Rheumatoid Arthritis
b. CRP, rheumatoid factor, radiograph of hands
c. Methotrexate and folic acid

Question 3:
a. Osteoporotic compression fracture.
b. Bone profile, blood count, CRP (+/- 25OH vitamin D level)
c. Vitamin D supplements, bisphosphonate (alternatively strontium ranelate)

Best of five answers:
Question 1: D
Question 2: E
Question 3: A

6. FALLS AND SYNCOPE

Data interpretation answers:
Question 1:
a. A fall in systolic blood pressure of 67mmHg and a period of asystole of 5.7 seconds
b. Mixed cardioinhibitory and vasodepressor carotid sinus syndrome
c. Stop any exacerbating medications eg. beta blockers, calcium channel blockers. Dual chamber pacemaker insertion

Question 2:
a. Orthostatic hypotension
b. Parkinson's disease
c. Postural related advice
Fludrocortisone or midodrine

Question 3:
a. Carotid sinus syndrome.
b. Ventricular tachy- and brady-arrhythmias
c. Atrial fibrillation
d. Stroke

Best of five answers:
Question 1: D
Question 2: A
Question 3: D
Question 4: A
Question 5: E
Question 6: D

7. ENDOCRINE AND METABOLIC DISORDERS

Data interpretation answers:
Question 1:
a. 3.12 mmol/l
b. Familial hypocalciuric hypercalcaemia
c. Conservative management. No benefit from parathyroidectomy

Question 2:
a. Plasma aldosterone; Plasma renin activity; CT/ MRI Adrenals; Adrenal vein sampling
b. Conn's syndrome (primary hyperaldosteronism)
c. Aldosterone-producing adrenal adenoma

Question 3:
a. ACTH; short synacthen test; Chest radiograph; CT abdomen
b. Addison's disease (adrenal insufficiency) secondary to carcinoma of the lung
c. Replacement hydrocortisone and fludrocortisone. Management of lung carcinoma

Best of five answers:
Question 1: B
Question 2: C
Question 3: E

8. ANAEMIA AND WEIGHT LOSS

Data interpretation answers:
Question 1:
a. Smoking history, weight loss and signs at left base are suggestive of underlying lung cancer
b. Marked hyponatremia with hyperkalaemia in setting of renal failure. These electrolytes imbalances combined with weight loss, pigmentation and abnormal CXR suggests adrenal metastases from a lung cancer causing hypoadrenalism

c. A short synacten test will confirm a low basal cortisol and blunted response to ACTH

Question 2:

a. Significant macrocytic anaemia

b Folate deficiency secondary to long term phenytoin therapy

c.Simple oral folate replacement combined with alteration of anticonvulsant

Question 3:

a. Polymyalgia Rheumatica

b. Commence 15mgs Prednisolone once daily and assess therapeutic response

c. Co-prescribing bone protection to prevent glucocorticoid induced bone loss

Best of five answers:

Question 1: C

Question 2: D

Question 3: D

---

9. DYSPNOEA AND CHEST PAIN

Data interpretation answers:

Question 1:

a. Renal impairment secondary to increased diuretics. Digoxin toxicity secondary to renal impairment

b. Digoxin level and cardiac enzymes to outrule myocardial ischaemia and TFTs to check thyroid status

c. Withhold digoxin, reduce diuretics and restart once heart rate has increased and renal function returns to normal

Question 2:

a. Hypercholesterolaemia. Raised transaminases secondary to statin therapy

b. CPK to ensure that patient is not developing myopathy or rhabdomyolysis secondary to statin therapy

c. Myalgia is common after commencing statins and often symptoms will abate after a couple of weeks. However the concern is that patients may develop myopathy and rhabdomyolysis and so it is necessary to check CPK. If levels rise to more than 5 times normal then the drug must be stopped. Likewise if muscle symptoms are severe then the medication must be stopped. For minor symptoms reducing dose or changing to another drug in the same class may be enough

Question 3:

a. Patchy consolidation affecting right upper lobe

b. TB. Community acquired pneumonia. Pneumonia with bronchial carcinoma

Best of five answers:

Question 1: B

Question 2: D

Question 3: C

---

10. ABDOMINAL PROBLEMS

Data interpretation answers:

Question 1:

a. Macrocytic anaemia and hypocalcaemia

b. Alcohol excess

Coeliac disease

Myelodysplasia

B_{12} or folate deficiency

c.Anti-endomysial antibodies or D2 biopsies

Question 2:

a. Iron deficiency anaemia

b. Gastroscopy

c. Proton pump inhibitor plus triple therapy if H. pylori positive

Question 3:

a. Clostridium difficile infection

b. Fluid resuscitation and oral metronidazole

c. Early consultation with the general surgeon regarding emergency colectomy

Best of five answers:

Question 1: C

Question 2: D

Question 3: B

---

11. CONTINENCE

Data interpretation answers:

Question 1:

a. Benign prostatic hyperplasia

b. Commencement of alpha-adrenergic blockers

c. Cystoscopy, urodynamic studies and possible transurethral resection of the prostate depending on results

Question 2:

a. Dehydration
b. Intravenous high volume hypotonic rehydration
c. Review of the indication for the thiazide diuretic and angiotensin receptor blocker, both of which should be held in the initial period

Best of five answers:
Question 1: C
Question 2: C

---

12. DRUGS AND AGEING

Data interpretation answers:
Question 1:
a. Transient Ischaemic Attack
b. Diabetes Mellitus with proteinuria, hypercholesterolaemia
c. Warfarin (discontinue aspirin), statin, metformin and angiotensin converting enzyme inhibitor for poorly controlled hypertension. An ACE inhibitor would also be indicated if the urinary microalbumin-creatinine concentration > 3mg/mmolCr/ml (diabetic nephropathy)

Question 2:
a. Microcytic anaemia, acute kidney injury, hyponatraemia
b. The anaemia is most likely caused by upper gastrointestinal blood loss secondary to the combination of NSAID and steroid without concomitant use of proton pump inhibitor. The acute kidney injury is most likely secondary to the NSAID and volume depletion due to reduced oral intake. Anorexia and nausea may be secondary to upper gastrointestinal symptoms and/or to tramadol. Confusion may be secondary to tramadol. Chronic steroid use is a risk factor for osteoporosis. Steroids and NSAIDs can cause fluid retention, which may have caused the lower limb oedema. Bendrofluazide can cause hyponatraemia
c. Discontinue all medications, being careful to wean steroid gradually. Commence proton pump inhibitor. Review analgesic requirements. Consider calcium and vitamin D supplementation and bisphosphonate (provided glomerular filtration rate is above 30ml/min)

Question3:
a. Hypothyroidism secondary to amiodarone

b. Thyroxine replacement

Best of five answers:
Question 1: E
Question 2: B
Question 3: C

---

13. MOVEMENT DISORDERS

Data interpretation answers
Question 1:
a. Idiopathic Parkinson's disease
b. Levodopa with decarboxylase inhibitor, physiotherapy, occupational therapy
c. No investigations are essential

Question 2:
a. Restless leg syndrome
b. Iron studies, serum ferritin, renal function with estimated glomerular filtration rate, full blood count, thyroid function tests
c. Replacement of iron if deficient and optimise renal function. If symptoms persist prescribe a dopamine agonist eg, pramipexole or levodopa at night

Question 3:
a. Benign essential tremor
b. Family history of similar symptoms, relief by alcohol intake, absence of clinical PD features
c. DAT scan

Question 4:
a. Huntington' s Chorea
b. Counselling of patient, relatives, (including genetic counselling), check genetic marker
c. Stop levodopa. Add tetrabenazine or low dose haloperidol

Best of five answers:
Question 1: D
(Probably related to treatment with Betahistine, Prochlorperazine etc.)
Question 2: C
Question 3: D
Question 4: E

14.   ETHICAL ISSUES

Data interpretation answers:
Question 1:
a. Despite the cognitive difficulties, every attempt should be made to ascertain the patients wishes and/or any declared wishes prior to his deterioration. A full discussion with his next of kin is also important
b. Given the data showing the absence of significant benefit to patients following insertion of PEG tube in the context of advanced dementia, the focus should be on encouraging oral intake. Speech and language therapy will have a major role in the ongoing management of his dysphagia

Question 2:
a. Repeated discussion with this patient will give a greater opportunity for her to understand her prognosis. The priority is to ensure that she has total insight into her condition, the effects of various treatments and her prognosis
b. Discontinuing her cardiac medications may result in a worsening of symptoms of heart failure. Symptomatic treatment may be most appropriate if an infection develops and any escalation of treatment should be carefully considered. Patient comfort is paramount and, to this end, involvement of the palliative care team is essential

Best of five answers:
Question 1: D
Comment: There are no grounds here for overturning the basic presumption that an individual has capacity to decide for themselves. Mild dementia is no grounds for deciding otherwise. Similarly, the wishes of a family member do not take precedence and they cannot provide 'consent' for someone else in any case. Note that even if there were doubt about the capacity of the patient here, the operation is undoubtedly in the best interests of the patient
Question 2: D
Comment: It is extremely difficult to judge another person's quality of life. There is much evidence from those with severe disability that doctors and family members are prone to underestimating a patient's quality of life. In this case, it sounds as if the patient is reasonably well between bouts of illness, and that treatment, albeit with the inconvenience of hospital admission, succeeds in restoring the status quo. When family

disagreement occurs, adhering to the majority view is not an acceptable way of reaching an ethical decision in the best interests of the patient. Using wardship would also seem an excessive and unwieldy approach. Instead, it is preferable to keep communication lines open, accept that everybody is trying to do their best to reach the right decision and defer making ultimate decisions until the situation is clearer and people have had a chance to consider the options
Question 3: A
Comment: Seeking patient consent is a process and the critical aspect is that sufficient information is provided to allow the competent patient to make an informed choice. While the actual signing of the form provides some documentary evidence that this process occurred in the event of later disagreement, it is not of itself critical to the process. In this case, the patient's verbal agreement to proceed is well informed and voluntary, and his refusal to sign the form is a minor issue and one that is adequately compensated for by a careful documentation of the process that has been followed

---

15.   INFECTIOUS DISEASES

Data interpretation answers:
Question 1:
a. The radiograph shows a cavitating mass in the right upper lobe
b. Infectious causes of cavitation include mycobacterium tuberculosis, mycobacterium avium, anaerobic organisms, staphylococcus aureus, enterobacteriae, haemophilus influenza B, pseudomonas, legionella pneumophilia and fungal infections due to aspergillus, histoplasma or cryptococcus. Non-infectious causes include neoplasm, infarction, vasculitis, empyema, emphysema and pulmonary sequestration
c. Sputum should be sent for cytology and culture and stained for bacteria, acid fast bacilli and fungi. Blood cultures should be performed along with a Mantoux test. Bronchoscopy and CT scans of thorax, including a CT pulmonary angiogram and CT guided biopsy, should be considered. An autoantibody screen may be helpful

Question 2:
a. Erythema chronicum migrans

b. Complete heart block / third degree atrioventricular block

c. Lyme disease caused by the spirochaete, Borrelia burgdorferia transmitted by Ixodes tick bites

d. This patient has symptomatic heart block and therefore will require temporary pacing. Serology will confirm Lyme disease. Suitable antibiotics are doxycycline, benzylpenicillin, cefotaxime, azithromycin or amoxicillin

e. Other potential complications are cardiac disease, meningoencephalitis, cranial nerve palsies, Borrelia lymphocytoma and a chronic Lyme disease which can occur years later with acrodermatitis chronica atrophicans or an erosive oligoarthritis

Question 3:
a. Staphylococcus aureus

b. This organism is likely to be sensitive to flucloxacillin. In the event that it is MRSA, an alternative agent such as teicoplanin or vancomycin should be used. Assuming the renal function is normal, gentamicin may be of benefit for the initial few days of therapy with careful monitoring of renal function.

c. MRI findings: In the thoraco-lumbar spine there is severe disc and facet joint arthritis with degenerative changes throughout. There is abnormal disc signal at L4/L5 and in particular T9/10 and L1/2 discs. There is a small abscess in the left psoas at the L2 and L3 level. Findings are consistent with discitis

Best of five questions:
Question 1: C.
Comment: Fungal emboli to the eye are important considerations in patients similar to that outlined. Her risks were a prolonged intensive care unit admission, antibiotic use, invasive central lines and a confirmed fungal infection

Question 2: B

Question 3: E
Comment: Herpes simplex encephalitis typically presents with headache, fever, focal neurology and occasionally impaired consciousness or seizures. After the virus enters the system it causes necrosis in the temporal lobes. Behavioural abnormalities have also been reported. To confirm the diagnosis, cerebrospinal fluid should be sent for viral PCR. Treatment is with fourteen to twenty-one days of intravenous aciclovir

Question 4: E
Comment: Campylobacter is the most likely cause

in this lady. The incubation period ranges from 1-7 days. Infection then becomes established in the jejunum, ileum, and often the colon and rectum. It can be contracted from water or from infected raw or undercooked meat or poultry. It is also associated with extra-intestinal complications such as pericarditis, haemolytic uraemic syndrome, IgA nephropathy, glomerulonephritis and Guillain Barre syndrome. Campylobacter gastroenteritis is treated with erythromycin

---

16.   DRIVING

Data interpretation answers:
Question 1:
a. Left homonymous hemianopia – assessed by clinical examination of visual fields
b. Perimetry performed by an optometrist
c. The problem is likely to persist and, if so, is a contraindication to driving
Question 2:
a. Full history required (including collateral) to establish the extent of the cognitive problem. A physical examination should be aimed at identifying any impediment to driving eg. power loss, agnosia, dyspraxia etc
b. She should be able to continue driving but should be accompanied particularly if she is venturing outside her neighbourhood and especially at night
Question 3:
a. Stop driving, inform insurance company pending final assessment
b. Full physical assessment and multidisciplinary assessment particularly occupational therapy to optimise hand function. A formal driving assessment is required hopefully to identify modifications which will facilitate a return to driving for this lady

Best of five answers:
Question 1: E
Question 2: E
Question 3: C
Question 4: E

17. ONCOLOGY

Data interpretation answers:
Question 1:
a. Anaemia, neutropaenia and renal failure
b. Neutropaenic sepsis secondary to chemotherapy.
Pre-renal failure secondary to volume depletion.
Bone marrow involvement with malignancy
c. Broad spectrum antibiotics, intravenous fluids and reverse barrier nursing

Question 2:
a. Anaemia, hyponatraemia, renal failure, hypercalcaemia with elevated alkaline phosphatase
b. Hypercalcaemia secondary to bony metastases from prostate cancer
c. Intravenous saline with or without a loop diuretic is vital as hydration helps decrease calcium levels through dilution.Bisphosphonates can be used at a later stage to address hypercalcaemia by inhibiting osteoclast activity

Best of five answers:
Question 1: C
Question 2: D
Question 3: C
Question 4: B
Question 5: E

---

18. SKIN PROBLEMS

Data interpretation answers:
Question 1:
a. Seborrhoeic keratoses
b. Reassurance regarding the benign nature of the lesions. If a particular lesion is troublesome or catching and becoming inflamed, cryotherapy or curettage can be considered
Question 2:
a. Malignant melanoma
b. Examine for local lymph nodes.
 Refer to a dermatologist urgently for assessment and primary excision with 2mm surgical margins. Further management will be based on Breslow thickness
Question 3:
a. Bullous pemphigoid
b. Lesional skin biopsy for histology and perilesional skin biopsy for direct immunofluoresence

c. Treatment is based on the extent of disease. Localized disease can be treated with a topical super potent steroid (0.05% clobetasol propionate). More extensive disease usually requires the administration of systemic steroids. Most patients are treated with doses of 0.5 mg/kg with a slow taper over a number of months

Best of five answers:
Question 1: D
Question 2: D
Question 3: E

---

19. SENSORY PROBLEMS

Data interpretation answers:
Question 1:
a. Opacities in the anterior lens. Cupped disc on fundoscopy. Peripheral and central visual field defects
Normal or raised intraocular pressure
b. Simple chronic glaucoma
c. Topical prostaglandin

Question 2:
a. Age related macular degeneration
b. 'Dry' and 'wet'
c. Intra-vitreal injection of VEGF inhibitor and lutein

Question 3:
a. Dix-Hallpike manoeuvre
b. Repositioning manoeuvre eg. Epley

Question 4:
a. Meniere's disease (cochlear)
b. Acoustic neuroma. Migraine. TIA. Demyelinating disease
c. No cure – 90% maintain remain independent with medical management

Best of five answers:
Question 1: C
Question 2: B
Question 3: C
Question 4: C

20. PALLIATIVE CARE

Data interpretation answers:
Question 1:
a. Anaemia, neutropaenia, renal failure, hyponatraemia
b Opiate toxicity due to fentanyl. A fentanyl '25' patch approximates a daily morphine dose of 90mg. A sudden increase in daily equivalent morphine dose from 20mg to 90mg in an older person with renal dysfunction is quite likely to result in toxicit
Question 2:
a. Oral morphine and a non-steroidal anti-inflammatory drug
b. 80mg daily
c. Oral bisphosphonate and radiotherapy

Best of five answers:
Question 1: C.
Comment: Non-steroidal anti-inflammatory drugs can induce cardiac failure in older patients, even at low doses
Question 2: E
Comment: In chronic kidney disease, particularly in older people, the dose and frequency of administration of morphine should be decreased
Question 3: D
Comment: Haloperidol is the anti-emetic of choice in nausea from chemical causes such as hypercalcaemia and uraemia, both of which are present here

when the metabolising enzymes become saturated at higher doses, with resultant sharp rise in serum concentration and toxicity. It would have been more appropriate to increase the dose by 25mg, rather than 50 mg
Question 3:
a. Underlying alpha rhythm
b. Epilepsia partialis continua secondary to previous left middle cerebral artery infarct
c. Lorazepam 2 - 4mg IV/orally stat

Best of five answers:
Question 1: B
Question 2: E
Question 2: C

21. SEIZURES

Data interpretation answers:
Question 1:
a. Hyponatraemia
b. Symptomatic hyponatraemia secondary to carbamazepine and/or thiazide diuretic
c. Change from carbamazepine to another AED eg. lamotrigine, as symptomatic hyponatraemia may be temporally related to introduction of carbamazepine. Also consider changing diuretic to another anti-hypertensive agent
Question 2:
a. Serum phenytoin concentration is in the toxic range. Mild hyponatraemia
b. Phenytoin toxicity
c. Phenytoin displays saturable kinetics ie. it changes from first-order to zero-order kinetics